Meddling with mythology

Now that the intial panic surrounding the predicted AIDS epidemic has abated slightly, it is time to take stock of the body of knowledge and theoretical frameworks developed through AIDS research. The applied nature of this work and its separation from mainstream social science disciplines has meant that much of the data collected remained unmined. Such data, however, is crucial to understanding the ways in which research contributes to the social construction of knowledge. *Meddling with Mythology* offers a perspective on the politically, historically and socially situated nature of research and examines its role in the construction of the modern mythology surrounding AIDS.

The collection is framed within theories of story-telling and narrative exchanges. Issues discussed include:

* power;
* representation;
* the politics of text;
* understanding research relationships;
* impact of research on researchers and responders;
* potential for change.

Meddling with Mythology explores representations of AIDS, taking the reader from the theoretical to the practical and from the public to the personal. The issues raised here have significance for everyone who is interested in the social construction of knowledge, theory building and the research process more generally.

Rosaline S. Barbour is Senior Lecturer in Health Services Research at the University of Hull. **Guro Huby** is a Research Associate at the University of Edinburgh.

Meddling with mythology

AIDS and the social construction of knowledge

Edited by Rosaline S. Barbour
and Guro Huby
Foreword by Ronald Frankenburg

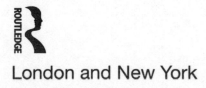

London and New York

First published 1998
by Routledge
11 New Fetter Lane, London EC4P 4EE

Simultaneously published in the US and Canada
by Routledge
29 West 35th Street, New York, NY 10001

Typeset in Times by Routledge
Printed and bound in Great Britain by Clays Ltd, St Ives PLC

British Library Cataloguing in Publication Data
A catalogue record for this book is available from the British Library

Library of Congress Cataloguing in Publication Data
Meddling with mythology: AIDS and the social construction of
knowledge/edited by Rosaline S. Barbour and Guro Huby;
foreword by Ronald Frankenberg.
Includes bibliographical references and index.
1. AIDS (Disease) – social aspects. 2. Knowledge, sociology of. I. Barbour,
Rosaline S. II. Huby, Guro.
RA644.A25M428   1998   97-49216
362.1'969792–dc21   CIP

ISBN 0–415–16389–7
ISBN 0–415–16390–0

This book is dedicated to the memory of Phil Strong. We hope that this collection will serve, in a small way, as a tribute to an inimitable scholar and colleague whose untimely death has left a gap in so many of our lives.

Amongst other things, this collection is about narratives and AIDS. Many of the people who have contributed to the stories told here are now dead. The book is also dedicated to the memory of Audrey, a great storyteller, who made her stories into an art of survival in the midst of so much myth about her.

Contents

Notes on contributors   ix
Read me first   *Ronald Frankenberg*   xiii
Acknowledgements   xx

1   Introduction: AIDS: from the specialised
    to the mainstream   1
    Rosaline S. Barbour and Guro Huby

Part 1   Power

2   Silence and strategy: researching AIDS/HIV narratives
    in the flow of power   21
    Brian Heaphy

3   Power, culture and the 'hard to reach': the marginalisation of minority
    ethnic populations from HIV prevention and harm minimisation   37
    Dima Abdulrahim

4   Policing boundaries: linking the theory and experience of
    psychotherapy in HIV/AIDS research   54
    Philip Gatter

Part 2   Boundaries and identities

5   It's a family affair: on public and private accounts of HIV/AIDS   75
    Hugh Masters

6   Researchers experience emotions too   90
    Jill Bourne

7   Fact-finder, fag hag, fellow and funambulist:
    research as a balancing act   104
    Katie Deverell

Part 3 Narrative exchange

  8 The story as gift: researching AIDS in the welfare marketplace   127
     Neil Small

  9 Of tales, myth, metaphor and metonym   146
     Clive Foster

10 On networks and narratives: research and the construction
    of chaotic drug user lifestyles   162
    Guro Huby

Part 4 Representation and agency

11 Engagement, representation and presentation in research practice   183
    Rosaline S. Barbour

12 Carrying out HIV-related research in an area of low prevalence:
    issues for researcher and researched   201
    Cathy Stark

13 Evaluation within a policy-making and contracting culture:
    reflections on practice   218
    Edwin van Teijlingen and Guro Huby

Part 5 A tribute to Phil Strong and an overview

    Introduction to Chapter 14   237
    Anne Murcott

14 The pestilential apocalypse: modern, postmodern and
    early modern observations   244
    Philip Strong

15 Conclusion: from meddling to mastery?   259
    Rosaline S. Barbour and Guro Huby

    Name index   268
    Subject index   273

Contributors

Dima Abdulrahim is currently working as a freelance health researcher. A Graduate of the American University of Beirut, she studied for a Ph.D. at the University of Exeter and her previous post was Senior Research Fellow at Staffordshire University/Drugs Advisory Service, Haringey. She has researched and published on the social anthropology of Palestinians in Berlin; gender and identity; and HIV, ethnicity and drug use.

Rosaline S. Barbour is Senior Lecturer in Health Services Research in the Department of Public Health and Primary Care, University of Hull. Her involvement in AIDS research began when she was employed as a Research Fellow at the MRC Medical Sociology Unit in Glasgow. Research experience and publications span both health and social services research. She is author of *A Professional Response: Health Care Workers and HIV/AIDS* (Taylor and Francis, forthcoming) and co-editor (with Jenny Kitzinger) of *Developing Focus Group Research* (Sage, forthcoming). Current interests include professionals' responses to change, users' experiences of sub-fertility services, strengthening the rigour of qualitative methods, and combining qualitative and quantitative methods.

Jill Bourne is Lecturer in Research Methods, Health and HIV/AIDS at the Sir David Owen Population Centre, University of Wales, Cardiff. Prior to this she carried out her Ph.D. research into carers of PWAs at SOCAS, University of Wales. Her main interests are social aspects of HIV/AIDS, reproductive technologies, death, dying and bereavement.

Katie Deverell has worked in the HIV prevention field for nine years as a researcher, trainer and volunteer. She has recently completed a part-time Ph.D. exploring issues of professionalism and boundary making in HIV prevention outreach. Her publications include *Working with Diversity: Building Communities* (an evaluation of the MESMAC Project – with Alan Prout: Health Education Authority, 1995) and 'Professionalism and sexual identity in gay men's HIV prevention' (in P. Aggleton *et al.* [eds], *Activism and Alliances*). Katie was Senior Research Officer at the HIV Project, London, but has recently left the field to pursue a career in industry. She is a Trustee of the LADS (gay men's HIV prevention) Project, London.

Clive Foster is qualified as both teacher and social worker, and has spent some twenty years working with youngsters brought before the courts and subsequently placed in residential schools. Having taken early retirement and having returned to university, these experiences provided an awareness of the culture he was to study for a Ph.D. in Social Anthropology.

Philip Gatter is a social anthropologist working as Senior Research Fellow in the Social Sciences Research Centre, School of Education, Politics and Social Science, South Bank University, London. His work has focused on sexuality and health, through evaluation research on HIV prevention and AIDS care organisations and services. He is currently exploring relationships between identity, sexuality and health in 1990s Britain via empirical studies of gay men's social and sexual networks.

Brian Heaphy is a Research Fellow in Sociology in the School of Education, Politics and Social Science, South Bank University, London. He has carried out research in the areas of intimate relationships, sexuality and AIDS/HIV. He is currently working (with Jeffrey Weeks and Catherine Donovan) on research which is investigating the structure and meaning of non-heterosexual relationships.

Guro Huby is an anthropologist currently employed as a Research Associate in the Department of General Practice, University of Edinburgh. She has recently completed a Ph.D. on co-ordination of care for people with HIV and AIDS in the Department of Anthropology, University of Edinburgh. Other research experience and publications cover problem drinking, gender and urbanisation in Africa; the management and prevention of alcohol problems in British urban settings; and self-help in primary care.

Hugh Masters is currently employed as a part-time Lecturer (Mental Health) at Napier University in Edinburgh, he is also a freelance health and social science researcher. From a background in mental health nursing, he has worked on a number of HIV-related community initiatives and was a Charge Nurse at Milestone House (AIDS hospice) from its opening until 1995. Having been awarded a Scottish Office Health Services Research Training Fellowship, he completed an M.Phil. at Edinburgh University in 1996. In addition to this study of parents, HIV and drug use in Lothian he has worked on a variety of mental health, public health and health promotion research projects.

Anne Murcott is Director (1992–8) of the Economic and Social Research Council (UK) Research Programme 'The Nation's Diet: The Social Science of Food Choice'. An MA in Social Anthropology and Ph.D. in Sociology, she is author of numerous articles on various aspects of health and on diet and culture. One of her more recent publications is *The Sociology of Food: Eating, Diet and Culture* (co-authored with Stephen Mennell and Anneke van Otterloo,

Sage, 1992). From 1982 to 1987 she was editor of *Sociology of Health and Illness* and is currently a co-executive editor of *Appetite*. Having taught both social science and medical/health professional students at the University of Wales (Cardiff) for more than twenty years, she now holds a research post as Professor of the Sociology of Health at South Bank University, London.

Neil Small is Senior Research Fellow at the Trent Palliative Care Centre and the University of Sheffield. He is the author of *Politics and Planning in the NHS* (Open University Press, 1989); *AIDS – The Challenge: Understanding, Education and Care* (Avebury, 1993) and co-editor (with David Field and Jenny Hockey) of *Death, Gender and Ethnicity* (Routledge, 1997). His current research interests include the way people are cared for at the end of their lives and the history of the hospice movement.

Cathy Stark is currently employed as Research Associate in the Centre for Family Studies, University of Newcastle. Her interest in HIV was sparked by an undergraduate health course whilst studying for a degree in Combined Studies at Newcastle. This led to her Ph.D. research on the experience of informal carers of people with HIV/AIDS. She has carried out research on several projects on homelessness, HIV counselling, IVF and assisted conception.

Philip Strong was Senior Lecturer in Sociology and Co-Director of the AIDS Social History Programme at the London School of Hygiene and Tropical Medicine. His research interests included medical consultations; variations in clinical practice; professions, organisations and NHS management. His publications include *The Ceremonial Order of the Clinic* (Routledge & Kegan Paul, 1979) and he was co-author (with Jane Robinson) of *NHS Under New Management* (Open University Press, 1990). He was academic editor, deputy chair and a co-author of the Open University course (U205) *Health and Disease* (Open University Press, 1985).

Edwin van Teijlingen is a Lecturer in the Department of Public Health, University of Aberdeen. Prior to that he worked as a researcher on several evaluation projects whilst employed at the Centre for HIV/AIDS and Drug Studies (CHADS). He has published on maternity services, HIV/AIDS and smoking. His current interests include young people and drugs (including tobacco), the organisation of maternity care and social aspects of HIV/AIDS.

Read me first

The *Simple Text* document has been read and the conditions of licensing consented to, the database loaded, the keywords AIDS, UK, Sociology, typed in, the book titles are shown on screen by date of appearance and Barbour and Huby 1998 is now visible. Were I a member of most world governments, or indeed if I had been a supporter of the governments that presided over the AIDS epidemic in the English-speaking nations, I would insist that a health warning should now be flashed onto the screen:

THIS IS NOT JUST ANOTHER BOOK ABOUT AIDS!

THIS IS NOT JUST ANOTHER BOOK ABOUT AIDS!

THIS IS NOT JUST ANOTHER BOOK ABOUT AIDS!

It is, in fact, a unique book of much wider general and global interest than its title might at first suggest, although it arises, somewhat guiltily, out of the personal tragedies of many individual men and women and the social tragedy of many neighbourhoods, districts and whole countries and continents – tragedies and a tragedy which although they have been pushed or fallen out of sight are still continuing unabated, their world significance unrecognised against the many generalised horrors of a murderous and now dying twentieth century.

But to see all is to understand nothing; the trick is 'to catch infinity in the palm of the hand', to see the universality in the particularity, to relate the social consequence to the individual experience, not only that already suffered, albeit with combative spirit, but that which might come if lessons are not analysed and learned.

The book derives its unique importance, among the many thousands across the world that make up the bibliography of the epidemic, from the fact that it focuses down on the research experiences of a collection of scholars, relatively privileged, and predominantly relatively young, neither adolescent nor mortescent, neither predominantly doctors nor even patients, and, as is to be expected in the late modern world, a network rather than a group. They almost parallel, even if in limited ways, the characteristics of those generations apparently most directly affected by the epidemic. They were first thrown together by a relatively rare set of circumstances which for a moment gave sociology and socio-cultural anthropology a privileged status and some economic advantage in being believed to be able to contribute to the solutions of problems which had taken the facile, triumphalist optimism of hard science and evidence-based medicine by surprise: 'Take care of the viruses; social reality can take care of itself'; 'Today we rule smallpox; tomorrow the world'; 'Health for all by the year 2000'.

These last scholars, for a short period, almost abandoned the field, to which they soon returned within the Trojan (US ™) Horse of statistical modelling. Those like myself, normally politically suspect, (fashionably) marginal to hard science and clinical medicine, marginal as well to the authors of this book, by virtue of chronological age and academic seniority (and in my case disciplinary focus), found themselves to their surprise suddenly in demand. We were asked to attend international conferences of governments, receptions at embassies, and to give private briefings for the great and the good (Berridge and Strong 1993), and even, sometimes, the royal. For us if only temporarily, the semantic value of the word 'protocol' was doubled overnight.

It was a new experience for my generation but not entirely for those even more senior, some of whom had written of the historical origins of the public health education movement in general and, in particular, of the Scottish and English Health Education Councils (which were to die from the terminal disease of incurable honesty and integrity in the epidemic and to be raised from the dead by an unduly optimistic and hostile government in a hopefully more amenable form as the Health Education Authority). They charted the rise of health education from its origins in the moral and military panic concerning the ironically named social diseases which from the late nineteenth century enabled a 'blameless' male elite to castigate what they saw as the anti-social sexual behaviours of the lower orders, who had replaced in England the urban Irish poor and in the US, immigrants in general. They described them as the precipitating and intensifying factors in epidemic disease. Others had participated, more or less willingly, in helping to devise such Second World War public lavatory poster campaigns as 'Clean Living is the Only *Real* Safeguard'. Anthropologists especially, even in my time, had been urged to create and then to describe in simple terms reified cultures (Frankenberg 1995) allegedly brought, fixed and unchanged, from such places as 'the West Indies' and the 'Indian subcontinent'. If they were not seen as actually causing disease, people assigned to these 'cultures' were certainly seen as obstacles to the rational application of scientific medicine and the destruction of forms alternative to it, then affectionately known as quackery.

This, then, was the first alchemy required of the sociologists whose work is reflexively analysed in the book. They were faced with the dross of victim-blaming and over-organising, mythologising health ideologies which their funders often expected them to reproduce and confirm. Could they instead turn it into gold of understanding rather than leaden and always partial explanations? How much did they have to change their own identity and practice in order so to do?

In order to restore a needed diversity of understandings in clinical situations, they certainly had to recognise the diversity within their own shared and/or individual narratives and its origins. Their experience has taught them that epistemology, the construction/validation of social knowledge, arises from a continuing cycle of experiences, formal and informal, rational and emotional, social and individual. Textbooks of research methodology often fail to remind us that field research neither begins nor ends in the field, let alone the study. Knowledge is transformed and re-ordered through conversations not only with the ambiguously named subjects of research but also with colleagues, friends and even more ambiguously named 'partners'.

While to understand a specific *disease-form* in relation to its specific curative technology, it may be an adequate approximation to generalise from tightly controlled, laboratory-type research processes, to understand the impact of experienced *illness-content* on the individual and of *sickness-process* on society, especially in epidemic conditions, one has to recognise different principles. These were set out clearly by Allan Young in his now classic paper (1981; see also 1995). This is that scientific analysis must be predicated on the principle that *all* empirical observations that *can* be connected through theory *should* in fact be connected and that the most useful theories adopted are of the kind which makes such connection possible. A researcher's empirical observations, theoretical orientations, rationalised knowledge, the way s/he presents her/his material to make it intelligible to others (intersubjectivity) and the meanings s/he negotiates with others all have to be related in this way (Young 1981: 176). Given time and opportunity, we all do this fairly easily in the context of conversation during conferences, speaking at seminars and discussions over dinner (providing, of course, that we choose our companions with care). We are lazier, more cautious and often settle for more partial analyses in print.

The urgency of the situation; the epidemic and, therefore, the overtly social nature of the disease complex; the vocal presence of the affected and the shared intimacy at once of the nature of the affliction, of the styles of research necessarily adopted and of the internal and external personal relations of the researchers all enabled, even compelled, the writers of the chapters in the book to demonstrate this in their accounts of practice. Is this perhaps still only possible in book collections rather than in the more prestigious and professionally rewarded form of journal publication? Read the book to understand and to be able to use the thinking behind the journal article!

Medical anthropologists lagged many years behind sociology in recognising that the experience of illness was different from the diagnosis of disease. They were slow to see the ways that illness and disease were trapped within what Phil Strong (1979) named 'the ceremonial order of the clinic'. They ignored the power rituals of an era marked by imperialism, total war and genocide, and their impact on attitudes to death and medical expertise. British sociology in general was similarly slow in taking account of problems of power and representation, which by the early 1980s was the stock in trade of US anthropology. All the writers in this book are conscious of power difference, but in the discipline at large it is still very often too easy in research merely to identify the apparently powerless and even the vulnerable in relation to the relatively powerful researcher. Clearly Gatter and Deverell, amongst others writing here, were made very conscious of their own limited power over their research subjects and therefore the process of their research. By the imaginative use of self-naming and exploiting the inherent ambiguity of language, Persons Living With AIDS (PLWAs) and persons living positively (at first in the US and then world-wide) rejected both the powerlessness of victimhood and the acceptance of being merely patient patients. They dared to question the moralities of methodology and forced researchers to do likewise. Heaphy's demonstration of the denial of speech to the seropositive in his small-scale British situation is complementary to Odets' moving (1995) account of the difficulties of the HIV negative gay survivors in San Francisco, reminiscent, if only by analogy, of those who went through but survived the Holocaust.

Classical anthropological theory, however far short it fell in practice, was designed to force the tyro to submit to cultural and linguistic pupillage at the hands of those they studied. Perhaps, in later publications concealed at the time, they revenged themselves in their diaries (Malinowski 1967) (cf. the patients' anecdotes described in Stimson and Webb 1975), in their choices about the use or not of their status as members of the colonial power (see Pat Barker's [1995] use of the Rivers Archive), and in the last analysis in their books and jokes (Evans-Pritchard's [1940] introduction, *Neurosis*). After AIDS research, sociologists in general ought to, and may be will, hesitate to stand outside and metaphorically above the social institutions which they study in quite the way many once did. Foucault (1983) demonstrated that the exercise of power is action to control the actions of others and cannot therefore be exercised on the subjectivity-lacking powerless. Most researchers here began their studies by empowering their subjects. They indicated that at least in this situation they could speak for themselves: a small step but one denied to those subjected to pre-coded questionnaires, and one which opens possibilities of wider escape from powerlessness. PWLAs and those living positively were quick to seize and extend these opportunities.

Conference speakers ignored this at their peril. In many international conferences and seminars, the AZT pill box in front of the delegate symbolised who really had the right to speak. Nor are PLWAs alone in this; the disabled and practitioners of Asian Medicine (Cohen 1995) are two other categories who have behaved similarly

Representation as even partial advocacy has been firmly rejected by many adopting the slogan 'These Natives *can* speak for themselves'. In my view, however, this book demonstrates once again the possibilities of what might be termed 'reflexive representation': the accurate and self-critical analysis of dialogic exchange between truly participant researcher and self-conscious subject. This analysis is used as a medium through which to refract rather than to reflect the subjects' accounts of interaction with others, in ways perhaps more personally significant than the current researcher-as-observer roles allow. This is achieved by representing dialogue rather than artificially isolated monologue treated as if narrative (as if even monologue is any more audience-free than more overt performance) (Favret-Saada 1980). No one can, of course, ever really talk to themselves; it does not require a computer to generate the virtual in this context. The anthropologist Robert Pool (1994) has explored this approach most fully his book-length study of illness in Cameroon, while Rabinow's (1996) *Making PCR* uses it within industrial society. An example nearest to its specific use in this book is Judith Monks' (1997) study of talk and narrative performance amongst persons with multiple sclerosis. Like some of the writers in this book, she is talked to not as someone who has actually directly shared the experience of the subject, but as someone who can be talked to as if she had. Perhaps, as Sally Gadow's (1980) work suggests, her achievement of empathy is in part derived from her earlier nursing experience.

One would at least like to think that if not all epidemiologists have yet become properly cautious about such concepts as risk, risk behaviour and risk group, at least the clinical and social analytic view of their usefulness will never be quite the same again. These chapters provide, even when not a direct contribution, certainly a commentary on a literature which is only just beginning to take account of AIDS and its multifaceted impact on perceptions of risk. It is not necessary here to rehearse at any length the arguments about risk groups really being categories and risk behaviours being more appropriate. In terms of supposedly quantitatively sophisticated methodologies, there is not only the problem of adapting methods intended to predict incidence in large populations to outcomes in individual cases, but also the fact that outside observers are thinking in terms of what s/he does that others don't, whereas the subjects of their concern may be comparing themselves to more narrowly defined others or indeed comparing their past to their present or their future. Disease asks, 'How do I differ from other possible diseases?' Illness, 'In what respect am I not myself?'

There is also the moral ordering of behaviour that makes some behaviours seem more prominent than others (and therefore figure more prominently in the statistics) and some disappear from view altogether and therefore never get counted at all. There is an unshared set of certainties about what is normal, and a sneaking suspicion that since I am rational and do not do that, it must be not only abnormal but also dangerous. There is a tendency for actions that seem natural, whether morally judged or not, as the editors of this volume suggest, either to pass unnoticed or to be seen as trivial. One of our problems as sociology has grown and fragmented is overlooking of what our colleagues in other areas of the discipline have profitably focused upon.

Anthropologists are drawn towards the trivial on the theoretical grounds that it is possibly symbolic; ethnomethodologists because its taken-for-grantedness might be indexical. Ethnographers of science, independently and influenced by

both of the above, have been driven to the trivial by the realisation that unconsciously embodied movements may make experiments possible and that
addressing, naming or cursing the apparatus helps to make it work! Qualitative
and quantitative researchers have complementary faults: the former, as is
suggested in the Introduction, fail to understand the shortcomings of often
partially or badly translated philosophy; the latter may fail sufficiently to understand the limitations of the mathematics that they use.

Finally, I think that all those social scientists who were concerned to
contribute both to the understanding and to the welfare of persons living with
AIDS and those infected with HIV were caught out by matters of specificity of
place, time and, as often happens to even the most scientific of clinicians, the
uniqueness of the particular. We fell into closure, to the feeling that now we
knew. Sophie Day and I both received plaudits at an early conference: Sophie,
because she defended female sex workers from victim-blaming by showing that
they used condoms with clients; I because I suggested that social science should
not focus exclusively on preventing new infection, but should also pay attention
to the social circumstances of progression from seropositivity to overt disease. We
were both criticised a decade later for our original analyses: Sophie because her
results had led to a reduction in funding for the care of street workers and I
because I was felt, quite correctly, to be underestimating the ability of those
living positively to think, analyse and act for themselves. Similarly, although it
was known from the beginning that the social aetiology of HIV infection was
different at different sites, scholars felt driven either to global generalisation or,
notoriously, to adaptations of familiar orientalist grand theories about Africa,
Asia and the West. As various authors have already pointed out – most notably
and most recently, Steven Epstein (1996), William Haver (1996), Steven Kruger
(1996) and Edmund White (1997) – a set of understandings have been generated
which are of equal value to those provided by biological and social sciences and
which chart the personal individual experience of people during the epidemic
through music, drama, story, poem and biography as well as through sculpture,
collage, painting and quilt-making and other crafts.

The value of this book is its emphasis on the particular in the context of the
universal. From it we can learn what questions the writers formulated and how
they developed them to produce more or less satisfying and useful answers. The
book is, as I suggested at the outset, uniquely important not just because the
answers they found *were* specific to place and time but also in the long run
because the processes by which they arrived at their conclusions have significance far beyond the bounds of a specific epidemic or even the specific
sociological field of health, sickness, death and suffering.

Ronald Frankenberg
University of Keele/Brunel

REFERENCES

Barker, P. (1995) *The Ghost Road*, London: Viking.

Berridge, V. and Strong, P. (eds) (1993) *AIDS and Contemporary History*, Cambridge, Cambridge University Press.

Cohen, L. (1995) 'The epistemological carnival: meditations on disciplinary intentionality and Ayurveda', in D. Bates (ed.) *Knowledge and Scholarly Medical Traditions*, Cambridge: Cambridge University Press.

Evans-Pritchard, E.E. (1940) *The Nuer*, Oxford: Clarendon Press.

Epstein, S. (1996) *Impure Science: AIDS, Activism and the Politics of Knowledge*, Berkeley: University of California Press.

Favret-Saada, S. (1980) *Deadly Words: Witchcraft in the Bocage*, Cambridge: Cambridge University Press.

Foucault, M. (1983) 'Afterword: the subject and power', in H.L. Dreyfus and P. Rabinow (eds) *Michel Foucault: Beyond Structuralism and Hermeneutics*, 2nd edition, Chicago: University of Chicago Press.

Frankenberg, R. (1995) 'Learning from AIDS: the future of anthropology', in A.S. Akbar and C. Shore (eds) *The Future of Anthropology: Its Relevance to the Contemporary World*, London: Athlone Press.

Gadow, S. (1980) 'Existential advocacy: philosophical foundation of nursing', in S.F. Spicker and S. Gadow (eds) *Nursing: Images and Ideals. Opening Dialogue with the Humanities*, New York: Springer.

Haver, W. (1996) *The Body of this Death: Historicity and Sociality in the Time of AIDS*, Stanford: Stanford University Press.

Kruger, S.F. (1996) *AIDS Narratives: Gender and Sexuality, Fiction and Science*, New York: Garland.

Malinowski, B. (1967) *A Diary in the Strict Sense of the Term*, London: Routledge & Kegan Paul.

Monks, J. (1997) *Describing Sickness: Talk, Social Relations and Personhood Following a Diagnosis of Multiple Sclerosis*, unpublished Ph.D. dissertation, Brunel University.

Odets, W. (1995) *In the Shadow of the Epidemic: Being HIV-Negative in the Age of AIDS*, London: Duke University Press/Cassell.

Pool, R. (1994) *Dialogue and the Interpretation of Illness: Conversations in a Cameroon Village*, Oxford: Berg.

Rabinow, P. (1996) *Making PCR*, Chicago: University of Chicago Press.

Stimson, G. and Webb, B. (1975) *Going to See the Doctor*, London: Routledge & Kegan Paul.

Strong, P. (1979) *The Ceremonial Order of the Clinic*, London: Routledge & Kegan Paul.

White, E. (1997) *The Farewell Symphony*, London: Chatto & Windus.

Young , A. (1981) 'The creation of medical knowledge: Some problems in interpretation', *Social Science and Medicine*, 15B: 379–86.

Young, A. (1995) *The Harmony of Illusions: Inventing Post-Traumatic Stress Disorder*, Princeton: Princeton University Press.

Acknowledgements

This book is the product of many people. We wish, firstly, to thank the contributors to this volume for their enthusiasm and support – and patience in the face of what were sometimes long editorial silences. Apart from their individual chapters, many have also provided comments, advice and suggestions about the book as a whole. In accepting our invitation to write an introduction to Phil Strong's chapter, Anne Murcott took on an unusual academic assignment; our heartfelt thanks to her for her unwavering scholarship and commitment to the project. We are also very grateful to Ronnie Frankenberg for his inspiring Foreword. As usual, we are indebted to our families for their support: Alasdair, Sarah, Joachim and Jenny, who have suffered maternal neglect with fortitude and patience (and now swear *never* to get an academic job which involves editing books in their spare time); also our partners, Mike and Chris, who have given moral and practical support and intellectual input. We are grateful to current colleagues for their tolerance in the face of our inevitable preoccupation and the demands which the project has made on our time. Thanks are also due to Maria (Winnie) Wilson for her invaluable support and help when our word-processing skills have faltered. Heather Gibson and Fiona Bailey at Routledge are to be thanked for their continuous encouragement and faith in the project. Last, but by no means least, we would like to acknowledge our respondents and our colleagues – past and present – who have provided so many insights over the years in 'the dark corners of the bar'.

Rose Barbour and Guro Huby
Hull and Edinburgh, October 1997

Chapter 1

Introduction

AIDS: from the specialised to the mainstream

Rosaline S. Barbour and Guro Huby

BACKGROUND TO THIS VOLUME

The official conference programme has drawn to a close, the academic debris of overheads and projectors, presenters' notes and papers has been tidied away and we drift towards the bar. We seat ourselves around a table, drinks are bought and distributed and the odd cigarette is lit. 'Of such situations is the telling of tales begun' (Clive Foster, Chapter 9). Confessions, gossip, tales of woe, sensation, boasting and one-upmanship blend with theoretical and political commentary, teasing and joking as the evening wears on. Invitations to seminars are extended, references are exchanged and new contacts made.

Thus, also, in our own case, were tentative ideas for this collection outlined and developed, invitations to contribute made and expressions of support, doubt or interest exchanged. It has long been recognised that informal networking at conferences is just as important as attending the formal sessions. It is often in this forum that information about anything from job opportunities to emergent theoretical perspectives is shared. Discussion and analysis of data and research findings are often embedded in informal exchange of experiences and anecdotes, especially in a context where we keep meeting the same individuals. In the case of the 'Scottish AIDS contingent', we have frequently realised that our anecdotes – even with due observance to the requirements of confidentiality – relate to the same clients, professionals, agencies or situations. What has, however, been intriguing is the somewhat different 'spin' on the story, depending on who is telling it, where they heard it, to what purpose they are retelling the tale to members of their own professional peer group, and whether or not they are conscious of the 'sociologising' involved (Horobin 1985; Barbour 1987). The contributors to this volume are part of a close-knit network of British researchers involved in research into the social aspects of AIDS. We meet regularly, in various permutations and wearing slightly different hats, both in and around formal meetings of social scientists and AIDS specialists. We write from the conviction that this material (a by-product of conferences and meetings) is as interesting, engaging and politically significant – and therefore relevant – as formal sessions where we present the substantive findings from our research. Indeed, it was in this context that the seeds of this particular edited collection were sown.

Although we never quite cast aside our professional selves, we need not, necessarily, be aware at the time of the impact of these playful and enjoyable episodes on our conceptualising and theorising. Such pleasurable social interaction with like-minded individuals accounts for much of the 'buzz' which most of us confess to experiencing at conferences. However, we seldom scrutinise our own interactions with the eye for detail that we cast over those of others in the research context. The aim of this edited collection is to make explicit and to begin to theorise this aspect of knowledge construction around AIDS, thus applying the tools of reflexivity to our own role in the production of AIDS and AIDS-related knowledge

Our current enterprise of putting this collection together would have been unthinkable during the early days of the AIDS epidemic. The circumstances surrounding the emergence of AIDS as a social event were extraordinary and it is hard for those who joined the 'AIDS bandwagon' at a later stage to imagine the early 1980s' sense of wartime emergency and the creativity which this unleashed. This impacted upon and shaped our contribution as researchers, caught up in this urgency and the need to produce our findings within a time-scale and format amenable to the policy process. Mick Bloor (1995) has observed that very few social science AIDS projects have published in mainstream socio-logical journals.

AIDS is no longer viewed as an apocalyptic threat, but rather as another chronic disease. HIV/AIDS is no longer a protected and ring-fenced item on service development and research budgets; instead the topic – and the researcher seeking funding – has to compete for attention with many equally pressing social and health concerns. This shift, however, also creates opportunities for developing new perspectives and knowledge about AIDS. Removed from the pressure of producing ever new and useful research we can afford ourselves the luxury of mining data which have otherwise not been used (Barbour 1987).

Now is, therefore, an appropriate point to take stock of and learn lessons from the body of knowledge which has been both employed and produced by research into AIDS. Although research into the social aspects of AIDS has been perceived as a special field producing its own body of knowledge, much of this work is of general theoretical interest which applies more widely. The topic throws into particularly sharp focus broader questions facing both researcher and practitioner with respect to understanding risk, power, representation and the politics of text. The lessons from AIDS work, in terms of both theory and method, are being pondered in a variety of fora and contexts, and this volume will add to these emergent debates. More specifically, however, we wish to take the opportunity afforded by the change in the circumstances surrounding AIDS research to 'step back' and reflect upon the politically, historically and culturally situated nature of the research enterprise itself.

Our reflections may conveniently begin with the chequered history of the title of the collection itself. The first proposal for a book carried the title *Meddling with Mythology: The Social Construction of AIDS Knowledge*. The lack of response from publishers made us revise both proposal and title to move the emphasis away from AIDS and our second draft was headed *Meddling with Mythology: Social Construction of Knowledge 'Post-AIDS'*. The 'Post-AIDS' was not intended either to imply that the crisis is over or to deny the poignancy of the experience of those with HIV or AIDS, their friends, families and their carers. Rather, it pointed to the vantage point offered us more than a decade on from our initial exposure to AIDS to examine the social constructions which have been created around it. We also wanted to look ahead and to consider the contribution which such an examination may yield for understanding the social construction of knowledge more generally. That it also proved necessary to take this wider perspective in order to convince potential publishers of the viability of our project – at least in terms of sales – affords a salient reminder and practical demonstration of the principal thesis of this book: that 'knowledge' and analyses are themselves the product of the intersection of social, political, cultural and professional preoccupations, dialogues and myths in the making. In the final product, we have removed 'Post-AIDS' from the title as both contributors and friends pointed out to us the ambiguity of this phrase.

EXPLORING THE 'SIGNIFICANT' AND THE 'TRIVIAL'

The boundaries of what can and cannot be said are shifting and are socially, culturally and historically contingent. As Plummer (1995) outlines the history of changing 'truths' and norms about sexual orientation and behaviour, so Armstrong (1987) highlights the changes in medical practice and discourse which have impacted upon the articulation of death – whose juxtaposition with sex, incidentally, makes AIDS such a potent symbol (Wallman 1988). Armstrong challenges the idea that the changing practice of terminal care in the 1960s liberated death from the silence and secrecy imposed on the event during the Victorian era. Rather, 'the truth' about death shifted with changes in the organisation of medical care. Whereas, before, 'the truth' about death was to be found in the physical act of dying, it is now found in the psychological and social processes which surround it. With it has come the idea of the 'good death', which poses stringent norms about the social and emotional reactions to the event. The norms concern openness about death and are policed by health and social care professionals. While they no doubt liberate experience from the silence and taboo which used to surround the topic of death, they also oppress those who are reluctant to conform to a new ideal of openness and disclosure. Refusal to talk about death in language which is currently acceptable does not necessarily denote lack of awareness (Huby 1997).

The research enterprise is similarly a historical and social product. The boundaries between what research should or should not legitimately and usefully address, together with the professional standards of conduct, shift with the times. These patterns reveal themselves particularly in the study of taboo or sensitive topics. Current trends in reflexivity provide tools for our understanding of ways in which history and wider social contexts impact on our professional practice and the result of our work. However, the term 'reflexivity' covers a multitude of uses and therefore needs to be examined and unpacked. In an age in which reflexivity is *de rigeur* in the social sciences, our own cultural work merits closer scrutiny than has previously been accorded it and is, in fact, a subject worthy of investigation in its own right.

Whilst we might once have expunged all mention of ourselves from our writings in the name of 'objectivity', of late some commentators have suggested that we have now taken reflexivity too far (see, for example, the discussion in Tierney 1995). Although much attention has been devoted to reflexivity, it has been pursued in practice as a largely individualistic rather than collective academic activity. For example, however much researchers have pondered over and disclosed their innermost experiences whilst negotiating access, carrying out fieldwork, analysing data and writing up their research, their gaze has been firmly locked on the research enterprise in the form of specific projects. Rarely do we build cumulatively on our experience through successive projects (although Edwin van Teijlingen and Guro Huby, Chapter 13, make a valiant attempt). Similarly, relationships with gatekeepers and respondents are dissected at the expense of those other minutiae of research activity which can be just as vital in the production of our final analyses and findings, for example the practical and political circumstances surrounding a project and likewise the day-to-day relationships which were formed with other researchers and through which analyses and theoretical arguments were produced.

Such details are generally considered trivial and, therefore, elude our published findings, the papers and the literature reviews. Whilst it is customary to acknowledge academic debts to those who have attended our seminars or who have commented on earlier drafts of published papers, our more informal and intimate – but equally formative – exchanges with members of our peer group form part of the taken-for-granted and unsung backdrop to academic endeavour.

Herzfeldt's (1997) discussion of the anecdotal highlights the importance of the apparently 'trivial' as a rich source of data on the ways in which 'the significant' is constructed. In an earlier book he suggests that it is only through a detailed examination of the minutiae of relationships that we can aspire to moving beyond the categories and classifications of the day:

> ... sensitivity to immediate context ... helps shift the focus away from perspectives that are already, to some extent, determined by the structures they were set up to examine.

(Herzfeldt 1992: 15)

The same perspective may be applied to research and the relationships it engenders and works through.

Clive Foster (Chapter 9) writes about narrative exchange on an Edinburgh housing estate as a way for the inhabitants to impose a moral and social order on an existence disrupted by heroin dealing, drug addiction and HIV/AIDS, and also as a form of challenge to the power of the police and medical and social services which structure so much of their existence. Foster vividly portrays the creativity, mischief and wishful thinking that his research participants unleashed in the drawing and shifting of boundaries between 'us' and 'them'.

The exchange of tales amongst researchers can be seen to serve the same purpose as does storytelling amongst the people we typically study. The neglect of our own storytelling and 'myth-making' as researchers can be explained, in part, by the widespread perception that such informal exchanges are the stuff of 'anecdotes', or 'gossip', as opposed to 'real data'. Writing in 1985, Gordon Horobin commented on our reluctance to present and publish such material:

> Although we all use personal anecdote in our sociologising between consenting adults in private, only the most secure or arrogant of us treat our experience as data in public.
>
> (Horobin 1985: 95)

Herzfeldt (1997) gives us ground to argue that the distinction between 'anecdote' and 'real research' is as much a political issue as it is an epistemological one. The invisibility of such anecdotes from our research accounts belies their importance and significance, belonging as they do to that domain where we engage with the bases of power that structure our own existence as researchers and challenge, invert and confirm boundaries and identities.

A firm intellectual grasp of our own work in this sphere has implications for reflexivity. It will allow us to move beyond the menace of 'essays laced with trendy amalgams of continental philosophy and autobiographical snippets' (Rosaldo 1989: 7 – cited by both Hugh Masters, Chapter 5, and Cathy Stark, Chapter 12) and come seriously, but also playfully, to grips with the historically and socially situated nature of our own intellectual products. As such it will give us a perspective on the political – with a small 'p' – effects of our work as researchers. In short, it will perhaps allow us to move on from 'meddling with mythology' to some sort of 'mastery'.

MYTHOLOGY

The 'Mythology' of our title refers to the many layers of meaning and experience which are segmented in past and present 'facts', figures, hypotheses, prognoses and emergent conventional wisdom concerning HIV and AIDS. As Susan Sontag (1989) so powerfully argues, some illnesses have come to be dramatised more intensely and carry a heavier symbolic burden than do others. In Europe and the USA, AIDS has become a symbolic marker on which we hang some of our most important fears, hopes, prejudices and beliefs about ourselves and the world which we inhabit. Sontag and other commentators have discussed the reasons for the symbolic status attached to AIDS: it is impervious to the powers of modern medicine and it poses the threat of social pollution and disintegration in the context of global interconnectedness and the vulnerability to foreign imports which this implies.

> AIDS is already one of the dystopian harbingers of the global village, that future which is already here and always before us, which no one knows how to refuse.
>
> (Sontag 1989: 3)

So compelling is the imagery surrounding AIDS and so resonant is this with our most central concerns in the late twentieth century that AIDS has become a potential 'apocalypse . . . made to seem part of the ordinary horizon of expectation':

> It seems that societies need to have one illness which becomes identified with evil, and attaches blame to its 'victims', but it is hard to be obsessed with more than one. . . . For several generations the generic idea of death has been a death from cancer, and a cancer death is experienced as a generic defeat. Now the generic rebuke to life and hope is AIDS.
>
> (Sontag 1989: 16, 24)

A central premise of sociological research into disease and its management is that the experience of biological events is socially mediated (Good 1994). The social construction of illness and the associated creation of meanings are important building blocks in the production of mythology. By seeking to understand AIDS with reference to mythology we intend not to deny the reality of AIDS and its impact on individuals or groups, but, instead, to provide insights into how the tales we are told – and, indeed, those which we as researchers tell – enable individuals 'to reflect on the conditions in which are grounded the hopes and beliefs of their world' (Clive Foster, Chapter 9, quoting Hannerz 1969: 115). Thus, such a perspective is not concerned with 'truth seeking' or distinguishing 'fact' from 'fantasy'. As Samuel and Thompson (1990) suggest – and as is borne out by the history of AIDS (Berridge 1996) – emotions, fears and fantasies do have a place in the shaping of history and the creation of what comes to be accepted as 'fact'. Samuel and Thompson argue that to ignore the role of 'myth' in this process is to rob ourselves as social researchers of much of our power to interpret the past – and, by implication, the present and future. They suggest that 'myth' may take us closer to (past) meanings and to subjectivity than 'thick description' and the 'painstaking accumulation of fact', and argue that myths can be understood only with respect to their relationship to other myths, rather than by reference to any underlying 'reality' (Samuel and Thompson 1990).

The symbolism around AIDS is constructed and mediated through various channels: the media, art, politics, research, and also through the machinery of bureaucratic intervention aimed at protecting society against the invasion of foreign bodies – be they viral or human 'others'. Berridge (1996) has outlined the UK policy response to AIDS as continuing the traditions of the post-war

British liberal welfare state. New themes developed out of old in ways which found resonance with current thinking around health and the allocation of responsibility between the state and the individual for its protection and nurturance. In similar ways, the symbolic work of AIDS happens and interacts at various structural levels and draws on a historical heritage which is refracted through the crisis created by AIDS, but by no means rejected through the process – apocalyptic imagery notwithstanding.

AIDS has come to be a moral and not a 'mere' natural event. From this interpretation flows the blaming of the people most affected – homosexual men, drug users and 'promiscuous' women – for that apocalyptic threat 'made to seem part of the ordinary horizon of expectation' (Sontag 1989 quoted above). Social scientists, such as the contributors to this book, have done a great deal to explore and explode the myths of moral attribution which makes HIV infection a double burden for those affected. However, as Philip Strong (Chapter 14) argues, the intellectual heritage on which we draw fits uncannily into the apocalyptic visions of AIDS as threats to a moral order. He talks of 'the noticeable tendency in so much nineteenth- and twentieth-century social theory to impose some form of metaphysical human meaning upon the world' and describes the acknowledged 'founding fathers' of modern sociology – Kant and Hegel, and through them Marx, Durkheim and Parsons – as seeming 'to lie within the Augustinian tradition of Christian apocalyptics – if in a secularised version rather than that of Henoch Clapham'. Critique involves transformation of thought, not its transcendence (Foucault 1973: 199) and 'postmodern' critics of these thinkers – on whom many contributors to this volume draw – necessarily operate within problematics of social and moral order. Although we may reject our forebears' notions of order, then, we do not transcend them. Contributions to this book suggest that we do operate with ideas of 'order' which, although more diffuse and refracted than 'modernity's', still are profoundly moral in the sense that they imply strong notions of 'rights' and 'wrongs' in doing research. As work with the book progressed, it became clear that the 'mythologies' to which the volume title refers concern not only those which envelop the policies and practices affecting people with HIV, but also the 'myths' shaping the role of the social scientist researching it all. Strong suggests that we revisit not only the epistemological and political underpinnings of our work, but also its moral foundation.

Although he is talking here about the social organisation of sexual storytelling, Plummer's (1995) questions are also pertinent to locating this edited collection within the large and wide-ranging literature to which HIV/AIDS has given rise:

What are the social conditions that have facilitated the emergence of the new stories being heard in the late twentieth century: how do these new stories come to be told and heard?

(Plummer 1995: 23)

The themes of this book and the process through which they came to be packaged together to form this collection reflect a number of different, but interrelated strands: the intellectual heritage on which contributors have drawn; the organisation of academic life; the ways in which personal biographies, history and politics have shaped the circumstances and contexts of our engagement as researchers – and hence, also, the products of our investigations. The contributors to this volume come from a number of different disciplines and sub-disciplines. This is reflected in the eclectic choice of literature utilised in our discussions, covering 'ethonography', 'anthropology', 'sociology', 'social science' 'interpretive sociology', and so forth. Whilst mindful that these disciplines and sub-disciplines have very different epistemological foundations, we have given ourselves licence to draw from these various literatures in attempting to illuminate the processes involved in the social construction of knowledge through the research enterprise.

AIDS AND SOCIAL SCIENCE RESEARCH

The social science response to AIDS itself became entangled in the bureaucratic and policy response to the challenge posed by a new potential epidemic. Until epidemiology allayed our fears of widespread AIDS epidemics in Western Europe and the USA, AIDS was a potential biomedical catastrophe without a technical biomedical 'fix'. The solution to the problem was, therefore, sought with respect to changing human behaviour. In the absence of a cure for, or vaccine against, HIV/AIDS, the only way to prevent – or limit – its spread was through persuading people to change intimate or stigmatised behaviours related to sexual encounters and drug taking. Social scientists revisited and dusted down earlier theories and perspectives on marginality, stigma and risk and sought to develop these, having found a ready market for their expertise. Suddenly topics, such as the practices of gay men or injecting drug users, which had previously been of interest to a relatively small and select band of 'consenting researchers', were deemed worthy of attention and funding in the governmental and policy arena (Barbour 1993). Both the MRC AIDS Programme and the ESRC Initiative made money available for social research, recognised the important contribution which it could make, and allowed methodological and theoretical development to flourish (Boulton 1994). Thus, not only has social science been influential in developing understandings of and responses to AIDS; AIDS has also been beneficial for social science (Berridge 1996).

For almost a decade service development and research in the AIDS field was protected by generous and ring-fenced grants. This field was cushioned from the encroaching market-oriented systems of health and social provision and the budget cuts witnessed in other areas of service provision (Bennett and Pettigrew 1991; Berridge 1996). AIDS provision and research developed a particular 'culture' where ideals of equality, non-discrimination and service users' rights to participate in decision-making around their care were crucial. These ideals are also a subtext of much social science medical research.

For a while, then, and within a limited and well-funded research and service-provision arena, the ideal of equity was fashionable. Apart from the funding, it was precisely this ideal of equality of access to services and the right of stigmatised and marginalised populations to a status of citizenship on a par with 'mainstream society' which attracted many of us to the field. For many of those whose research energies were thus harnessed, such involvement came about via the intersection of their academic interests and personal biographies and motivations (see, for example, Brian Heaphy, Chapter 2, Philip Gatter, Chapter 4, Hugh Masters, Chapter 5, Katie Deverell, Chapter 7). The ideals of equity and equality also permeated methodological approaches to the study of HIV/AIDS. Many projects sought to engage with participants in new ways which allowed them to have increased ownership of the research projects involved and sought also to include their voice and knowledge as co-researchers (Adam, 1992; Barbour, 1993).

Such developments notwithstanding, social scientists have also had to work within the conceptual and political frameworks constructed through the bureaucratic machinery which emerged in order to stem the spread and deal with the consequences of HIV/AIDS. AIDS has been described as a bureaucratic construct and an epidemiological/clinical classification of a range of disparate bodily symptoms conceptualised in terms of their progression through time towards death (Sontag 1989; Treichler 1992; Frankenberg 1995). This classification has structured the response to AIDS in numerous ways: the epidemiological mapping of incidence and spread in populations; the organisation and funding of clinical and social care (AIDS work attracted generous grants which were creatively allocated by cash-starved local authorities and health authorities); the administration of welfare (an AIDS diagnosis confers rights to welfare benefits); the access to insurance; and the restrictions on immigration.

The bureaucratic machinery has thus created and operationalised tight conceptual and social boundaries around categories of people – most notably, perhaps, through the assignment of membership of 'risk groups'. The concept of 'community' has been applied to people with widely divergent lifestyles, affiliations and notions of identity, the idea of a 'heterosexual community' being one of the more obvious examples of this tendency. Of course, social scientists have challenged such conceptualisations and stereotyping (Frankenberg 1992) – for example, by advocating that the term 'risk group' be replaced by 'risk behaviour' (Bloor 1995).

Regardless of our role in critiquing and challenging bureaucratic criteria and assumptions, researchers have themselves played a role in creating such classifications – not least since a challenge confirms the reality of that which is being challenged. Several of the contributors to this volume (Brian Heaphy, Chapter 2, Philip Gatter, Chapter 4, Jill Bourne, Chapter 6, Katie Deverell, Chapter 7, Neil Small, Chapter 8, Guro Huby, Chapter 10) illustrate vividly the difficulties researchers have faced in attempting to realise ideals concerning representation, equity and equality when entering social fields structured by competing and conflicting interests and perspectives. Neil Small explores the extent to which this is actually possible and suggests that, despite our good intentions and desire to facilitate change, we operate within a context where such research contracts are rendered, if not impossible, then, hard to realise. Challenges also have their own parameters which we inadvertently construct and reproduce. Therein lies a tension and a dilemma of social research which we highlight and elaborate in this volume: if research is a social act, then we operate under the conditions of social interaction where boundaries are both a prerequisite and an outcome. This predicament is especially pertinent for qualitative researchers. Although here commenting on methodological debates, Tierney's observations apply equally to our research 'findings' and how these can assume a life of their own:

> ... when our ... debates decontextualise issues to create 'rules of the road', we ironically create dogmatic generalisations in a field that resists generalisability.

> (Tierney 1995: 387)

Sophie Day (1990) reflects on the influence of her own earlier research in establishing the accepted wisdom that prostitutes neglect to use condoms when engaging in sex with non-commercial partners. Deconstruction is never context-free and so implies the construction of other structural contingencies to be deconstructed in turn.

POWER

This problematic echoes a long-standing debate within the social sciences about 'power', which is picked up on by several of the contributors to this book. Indeed, Plummer argues that personal accounts operate within the flow of power and that the 'power to tell a story, indeed not to tell a story, under the conditions of one's own choosing, is part of the political process' (Plummer 1995: 26). Brian Heaphy (Chapter 2) argues:

> If 'medical', 'activist' and 'personal' narratives of AIDS/HIV exist in the flow of power, so too do our social scientific research accounts. While many researchers may not aim to engage in questions of power, in our production of AIDS/HIV research accounts we are explicitly and/or implicitly involved in asserting, accepting or contesting what is rational, sane and true in the AIDS/HIV context. In this sense, we become involved in the production or reproduction of AIDS/HIV 'truths', and, therefore in the production (or reproduction) of what Foucault (1979) terms 'power-knowledge'.

'Power' is a useful tool for analysing and providing an understanding of social systems, but the precise nature and meaning of the term is difficult to pin down. Attempts to do so have sparked off a long and, some might say, inconclusive debate in the social sciences (for example, Lukes 1974; Foucault 1982; Fardon 1985; Turner, 1994). The lack of clarity around the term has been a factor in discussions and correspondence among the editors and contributors to the volume. In particular, the debate has revolved around questions of power as oppressive versus productive of individual and social truths and whether the terms exist by which we deem one truth more 'genuine' than others. Again, Brian Heaphy has articulated particularly well the outcome of our deliberations:

> A major point in the letter concerned my use of the term 'power' – I under-stand the points you were making. . . . For me to engage with questions of power is to be faced with contradictions, tensions *and* confusions – for the very reasons you point out in your letter. I employ Plummer's notion of 'the flow of power' as it has potential to conjure up a sense of this.
> I don't agree that my use of Foucault's sense of power . . . implies that there is a 'truth' out there to be known. Rather, I am concerned with the contests engaged in for the establishment (i.e. construction) of (contingent) 'truths'. In the end I have not expanded much further on the discussion of power in this paper – I think that doing so might make it into 'another' paper. If it's OK by you, I would prefer to allow my own tensions with the term to stand.
>
> (Brian Heaphy, letter to Rose Barbour and Guro Huby, August 1997)

Ritches (1985) sees power as a cultural construct, deeply rooted in the Western intellectual milieu. In drawing on the concept of 'power' to provide an under-standing of relationships and events are we merely importing our own cultural constructs without subjecting them to critical scrutiny which we reserve for and routinely apply to the accounts of all other parties touched by the research process?

Nevertheless, although the term 'power' as used in academic contexts may not carry meaning for all our respondents, some may be said to have intimate knowledge of what 'power' is and how it affects their lives. They have also devel-oped strategies of resistance which are described and discussed by several authors. Clive Foster (Chapter 9) shows how drug users on an Edinburgh estate are able to manage and harness their 'powerlessness'. In echoing the rhetoric of the authorities and the pejorative terms reserved for drug users, they are not confirming their lack of control over their own lives, but, rather, are engaging in a sophisticated process of exaggeration in order to confuse and reclaim control. Similarly, Dima Abdulrahim (Chapter 3) describes how 'ethnic minority' drug users are excluded from resources of care and prevention through a well-meaning but misplaced bureaucratic use of the term 'culture'. Her 'ethnic minority' respondents, on their part, reclaim the word 'culture' and define it in their own terms to create for themselves a space of autonomy and positive identities. Guro Huby (Chapter 10) describes how drug user respondents actively and strategically manage the 'chaos' which, although attributed to their lifestyles and patterns of service use, are also to a large extent created by the complexity of service provision and research on which they are forced to rely.

NARRATIVE

The study of narrative and narrative exchange has been used as a way of accessing the structurally contingent construction of individual experience (Good 1994). Seen from this perspective, it is the structural context in which stories are created and exchanged and the dynamic interplay of relationships between content and structural context which is of analytical and theoretical interest.

Research also has a part to play in this structural context as one of the protagonists in the exchange of tales. It reflects and reflects upon, but also actively contributes to, the production of stories. Talking about the personal sexual story Plummer (1995) describes narrative exchange as an interaction with three principal parties. These are, firstly, the producers of stories who tell or perform their personal stories; secondly, the audiences who consume the stories; and, thirdly, the 'coaxers' of stories who persuade and invite these personal performances. Researchers belong to this group – along with journalists and talk show hosts, amongst others.

The boundaries between the personal and the social in these stories are, however, difficult to discern. According to Plummer:

> All of these people – producers, coaxers, consumers – are engaged in assembling life story actions around lives, events and happenings – although they cannot grasp the actual life. At the centre of much of this action emerge the story products: the objects which harbour the meanings that have to be handled in social interaction.
>
> (Plummer 1995: 21–2)

The content of stories – even of the personal narrative – is not accidental, but draws on a backdrop of public and shared imagery and knowledge – that is, 'myth'. The personal and the public merge at a certain level of experience and so the personal stories told in a particular period or around a particular situation share common themes. Mick Bloor (1995), for example, points to the rehearsed nature of many of the accounts produced by rent boys to explain how they drifted into this work, noting that some would preface their tales by describing them as 'sob stories'.

Both the teller of stories and the researcher are selective, emphasising certain details or themes at the expense of others. Thus, in the 1980s Plummer (1995) looked for – and found – tales of normalcy in the stories of sexual deviance which he collected, whereas, a hundred years previously, Krafft-Ebbing looked for – and found – tales of pathology. The same story can be told for a very different purpose and to different effect. Rosaline Barbour (Chapter 11) discusses the ways in which we, as researchers, select stories and quotes with which to illustrate our arguments or presentations and she examines the ways in which our choice varies with our audience, whether it be fellow academics, policy-makers, practitioners, or our respondents. Although we might like to think that our analyses are always data-driven, we are influenced by the ever-shifting academic – and, indeed, funding – gaze, as it focuses on particular topics and debates, and this affects what we view as relevant amongst the large volume of data generated by many of our research projects.

STRUCTURE OF THE BOOK

Mick Bloor (1995) and Paul Atkinson (1996) have both cautioned against privileging certain accounts – in both cases narratives elicited from research respondents. In putting together and structuring a collection such as the present one we also run such a risk: it is difficult to communicate without either confirming old boundaries or erecting new ones which may be equally misleading or disabling.

Aldridge (1993) comments on how the conventions of academic presentation imply that research accounts were written in a particular temporal order. This observation applies equally to conceptual ordering of written work. As editors of this collection we had many discussions about how best to order the material presented in this introductory chapter: whether to open with a theoretical discussion of 'mythology'; whether to locate the collection firstly within the unfolding context of HIV/AIDS and AIDS-related research; or whether to start with an account of how we came to think about putting this collection together. In the end, bearing in mind the potential for distortion inherent in such a task, we opted for the most straightforward and, we hope, most 'honest' sequence, which charts our own emergent ideas which have culminated in this book. However, even this ordering involves a reconstruction of events.

The difficulty surrounding decisions about the ordering of material relates also to the order in which individual chapters are placed and the subheadings attached to them. We started out, as editors, with a structure which separated issues about the public and the private from issues of policy and practice. However, in discussion with contributors, it was pointed out to us that this was contrary to our intentions and aims. We were separating out those invisible aspects of the research enterprise which we considered a crucial dimension integral to its products. We thus risked marginalising them from the 'important' and 'significant' aspects such as policy implications. The boundary between the public and the private and between the individual and the social is blurred. The personal and the public intersect in many and complex ways and this is a theme which runs through all chapters. We, therefore, have employed a structure which attempts both to avoid distinctions rooted in the very discourses which we are examining and also to use the contributions to progress an argument about the role of research in the myth-making around AIDS.

The book is divided into five main parts and a conclusion:

I Power

Questions of 'power' and its impact on the research process have driven much of the development of this book and it opens appropriately with papers dealing with this problematic. Brian Heaphy discusses the 'dialogic ideal' and equality of relationship between researcher and researched. His chapter concerns the silences around which discourses about AIDS are constructed. The rules surrounding who can and cannot speak on AIDS in various capacities are powerful external checks on behaviour and speech. For example, the opinions of seropositive people and their knowledge of their medical condition and its management are not accepted. Similarly, he has been advised to keep silent about his seropositive status in a research context. However, this self-imposed silence becomes especially difficult when the researcher is faced with the dilemma of whether or not to question a respondent's approach to medication.

Dima Abdulrahim continues a discussion of 'power' in her chapter on the construction of Turkish Cypriots within British society as a 'hard to reach' ethnic minority in terms of harm minimisation strategies for tackling drug use. These strategies – if based on the reification of 'culture' as inherent in defined popula-tions – ignore the many and various boundaries across which communication and negotiations take place and effectively exclude ethnic minority drug users from help and support. She questions whether – and how – a community or cultural group can actively accept HIV-related issues when the resources and symbolic imagery are controlled by others.

Philip Gatter's chapter addresses public and private dimensions of research constructions from a theoretical perspective, suggesting that '[w]hat is noticeably lacking, in both anthropology and sociology, is an adequate *theoretical* account of the links between the subjectivity of the researcher and the field of research'. He recounts the ways in which he, as a researcher, became caught up in counselling staff's definitions as 'pathological' criticism levelled by clients at the agency he was evaluating. Then he goes on to discuss ways in which the treatment constructs the problems and the solutions around which the 'selves' of the clients then become constituted. This theme leads into issues of identity and boundary negotiations as they pertain to research and the construction of researcher roles and selves.

II Boundaries and identities

Hugh Masters transcends the confessional genre to provide an analysis of his own progress from professional health care provider to researcher and informal carer, and examines the many contradictions and conflicts inherent in such a multiplicity of roles and motivations. Reflecting on the implications of personal biography and respondents' expectations, he provides a thoughtful analysis of relationships between researcher and researched. This chapter also touches upon the nature of the research bargain.

Jill Bourne then looks at the impact for the researcher of engaging with emotionally sensitive topics. She suggests that we can enhance our analyses by treating our own feelings as a tool for ordering and understanding the data which we collect and she points out the dangers of merely putting these to one side as troublesome reminders of our vulnerability which threaten rigorous analysis.

Katie Deverell describes how she negotiated her many identities throughout her work on evaluation of the MESMAC project on health education among men who have sex with men. She discusses the boundaries researchers must create and negotiate in the field in order to interact with respondents and collect data. She highlights the distinction frequently made between the production of 'relevant facts' to be used by agencies in funding bids and 'insignificant or irrelevant' theoretical descriptions – including reflexive accounts. This chapter illustrates how discourse about research is shaped and constrained by political and social convention, with personal biography intersecting in significant ways to form the changing research climate in which we function.

III Narrative exchange

Neil Small uses economic and anthropological theory of exchange to consider the extent to which it is appropriate to view the research relationship as a gift exchange. He raises important issues with respect to the potential for reciprocity within a research and service provision context which is driven by a market ideology.

Clive Foster describes how the inhabitants of an Edinburgh housing estate employed stories to create social and moral order in an existence otherwise disrupted and marred by heroin and AIDS. He uses the terms 'myth', 'metonym' and 'metaphor' as analytical tools to understand how people in an economically and politically marginal locality use tales and storytelling to construct self and community.

Guro Huby develops the theme of narrative exchange in her discussion of the ways in which her research project became part of a set-up of service provision and research where the complexity of information exchange generated a sense of 'chaos' which, in turn, was projected onto drug users and their lifestyles. Research then reproduced 'facts' about the 'chaos' said to be incurred by such lifestyles. Research thus both reflected and contributed towards certain responses and behaviours. The chapter also reflects on both respondents' and researchers' reactions to the way classifications and stereotyping of 'drug users' affected relationships in the setting.

IV Representation and agency

'Facts' are constructed and contested within an exchange of stories in settings made up of intersecting and shifting constellations of interests and power. Rosaline Barbour looks at the functions served by the stories told by AIDS workers and explores researchers' conscious and unwitting involvement in the process of constructing contemporary AIDS folklore, through their recording and retelling of stories and through the presentation of their work. She also discusses the implications of selection of material for presentation to different audiences.

Cathy Stark describes her project aimed to produce accounts of her respondents' experience of caring for someone with AIDS in an area with very low HIV prevalence. She discusses how she maintained the 'facts' whilst distorting biographical detail in order to preserve the anonymity and confidentiality of her respondents.

Edwin van Teijlingen and Guro Huby explore the complex relationship between research, policy and funding decisions and the ways in which participants' contributions (both those of researcher and researched) may be distorted or ignored in this process.

V A tribute to Philip Strong and an overview

From conception to publication of an edited collection such as this is a long and difficult process. We have been relatively lucky in that most of the colleagues who expressed an interest in contributing to this volume have stayed with us, through our many revisions and reconceptualisations. This testifies, we hope, to the legitimacy and timeliness of addressing 'AIDS knowledge' – and indeed the social construction of knowledge more generally – from the standpoint outlined here. Sadly, however, we lost one of our contributors to an untimely death from a heart attack before our project could be realised. Philip Strong died on 11 July 1995. We were fortunate, however, in that Phil had already provided us with a first draft in the form of a paper which he had presented to colleagues at the History of the Present Seminar.

The collection ends with a tribute to Phil, whose paper, although submitted before he had had the chance to see how the book was developing, is an apt theoretical and historical commentary on the issues raised in the collection. Anne Murcott, herself a prominent sociologist and long-term partner of Phil's, has written a short introduction to his chapter, providing a commentary which places Phil's contribution within the context of his previous work and the ongoing work he was engaged in prior to his death. We hope that the resulting collection, in a small way, pays tribute to Philip Strong and the spirit of imaginative and scholarly inquiry which he so brilliantly exemplified and which he sought to encourage in the rest of us.

Philip Strong's historical analysis of the AIDS epidemic is also a critique of the cultural tools at our disposal for understanding the phenomenon of HIV/AIDS and, by implication, our own role as researchers in documenting them. Looking back beyond the traditional sociological gaze (encompassing theorists such as Marx, Weber and Durkheim), he argues that publicly available, reflexive commentary is a product of early modernism rather than postmodernism. He concludes that a Hobbesian perspective on human motivation and social behaviour is much more helpful than postmodern reflexive trends in explaining the social trajectories involved in the reporting and conceptualising of HIV/AIDS.

Conclusion

Rosaline Barbour and Guro Huby attempt to pull together the many strands which have emerged from the contributions and to propose a way forward from 'meddling' with mythology to 'mastering' it. We urge the deconstruction of boundaries between 'formal' and 'informal' theorising and suggest that the sociological gaze of reflexivity be directed at the latter as it focuses on details of practice. We introduce 'the Last Visible Dog' from Russell Hoban's story of the Mouse and his Child as a way of illustrating Phil Strong's and Anne Murcott's caution against a spiralling reflexivity which intellectualises, rather than reflects on, the practice of doing research and the ever-changing contexts in which this occurs. We end with Philip Strong's suggestions that we revisit early nineteenth-century moral philosophy to explore an existential basis for such reflections.

REFERENCES

Adam, B.D. (1992) 'Sociology and people living with AIDS', in J. Huber and B.E. Sneider (eds) *The Social Context of AIDS*, Newbury Park, CA/London: American Sociological Association Presidential Press/Sage.

Aldridge, J. (1993) 'The textual embodiment of knowledge in research account writing', *Sociology (Special Issue: Auto/Biography in Sociology)*, 27(1): 53–6.

Armstrong, D. (1987) 'Silence and truth in death and dying', *Social Science and Medicine*, 24: 651 7.

Atkinson, P. (1996) 'Narrative turn or blind alley? Reflections on narrative and qualitative health research', plenary paper presented at the Third International Interdisciplinary Qualitative Health Research Conference, University of Bournemouth, 30 October–1 November.

Barbour, R.S. (1987) 'The irritating sociologist: notes towards defining an occupational stereotype', in N.P. McKeganey and S. Cunningham-Burley (eds) *Enter the Sociologist*, Aldershot: Avebury, 114–26.

—— (1993) 'HIV/AIDS and medical sociology in the nineties', in M. Haralambos (ed.) *Developments in Sociology*, volume 9, Ormskirk: Causeway Press

Bennet, C. and Pettigrew, A.M. (1991) *Pioneering Services for AIDS: The Response to HIV Infection in Four Health Authorities*, Final Report for the Department of Health CCSC, University of Warwick.

Berridge, V. (1996) *AIDS in the UK: The Making of Policy 1981–1994*, Oxford: Oxford University Press.

Bloor, M. (1995) *The Sociology of HIV Transmission*, London: Sage.

Boulton, M. (ed.) (1994) *Challenge and Innovation: Methodological Advances in Social Research on HIV/AIDS*, London: Taylor & Francis.

Day, S. (1990) 'Anthropological perspectives in sexually transmitted diseases', In N. Job-Spira, B. Spencer, J.P. Moatti and E. Bouvet (eds) *Santé Publique et Maladies à Transmission Sexuelle*, Paris: John Libbey/Eurotext.

Fardon. R. (ed.) (1985) *Power and Knowledge: Proceedings of a Conference Held at the University of St Andrews December 1982*, Edinburgh: Scottish Academic Press.

Foucault, M. (1973) *The Birth of the Clinic*, London: Tavistock Publications.

—— (1979) *Discipline and Punish: The Birth of the Prison*, Harmondsworth: Penguin.

—— (1982) 'The subject and power', in R. Dreyfus and P. Rabinow (eds) *Michel Foucault: Beyond Structuralism and Hermeneutics*, Chicago: University of Chicago Press.

Frankenberg, R. (1992) 'The other who is also the same: the relevance of epidemics in space and time for prevention of HIV infection', *International Journal of Health Services* 22(1):73–88.

—— (1995) 'Learning from AIDS: the future of anthropology', in A.S. Akbar and C. Shore (eds) *The Future of Anthropology: Its Relevance to the Contemporary World*, London: Athlone Press.

Good, B.J. (1994) *Medicine, Rationality and Experience: An Anthropological Perspective*, Cambridge: Cambridge University Press.

Hannerz, U. (1969) *Soulside: Inquiries into Ghetto Culture and Community*, New York and London: Columbia University Press.

Herzfeldt, M. (1992) *The Social Production of Indifference: Exploring the Symbolic Roots of Western Bureaucracy*, Chicago: University of Chicago Press/Berg.

—— (1997) *Cultural Intimacy: Social Poetics in the Nation-State*, New York and London: Routledge.

Horobin, G. (1985) 'Review essay – Medical sociology in Britain: true confessions of an empiricist, *Sociology of Health and Illness*, 7(1): 74–107.

Huby, G. (1997) 'Interpreting silence, documenting experience: an anthropological approach to the study of health service users' experience with HIV/AIDS care in Lothian, Scotland', *Social Science and Medicine* 44(8): 1149–60

Lukes, S. (1974) *Power – A Radical View*, London: Macmillan.

Plummer, K. (1995) *Telling Sexual Stories: Power, Change and Social Worlds*, London: Routledge.

Ritches, D. (1985) 'Power as a representational model', in R. Fardon (ed.) *Power and Knowledge: Proceedings of a Conference Held at the University of St Andrews, December 1982*, Edinburgh: Scottish Academic Press.

Rosaldo, R. (1989) *Culture and Truth: The Remaking of Social Analysis*, London: Routledge.

Samuel, R. and Thompson, P. (eds) (1990) *The Myths we Live By* , London: Routledge.

Sontag, S. (1989) *AIDS and Its Metaphors*, New York: Farrar, Straus & Giroux.

Tierney, W.G. (1995) '(Re)presentation and voice', *Qualitative Inquiry* 1(4): 379–90.

Treichler, P.A. (1992) 'AIDS, HIV, and the cultural construction of reality', in G. Herdt and S. Lindenbaum (eds) *The Time of AIDS: Social Analysis, Theory and Method*, London: Sage.

Turner, T. (1994) 'Bodies and anti-bodies: flesh and fetish in contemporary social theory', in T.J. Csordas (ed.) *Embodiment and Experience: The Existential Ground of Culture and Self*, Cambridge: Cambridge University Press.

Wallman, S. (1988) 'Sex and death: the AIDS crisis in social and cultural context', *Journal of Acquired Immune Deficiency Syndromes* 1: 571–8.

Part I

Power

Chapter 2

Silence and strategy
Researching AIDS/HIV narratives in the flow of power

Brian Heaphy

INTRODUCTION

This chapter has had a relatively long history, which dates from the beginning of my Ph.D. research. It was at this time that I first experienced the contradictory ways in which the academic context in which I had begun to operate appeared to open up some spaces for the voices of people with AIDS/HIV (PWA/HIV), while simultaneously closing others off. Initially this contradiction was experienced at a personal level: while on the one hand I was encouraged in my endeavour to research 'ourselves' as PWA/HIV, on the other it was frequently suggested that my own HIV positive status should not become 'general knowledge'. While the encouragement I received was on the basis that my dual positioning might have something to offer in terms of providing greater insights into the lives of PWA/HIV, the advice on maintaining secrecy concerned the potential implications of 'coming out'. Such implications were mostly framed in terms of possible hostility from colleagues and students, the damaging effects on career prospects, and the extent to which disclosure might cause 'general uncomfortableness'. While the voices of PWA/HIV, it seemed, were acceptable in the academic space provided for the subjects of research, the voices of PWA/HIV as the producers of research might be more problematic.

The local impulse to silence or 'hide' the PWA/HIV can be understood in terms of the power of AIDS/HIV to mark PWA/HIV as 'dangerous' and 'problematic'. It is also consistent with powerful AIDS/HIV knowledge formations that can work to prevent PWA/HIV from speaking out of place (Patton 1990). In a research context, however, such impulses are at odds with more public attempts to address questions of power through 'revealing' the researcher. Within social scientific discourses on methodology there has been a growing emphasis on the need for reflexive approaches to research and an acknowledgement that the results of research are shaped and influenced by the positioning of the researcher. This positioning, together with the context of research, works to construct particular truths and knowledge on any given topic (Steier 1991). To adopt a reflexive approach can also be to acknowledge that research has a role to play in strategies of power (Söderqvist 1991) and to address the ways in which research itself can be employed as a strategy to question the ways in which power works and the ways in which our experiences are shaped (Harding 1987).

For PWA/HIV, as with feminist (Fonow and Cook, 1991) and ethnic minority (Stanfield, 1994) researchers, providing reflexive accounts of the dilemmas and tensions that arise in researching 'ourselves' may be one way in which our research may be of particular value. Although such narratives are of interest in their own right, they can be invaluable in throwing into sharp focus strategies in 'the flow of power' (Plummer 1995). While the accounts or 'stories' of PWA/HIV as research subjects can be important resources in questioning the ways in which power works in the context of AIDS/HIV, the narratives of PWA/HIV as researchers can also be useful in this regard.

The following discussion begins with an account of how AIDS/HIV narratives can be seen to exist in the flow of power. This is also the case for our research accounts of AIDS/HIV. Viewing research in terms of 'story' productions that are bound up with story actions such as 'conversations' and 'dialogues' opens up the possibilities of accounting for power in the research context (Schrijvers 1991; Steier 1991). Through a related focus on the notion of a 'dialogical ideal' we can question the extent to which researching PWA/HIV can be aligned to 'political' projects which aim to challenge existing power relationships. Seen in these terms, however, research also evolves and revolves around silences. In reflecting on my own silences as a researcher I outline the contradictions and tensions encountered between conceptualising research as an opportunity for dialogical communication but recognising that my role as a researcher, in effect, prevented me from realising this opportunity. In reflecting on the silences of PWA/HIV as research subjects I suggest that we are faced with the dilemma that while researchers may aim to *open up* possibilities for PWA/HIV, we may in fact collude with the power relationships we aim to challenge.

AIDS/HIV NARRATIVES AND THE FLOW OF POWER

> The AIDS narrative exists as a technology of social repression; it is a representation that attempts to silence . . . the people marginalised by AIDS.
>
> (Patton 1990: 131)

The present discussion is based on my experience of qualitative research focusing on the changing identities of men and women living with AIDS/HIV. While the research is, in part, concerned with the relationship between medicalisation and identity formation, it is also concerned with 'stories' or 'narratives' about the meaning of AIDS/HIV. In this sense, the research focus has been the stories that respondents tell of the personal meaning of AIDS/HIV, and accounts of the negotiation of 'expert' and 'local' narratives concerning the virus and syndrome.

In Plummer's (1995) terms it is possible to conceptualise these stories as emerging narrative forms that significantly shape the ways in which PWA/HIV conceive possibilities of living. As Plummer puts it:

> The ceaseless nature of story telling in all its forms in all societies has come to be increasingly recognised. . . . Society itself may be seen as a textured but seamless web of stories emerging everywhere through interaction: holding people together, pulling people apart, making societies work . . . the metaphor of the story . . . has become recognised as one of the central roots we have into the continuing quest for understanding human meaning. Indeed culture itself has been defined as 'an ensemble of stories we tell about ourselves'.
>
> (Plummer 1995: 5)

In sustaining and revising their biographical narratives in the face of diagnosis of infection and illness, PWA/HIV are faced with a multiplicity of stories regarding the meaning of the virus and syndrome. These can include accounts provided by 'AIDS professionals' such as doctors, scientists and counsellors, and accounts provided by those personally affected by AIDS/HIV, including other PWA/HIV. It has been suggested, however, that medical and scientific narratives dominate our thinking on the virus and syndrome, as the master narratives or discourses through which AIDS and HIV are given meaning (Treichler 1988; Patton 1990).

From Foucault (1979) and others, it is clear that medico-scientific discourses and narratives of the meaning of illness and disease are far from neutral accounts of the 'truth' . Rather, they are bound up with strategies of power, and have a crucial role to play in disciplinary society. Theorists such as Foucault (1979) have characterised power as it is productive, and partly operates in disciplinary society through an incitement to self-regulation and according to binary divisions of 'mad/sane' 'normal/abnormal' and 'sick/healthy'. Medico-scientific discourses on AIDS/HIV play a crucial role in investing PWA/HIV with a distinct sense of place, function and attribution, and positioning them within these binary oppositions. While AIDS/HIV can be productive of physical illness and disablement, the experience of being a PWA/HIV can also be productive of a self-knowledge of one's 'difference', 'abnormality' and 'otherness'. This self-knowledge of PWA/HIV can be understood as being bound up with medical and scientific constructions of the virus and syndrome and can be conceptualised as a strategy and effect of power (for detailed discussion see Heaphy 1996).

Other stories – such as those provided in 'alternative' medical accounts, moral accounts and activist accounts – interweave with dominant HIV/AIDS narratives and compete to establish what is rational sane and true in this context. As Plummer (1995) argues, with regard to 'sexual' stories, the *personal* accounts of those most closely affected also operate in this flow:

> . . . ultimately it [power] flows through the whole *negotiated social order* – controlling and empowering, closing and opening, making some things

possible and other things impossible. . . . *Sexual stories live in this flow of power.
The power to tell a story, indeed not to tell a story, under the conditions of one's own
choosing, is part of the political process.*

(Plummer 1995: 26; his emphasis).

From my own research it is clear that PWA/HIV stories are often connected
with strategies of power (Heaphy 1996). For example, in terms of knowledge
regarding AIDS/HIV and treatment, PWA/HIV and medical practitioners'
accounts of the role of 'expert' and 'PWA/HIV' are often in conflict. In many
cases, the PWA/HIV's narrative of her/himself as knowledgeable with regard to
her/his own treatment can be in tension with the practitioner's account of who
the PWA/HIV 'should' be as a patient. This is clear from Sue's account:

It was very much a case of, 'This is the drug we give for this and you'll have
it', and if you don't have it then we can't treat you and I felt that unless I
researched it I didn't have any argument to say why I didn't want to take their
drugs. . . . And then I felt that when I was offered something I could actually
say, 'Well I want to spend a week looking at the possible effects and whether
they outweigh – whether the pros outweigh the cons', which didn't go down
at all well. . . . I think it threatens them if you're informed because they've
only read the same things you have – you know? And that's what they don't
want. I think they were certainly threatened and they started seeing me as a
very awkward patient and someone who wouldn't fit in with what they
wanted. They were very unkeen on me finding out my own information. I've
had to really fight to maintain control of what I want and what I don't want.
And they didn't like it at all.

Accounts such as Sue's may highlight how some PWA/HIV reject notions of
themselves as the 'passive patient' in their narratives of self-identity,. They also
suggest that the power of the story is connected with the construction of appropriate and inappropriate storytellers. Patton (1990) suggests that, within
dominant AIDS narratives, the categories of 'PWA' and 'AIDS expert' have been
constructed as mutually exclusive. The voices of PWA/HIV are placed within
the space provided for stories of the personal meanings of living with the virus
syndrome, but not within that provided for 'expert' narratives:

The emerging social roles within the [AIDS] industry were each believed to
possess unique forms of knowledge – the 'experts' knew about the virus and
treatment, the 'person living with AIDS' knew about suffering and death, the
'volunteer' knew about the courage of the human spirit. In fact, the social
role categories which defined how to be an expert, or volunteer, or person
living with HIV/AIDS rarely corresponded with the lived multiple experiences of the epidemic; AIDS knowledge formations tended to silence people
speaking out of character. These silencing effects are grounded in the political
commitments which cordon off the knowledge of science into an unbreach-
able, unquestionable domain; people living with AIDS are not supposed to

become actively involved in treatment concerns and are considered highly biased.

(Patton 1990: 51)

Many PWA/HIV do, of course, resist and challenge such silencing effects in producing their own treatment narratives. Listening to PWA/HIV stories of their own management of infection and illness has allowed me to question the extent to which the medicalisation of AIDS/HIV and PWA/HIV is effective, and also to see the ways in which it is actively resisted. Stories such as Sue's suggest that PWA/HIV *are* often experts in their own treatment (as has been shown to be the case with people dealing with other chronic illnesses – Robinson 1988; Scambler 1989; Bury 1991). We must, of course, beware of privileging these alternative accounts and thereby slipping into what Atkinson (1996) describes as 'romantic reconstructions'. However, through opening up spaces for the voices of PWA/HIV, research can critically engage with medical/scientific claims to be *the* experts on AIDS/HIV and can, thus, have a role in challenging the assumption, found in much AIDS/HIV research, that medico-scientific constructions of AIDS/HIV and PWA/HIV are given and unproblematic.

Using AIDS/HIV narratives in this way is to see the research endeavour itself in terms of strategies of power. It is naive to assume that as researchers we simply document what is 'out there' (Pels and Nencel 1991; Steier 1991; Brewer 1994). As researchers we actively engage in the 'realities' of AIDS/HIV. If 'medical', 'activist' and 'personal' narratives of AIDS/HIV exist in the flow of power, so too do our social scientific research accounts. While many researchers may not *aim* to engage in questions of power, in our production of AIDS/HIV research accounts we are explicitly and/or implicitly involved in asserting, accepting or contesting what is rational, sane and true in the AIDS/HIV context. We become involved in the production or reproduction of AIDS/HIV 'truths', and, therefore, in the production (or reproduction) of what Foucault (1979) terms 'power-knowledge'.

REFLEXIVITY, CONVERSATIONS AND A DIALOGICAL IDEAL

In producing our research accounts we do not operate in a power-free zone (see Denzin 1989; Hammersley, 1989; Atkinson, 1990). Research methodologies can work to reproduce existing power relationships and can also be related to political strategies that aim at empowerment. As Ramazanoglu remarks with regard to feminist research:

Feminist methodologies are then new ways of knowing and of seeking 'truths', but they are also forms of political commitment to the empowerment of women. . . . There is no alternative to political commitment in feminist or any other ways of knowing. Since knowing is a political process, so knowledge is intrinsically political. . . . Other ways of knowing . . . are committed to other political goals.

(Ramazanoglu 1992: 210)

Research accounts themselves are currently conceptualised as stories or narratives (for discussion, see Denzin 1989; Atkinson 1990; Duncombe and Marsden 1996). This acknowledges the constructed and contingent nature of research results or 'truths' (Steier 1991). It is widely suggested that by providing the accounts of why and how we go about research, both the producers and audience of research can begin to separate out and clarify the forces at work in the production of research stories. As Pels and Nencel argue:

> We need these 'second-order narratives' . . . to become acquainted with the power relationships in which we move. If our own project is not clear, we will fail to recognise the project of others. If we keep silent about the motivations of our own statements, other voices will be muted by it.
>
> (Pels and Nencel 1991: 19)

Feminist researchers have long attempted to develop reflexive methodological strategies that acknowledge and deal with power potentials (see Oakley 1981; Harding 1987). As noted by Ramazanoglu (1992), such attempts are not simplistic efforts at 'neutralising' power. Rather, they are attempts to critically engage with existing power relationships and make visible the extent to which research is tied up with political strategies. Feminist researchers have often been concerned with both charting *and* changing the 'realities' of women's lives as an engagement with strategies of power (for discussion, see Gelsthorpe 1992; Hammersley 1992; Ramazanoglu 1992).

In attempting to account for my own involvement in the story actions that inform the results of the research, I have been drawn to a focus on 'conversations' and 'dialogue'. As Steier suggests:

> . . . taking reflexivity seriously in doing research is marked by a concern for recognizing that constructing is a social process, rooted in language, not located inside one's head. . . . It is precisely through such an orientation to languaging that the self to whom our reflexivity refers is most clearly a social self, who becomes 'that' self precisely through participation with others, and allows research to become understood as a conversation (or, rather, several).
>
> (Steier 1991: 5–6)

The formulation of the research topic, the approach adopted to research, the fieldwork and the writing up of research results can all be understood to develop through a wide variety of 'conversations'. These can include those we have with funders, supervisors, colleagues, friends, family, research participants, written materials, and so on. Hence, as Steier (1991) suggests, it is possible to recognise that research evolves and revolves around multiple conversations that work to construct the results of research which are, in effect, multiple 'realities' – with no one being 'the real conversation'. Implicit here is an acknowledgement that in the writing and presentation of results we are editing 'in' some realities while we are editing 'out' others. Our presentation of results by no means exhausts the wide variety of conversations we could have focused on. Rarely do we present, or are we even aware of, the multiple realities that could be presented.

For Steier (1991), adopting such an approach allows contradictions and paradoxes to appear. For researchers this can become 'a way of "unconcealing" our own tacit world, including the constraints we have self-imposed' (Steier 1991: 7). We can begin to see how our values enter our research, and by doing so, Steier suggests, they can become less so:

> Our reflexivity thus reveals itself as an awareness of the recognition that we allow ourselves to hear what our subjects are telling us, not by imposing our categories on them, but by trying to see how our categories may not fit.
>
> (Steier, 1991: 7–8)

Research projects involve complex sets of relationships and negotiations. Throughout the process of research, from the formulation of the topic to the presentation of results, we negotiate with ourselves and others the 'why', 'what', 'how' of research. It is through such interactions that the possibilities and limitations of the project are set – as they impact on decisions regarding what constitute interesting or appropriate aims, focuses, methods and findings. It is here, in developing my own approach, that the focus on conversation also appeared to be useful in considering questions of power. In an effort to disclose the enabling/disabling and empowering/controlling impulses at work we can ask: Which conversations (and, by implication, what and whose agendas) were most influential in defining the subject of research? Which dictated the course of the research? Which are represented in the results of research?

In providing reflexive accounts, and in questioning the research/power relationship, other researchers have also focused on conversation and dialogue. Indeed, in modern anthropology, Schrijvers (1991: 169) suggests that the notions of *dialogical* and *reflexive* research are interchangeable to a certain degree. In dealing with questions of power in terms of the researcher/researched relationship, Schrijvers herself uses the term 'dialogical' to refer to

> a specific, reciprocal manner of exchange and communication during research interaction, between the researcher and the subjects of research. It indicates a continuing process of actual communication between people who respect and value each other's contribution and in that regard are equals in their dialogical relationship. Throughout this communication the participants influence each other's points of view. This can lead to the transformation of the initial concepts and conceptions of the researcher and other participants.
>
> (Schrijvers 1991: 169–70)

Based on her own experience as an anthropologist engaged in 'action-research', and in an attempt to characterise the possibilities and limitations of a 'dialogical ideal', Schrijvers (1991: 170) distinguishes five aspects which characterise dialogical communication in anthropological research: *dynamic*, where the research focuses on change, and the results reflect the dynamics of life; *exchange*, where the terms 'researcher' and 'researched' lose their distinctive meanings; *ideal of egalitarian relations*, where researcher and research subjects become more acutely aware of power inequalities that separate them; *shared objectives*, where the objectives and priorities of research are determined by all participants; and *shared defining-power*, where all participants are empowered to determine the course and outcome of the research.

Dialogical communication, it is suggested in this account, is necessary to reduce inequality in the research context. Further, the researcher both implicitly and explicitly acknowledges that he or she is actively engaged in various sets of power relations and, to some extent, a political endeavour: 'action-research involves activists who are struggling against existing power inequalities' (Schrijvers 1991: 172–3).

A consideration of the 'dialogical ideal' allows us to question the extent to which research on PWA/HIV, particularly as it is carried out by PWA/HIV, can be aligned to political projects which aim to challenge the powerful boundaries between 'knower' and 'known'. To those of us concerned about the extent to which PWA/HIV may or may not have the power to voice their own stories of the meaning of AIDS/HIV – and situations where the terms 'researcher' and 'PWA/HIV' are mutually exclusive – the dialogical ideal, with its emphasis on egalitarianism and shared aims/objectives, is particularly attractive. After all, in cases such as my own the conversations and dialogues between researcher and respondents are also conversations and dialogues between PWA/HIV. The endeavour could be conceptualised as a 'political strategy' that aims to challenge the privileging of expert/professional knowledge and meaning over expert/local knowledge, but also as a strategy for the development of community or local knowledge and 'social' capital (see Wan 1995; Weeks, 1996).

The 'dialogical ideal' allows for a sense of the ways in which research can be conceptualised in terms of 'activist' engagements with power. The potential of such approaches is dependent on the understanding not only that is power productive of oppression, but also that it can be enabling. Yet, as noted earlier, self-reflexivity highlights and brings to the fore contradictions and paradoxes. One of the paradoxes that appears in attempting to 'locate' power by focusing on the 'discursive' is that we become confronted with what is *not* said.

SILENCE AND RESEARCH

Silence: the unspeakable, the perceived but best not said, the ignored, the space occupied by that which is ignored, the hidden, the safely tucked away, the camouflaged, the safety of camouflage.

(Patton 1990: 129)

The research process is also structured by *silences*. In AIDS/HIV research we need to address questions of who can/cannot speak, and what can/cannot be said, as this begins to address the limits of dialogical communication in the research context. In reflecting on the flows of power in which my own research has been produced, I have become concerned with stories that are not told, and conversations or dialogues we do not have. Anderson and Jack (1991) suggest that the development of interview strategies necessitates 'listening beyond' what is explicitly voiced. In order to chart the power of silence we need to '*reflect beyond*' the stories that are told and the conversations/dialogues that do take place.

In my own research, dilemmas regarding silence were experienced throughout the fieldwork in terms of the extent to which it was acceptable to engage 'as an equal' with respondents. In particular, tensions arose with regard to AIDS/HIV treatment stories. The study was informed by a broad range of sociological and activist work that has been critical both of medical interventions in the context of AIDS/HIV and of the medicalisation of PWA/HIV. Yet some respondents' accounts indicated an uncritical faith in medical approaches. Also, while my own strategy for dealing with my HIV status was developed in the context of a suspicion of drug trials, some respondents were keen to participate in these. While some respondents appeared to have faith in particular treatments, the effectiveness of these were widely challenged in other respondents' accounts. Many of those interviewed expressed a distrust with regard to drug trials and the prescription of drugs such as AZT:

> I think they're prepared to kill you off just to sell their drugs. I think they would, yeah. I think it's all political. It's these multinational companies who make AZT. Welcome and all that. I think you've got to be very very sceptical, and look after yourself.
>
> (Rose)

> I took AZT but it made me ill, for about a month or two months, so I didn't take it any more, so I stopped it of my own accord. I chucked it down the toilet. It was my choice – I wouldn't take those drugs again. I don't really trust them. I don't know, they're obviously not too sure about it, or they wouldn't be just trials, why give them to us and not someone else?
>
> (Simon)

Accounts of the 'politics' of drug trials and the effects of particular drugs were matched with accounts that located the taking part in such trials as the 'only hope'. The latter were common not only amongst respondents who were seriously ill, but also amongst those who were recently diagnosed and asymptomatic. Some respondents, like Sam below, sought these out and made great efforts to participate:

> . . . what I'm doing at the moment is that I'm taking part in a trial of a new drug that's up in London. I travel up, because [area] is too small . . . there just aren't enough people in this area for the drug companies, and they don't want to spend money for a small sample. Then this trial came up, and I fitted the profile, and I've always wanted to do something, not sit back and wait.

It could have been possible to have viewed accounts such as Sam's as evidence of the effectiveness of medico-scientific narratives, that imply that hope in the face of AIDS/HIV lies primarily in medical research. However, as the participation in trials *can* be the basis of much hope regarding the possibility of survival, decisions such as that made by Sam are based on more than an uncritical acceptance of the model of 'expert' medical knowledge. In such situations, ethical imperatives can work to silence the researcher who wishes to problematise respondents' decisions to take part in clinical trials. Of course, researchers can choose to accept accounts at face value in the interview, but go on to problematise them in their analyses. This is not necessarily a 'comfortable' choice (see Barbour, Chapter 11). In not challenging respondents' accounts, however, are researchers actually denying them the status of agents? (Huby, in Chapter 10, makes a similar point with regard to the 'forced' and perhaps ultimately 'patronising tolerance' which we extend to interviewees.)

In other cases, ethical dilemmas around intervention and silence were even more acute. This was particularly the case when some respondents felt that they had no choice with regard to treatment. This was not uncommon amongst those whose primary source of support and information came from the clinic, and who had little contact with other PWA/HIV. Some respondents' accounts, like Diana's below, suggested a lack of awareness that their illnesses might be related to the side-effects of the treatments prescribed for them:

BH: What drugs are you taking?

Diana: Do you really want a list? [*Laughs*] Do you really want a list?! I'm on the AZT obviously, I'm on steroids because I'm having eczema really bad, I'm on sleeping pills and another drug for my stomach. I've lost all my hair by the way – this is a wig. [*Laughs*] I don't know what else I'm on. I'm on twelve different pills, twelve lots of tablets.

BH: Do you know what they're all for?

Diana: The AZT – don't know what that's for – I suppose it boosts your immune system. Steroids, for the skin. Sleeping tablets. I'm on anti-itch ones. . . .

BH: Do you absorb them all well? Do you have any side-effects?

Diana: I don't know if I've had any side-effects. I couldn't tell you if I had – I just swallow what I'm given. Do you know what I mean?

Diana was in the relatively early stages of HIV infection. From her account it appeared that the radical decline of her health might be related to the treatment programme. As she had little contact with other PWA/HIV or self-help organisations, she was dependent on the clinic staff for both medical *and* emotional support. Problematising the faith she had placed in those treating her was ethically highly questionable. In fieldwork situations such as this the notion of a dialogical ideal is problematic.

In terms of both Sam's and Diana's treatment accounts, the dilemmas I encountered revolved around the professional and ethical tension between disclosing my own opinions and experience and the impulse to silence. Although the silence was 'self-imposed', I operated, as an individual researcher, within a research culture which has developed its own standards with regard to what are defined as 'acceptable' and 'unacceptable' roles and practices for researchers to adopt.

The political, policy and funding climate can produce silencing effects and can restrict or shape the focus of research. Few researchers today can afford to ignore the politics of resourcing (see also Neil Small, Chapter 8). Most of us are required to tailor our projects in terms of what is likely to be sponsored or funded. There are, however, more subtle forces at work which shape our research.. Given the exigencies of the funding and publication traditions within which we, as researchers, must work, we frequently find ourselves operating in contexts which value and privilege only certain approaches to research and certain kinds of knowledge.

The academic disciplines in which we operate play a crucial role in defining the appropriate topics and aims of research, together with the appropriate methodological approach (Smith 1987; Pels and Nencel 1991). There is a tension between the ethos of 'objectivity' (that is central to both scientific/academic claims of expertise and the privileged position of 'knower') and the characterisation of research as a political project. As Söderqvist notes with regard to the structures that shape the production of scientific/academic knowledge:

> The key element in the institutions of science and scholarship, and hence in the reproduction of knowledge-power, is the idea of objective knowledge. Objective knowledge consists of general mental representations which obtain their meanings exclusively through their capacity to correspond to things, properties, and relations which exist in an external world. Objective knowledge representing real world events has priority over personal experience in which representation of inner states cannot be excluded. Experiences that are not incorporated into the body of scientific, scholarly and professional knowledge are degraded as 'subjective', 'mere folk belief', etc. It is not what 'I feel' or 'I experience' that counts, but 'How things are'.
>
> (Söderqvist 1991: 146–7)

The power of our voices as researchers has traditionally relied on constructions and presentations of ourselves as *objective* knowers. There are two notable ways in which the claim to objectivity produces silence: in the presentation of research results the claim has often resulted in the 'editing out' of the motives of the researcher; in carrying out the fieldwork it has traditionally prompted the researcher to remain silent about his/her own opinions and experiences.

In terms of the motives for research, the notion of the 'pure' researcher who is unaffected by his/her social, cultural and political positioning has been widely challenged. Silverman (1985) suggests that most research is generated by a series of circumstances relating to the particular researcher and the economic, social and political context in which he or she works. Stacey (1991) notes that, in feminist research, personal interests and skills meld, often mysteriously, with collective feminist concerns to determine a particular research topic. In the end, the research endeavour can be influenced by a broad range of personal, professional and political motives (see also Marshall and Rossman 1995).

While social research on AIDS/HIV is often explicit in terms of *how* research is carried out, relatively few researchers are as explicit as to why *they* are engaged in such research. Inherent in the common reference to the 'urgency' of the 'crisis' of AIDS/HIV is the implication that the researcher's motivation is based on some assumed common AIDS/HIV agenda, and that the personal impetus behind the project 'goes without saying'. Also, while there are some notable exceptions, an explicit account of what the particular researcher's political project might be is often lacking. Audiences and subjects of research, however, do not necessarily share researchers' self-notions of integrity and the implicit worthiness of our endeavours.

In focusing on *how* we do research, and not *why* we do so, the illusion of objectivity remains intact while the claim to reflexivity appears to be accounted for. Yet this is to become actively involved in the reproduction of knowledge–power relations in a way that is at odds with the possibilities offered by reflexivity. At its most radical point, what is at stake in the reflexive project is not only the researcher's reflection on the history of the research, but also the revealing of this history, including the researcher's motives, in the results of research. In researching 'ourselves', PWA/HIV must interrogate and reveal our own motivations, not least of all in terms of who the research is strategic for – the individual researcher or PWA/HIV generally. With regard to my own work, this has meant addressing questions such as: To what extent is the focus on the changing identities of PWA/HIV an indication of this particular researcher's interest in his own changing identity? Is the focus on the meanings and personal implications of AIDS/HIV related to the researcher's own negotiation of the meaning of infection and illness? Does the concern with personal stories reflect the researcher's concern with his own story, and to what extent is the research autobiographical? To what extent is the researcher concerned with using the experience of other PWA/HIV as a means of accumulating academic capital?

It is often implied that PWA/HIV are 'too close' to the topic, and cannot be neutral. Such a perspective plays into other dynamics of power related to the notion of objectivity. While our motives for researching ourselves do not go without saying, the position of the non-PWA/HIV as researcher is *equally* problematic. Unlike the claim to be a feminist researcher which reveals an alignment to a broader 'political' project – even if what that might mean is by no means the subject of broad agreement – the label of AIDS/HIV researcher reveals very little. It tells us very little about the researcher's personal or political project and how it has influenced what, how and why s/he does what s/he is doing. Irrespective of their AIDS/HIV status, it is in revealing 'themselves' that researchers can begin to demonstrate an awareness of their involvement in the flow of power. In doing so, they may also resist some of the potential silencing effects of the claim to objectivity.

Yet, the claim to objectivity can limit the extent to which the researcher/ researched relationship can be an equal one. In terms of fieldwork, and the researcher/researched relationship, the claim can work to silence researchers in a way that is at odds with the empowering possibilities of dialogical communication. The possibilities, as outlined earlier, are dependent on a form of communication between equals that can lead to the transformation of concepts and conceptions of the researcher *and* participants. In this sense, the dialogical ideal is consistent with critiques of traditional notions of objectivity which have led some researchers to develop interview strategies based on an 'equal exchange of information' (see Oakley 1981). However, such characterisations of fieldwork underestimate the extent to which traditional notions of objectivity are publicly presented as the *defining* element of science and scholarship. As such they inform not only researchers' notions of acceptable practice, but also those of research subjects. In fieldwork such as the interview, both 'the discipline' *and* the respondents may expect that the researcher's objectivity will be manifest in her/his silence. Such expectations present the researcher with professional and ethical dilemmas that are not easily resolved.

We need to be aware that when PWA/HIV agree to be researched, even by other PWA/HIV, they rarely expect an equal conversation or dialogue. While researchers may conceptualise the research process as a chance for 'equal' exchange, respondents may have expectations of the process which do not include the possibility of decisions, or accounts, such as those relating to treatment strategies, being questioned. We are dealing not *only* with the extent to which researchers internalise the requirements of objectivity, the quest for knowledge, and assumptions about the necessity of disparities in power between researchers and researched and the ways in which this is used to justify silence and non-intervention. We must also recognise the importance of respondents' assumptions about researchers' silences and what these reveal with regard to their moral/medical decisions and practices. As researchers and academics we may have deconstructed traditional notions of objectivity; yet, the extent to which research subjects retain such traditional notions presents important limitations to the dialogical ideal and the notion of 'empowerment' that is implicit therein.

SILENCE AND PWA/HIV

Reflection on the silences of research subjects is also instructive in considering how research operates in the flow of power. This is particularly so when we consider *why* research subjects might actively choose silence over disclosure. From my own research it is clear that PWA/HIV often employ silence in an effort to resist medical practitioners' attempts to know and place them in terms of categories of normality (see also Huby 1997). As Maya says:

I mean it was a constant question, every time the doctor came round they would say 'Do you think you could tell us how you think you got it' and I would just say 'No'. . . . They like to feel that ordinary people do not go around getting HIV, you *have* to have done something that falls into what they call risk categories . . . and they just want to feel that it isn't suddenly breaking into the 'straight' community. I really do think that that's their agenda, that they want to see where it is . . . they were just interested to know what I was doing basically so that they could slip me into one of their categories.

Other respondents, such as Paul below, indicated that silence has been employed in the face of what they see as questionable research interests:

BH: One question I wanted to ask is why you agreed to take part.
Paul: Well, I don't usually! I suppose because your advert said that you were positive – I just thought 'That's interesting'. . . . To be honest I think a lot of it can be quite dodgy. [*Laughs*] You know, especially when it's. . . . Like I never fill in those forms they give you about your sexuality and race and things – or when they ask you if you've recently been to Africa or whatever, I just think 'Mmm?'

Silence may reflect the mistrust with which some PWA/HIV view researchers' motives and the possible implications of our research. In one study of the sexual lives of HIV positive men, which aimed to explore strategies which enable PWA/HIV to maintain having safer sex, the authors report that 'Potential respondents voted with their feet and refused to get involved' (Donovan *et al.* 1995: 18). The authors suggest that the lack of success in recruiting interviewees can be understood in terms of death and illness of the study population, study fatigue and sensitivity of the topic:

> The very poor response to the researcher's attempts to attend meetings to speak about the project . . . led us to the conclusion that sex and especially risky sex was a threatening topic for research.
>
> (Donovan *et al.* 1995: 18)

It is crucial that we interrogate such silences further. Whatever the aims of researchers, our projects exist in flows of power, where intentions and effects do not necessarily mesh in the ways which we intend. It may be not so much that the 'sensitivity' of our research topics is threatening. Rather, the research endeavour to know PWA/HIV, as it is potentially part of pathologising and disciplining strategies, poses a threat to PWA/HIV. In these terms the silence of PWA/HIV can be understood as a *strategy of resistance* (see also Abdulrahim, Chapter 3).

The silences of research subjects have much to say to us about our research endeavours. In over-emphasising the empowering aims of AIDS/HIV research we risk silencing the extent to which the research exercise can be bound up with power/knowledge in other ways. Reflecting beyond the explicit aims and possibilities of research we can see that we may be actively engaged in the production of silences regarding the unintended effects of our research. In researching the experiences of PWA/HIV, researchers – whether PWA/HIV or not – work with the tension that while we may *aim* to open up possibilities for PWA/HIV, we may, in fact, silence important stories and may thus collude with disempowerment.

Whilst it is possible to characterise clinical experts' concerns with 'knowing' people with AIDS/HIV in terms of disciplinary and regulatory impulses (Patton 1990; Heaphy 1996), as researchers we are often silent about the potential of our own work in these terms. In this sense one of the questions we *could* address relates to the extent to which our concerns with who PWA/HIV are can fuel the very power relations we attempt to challenge. As noted earlier, Foucault (1979) has emphasised the power of the 'normative' within disciplinary society. In doing so, he has also suggested that the judges of normality are everywhere: the teacher judge, the doctor judge, the educator judge, the social worker judge on whom 'the universal reign of the normative is based' (Foucault 1979: 304). We must acknowledge that our own endeavours to know PWA/HIV are potentially bound up with judging, policing and disciplining strategies. If we are truly interested in addressing the power/research relationship we must therefore interrogate, and voice, how our research benefits the populations we study *and* how it does not.

ACKNOWLEDGEMENTS

My thanks to Kevin Eisenstadt and Rachel Thomson for invaluable conversations relating to this chapter.

REFERENCES

Anderson, K. and Jack, D. (1991) 'Learning to listen: interview techniques and analyses', in S.B. Gluck and D. Patai (eds) *Women's Words: The Feminist Practice of Oral History*, London: Routledge.

Atkinson, P. (1990) *The Ethnographic Imagination: Textual Constructions of Reality*, London: Routledge.

—— (1996) 'Narrative turn or blind alley? Reflections on narrative and qualitative health research', plenary paper presented at the Third International Interdisciplinary Qualitative Health Research Conference, University of Bournemouth, 30 October–1 November.

Brewer, J.D. (1994) 'The ethnographic critique of ethnography: sectarianism in the RUC', *Sociology*, 28(1): 231–44.

Bury, M. (1991) 'The sociology of chronic illness: a review of research and prospects', *Sociology of Health and Illness*, 13(4): 451–68.

Denzin, N.K. (1989) *Interpretive Interactionism*, London: Sage.

Donovan, C., Sugden, N., Mearns, C. and McEwan, R. (1995) *Keeping On, Keeping On: A Study Looking at Ways of Enabling People with HIV and Their Partners to Keep on Having Safer Sex*, Newcastle upon Tyne: Northern & Yorkshire Regional Health Authority.

Duncombe, J. and Marsden, D. (1996) 'Can we research the private sphere? Methodological and ethical problems in the study of the role of emotion in personal relationships', in L. Morris and S. Lyon (eds) *Gender Relations in Public and Private: New Research Perspectives*, London: Macmillan.

Fonow, M. and Cook, J. (eds) (1991) *Beyond Methodology: Feminist Scholarship as Lived Experience*, Indianapolis: Indiana University Press.

Foucault, M. (1979) *Discipline and Punish: The Birth of the Prison*, Harmondsworth: Penguin.

Gelsthorpe, L. (1992) 'Response to Martyn Hammersley's paper "On feminist methodology"', *Sociology*, 26(2): 213–18.

Hammersley, M. (1989) *The Dilemma of Qualitative Method*, London: Routledge.

Hammersley, M. (1992) 'On feminist methodology', *Sociology*, 26(2): 187–206.

Harding, S. (1987) 'Introduction: is there a feminist method?', in S. Harding (ed.) *Feminism and Methodology*, Milton Keynes: Open University Press.

Heaphy, B. (1996) 'Medicalisation and identity formation: identity and strategy in the context of AIDS and HIV', in J. Weeks and J. Holland (eds) *Sexual Cultures: Communities, Values and Intimacy*, London: Macmillan.

Huby, G. (1997) 'Interpreting silence, documenting experience: an anthropological approach to the study of health services users' experience with HIV/AIDS care in Lothian, Scotland', *Social Science and Medicine*, 44(8): 1149–60.

Marshall, C. and Rossman, G.B. (1995) *Designing Qualitative Research*, London: Sage.

Oakley, A. (1981) 'Interviewing women: a contradiction in terms', in H. Roberts (ed.) *Doing Feminist Research*, London: Routledge & Kegan Paul.

Patton, C. (1990) *Inventing AIDS*, London: Routledge.

Pels, P. and Nencel, L. (1991) 'Introduction: critique and the deconstruction of anthropological authority', In L. Nencel and P. Pels (eds) *Constructing Knowledge: Authority and Critique in Social Science*, London: Sage.

Plummer, K. (1995) *Telling Sexual Stories: Power, Change and Social Worlds*, London: Routledge.

Ramazanoglu, C. (1992) 'On feminist methodology: male reason versus female empowerment', *Sociology*, 26(2): 207–12.

Robinson, I. (1988) *Multiple Sclerosis*, London: Routledge.

Scambler, G. (1989) *Epilepsy*, London: Routledge.

Schrijvers, J. (1991) 'Dialectics of a dialogical ideal: studying down, studying sideways, studying up', in L. Nencel and P. Pels (eds) *Constructing Knowledge: Authority and Critique in Social Science*, London: Sage.

Silverman, D. (1985) *Qualitative Methodology and Sociology*, Aldershot: Gower.

Smith, D.E. (1987) 'Women's perspectives as a radical critique of sociology', in S. Harding (ed.) *Feminism and Methodology*, Milton Keynes: Open University Press.

Söderqvist, T. (1991) 'Biography or ethnobiography or both? Embodied reflexivity and the deconstruction of power-knowledge', in F. Steier (ed.) *Research and Reflexivity*, London: Sage.

Stacey, J. (1991) 'Can there be a feminist ethnography?', in S.B. Gluck and D. Patai (eds) *Women's Words: The Feminist Practice of Oral History*, London: Routledge.

Stanfield, J.H. (1994) 'Ethnic modeling in qualitative research', in N.K. Denzin and Y.S. Lincoln (eds) *Handbook of Qualitative Research*, London: Sage.

Steier, F. (1991) 'Introduction: research as self-reflexivity, self-reflexivity as social process', in F. Steier. (ed.) *Research and Reflexivity*, London: Sage.

Treichler, P. (1988) 'AIDS, homophobia and biomedical discourse', in D. Crimp (ed.) *AIDS: Cultural Analysis, Cultural Activism*, London: MIT Press.

Wan, M. (1995) *Building Social Capital: Self Help in the 21st-Century Welfare State*, London: IPPR.

Weeks, J. (1996) 'The idea of a sexual community', *Soundings* 2: 71–83.

Chapter 3

Power, culture and the 'hard to reach'

The marginalisation of minority ethnic populations from HIV prevention and harm minimisation

Dima Abdulrahim

INTRODUCTION

The success of the British strategy in tackling HIV amongst injecting drug users has been well documented (see, for example, Stimson and Hunter 1996). It has been argued that interventions such as sterile syringe distribution would not work unless the target population was amenable (Stimson and Donoghoe 1996). However, and although it is insufficiently substantiated, it is widely believed that minority ethnic dependent drug users may be reluctant to establish contact with drug agencies (Task Force to Review Services for Drug Misusers 1996: 89) and that their needs may not be adequately met by services. Collectively, they have been construed as possibly the hardest to reach of a wider category of 'hard to reach' groups: a label applied to illicit drug users in general because of their reluctance to establish contact with specialist agencies or researchers. However, and despite the increased use of alternative strategies such as outreach work and peer education, mainstream policy and practice is still generally based on the premise that educating drug users about HIV and changing their behaviour involves first bringing individuals into contact with specialist agencies.

Relationships between these agencies and people classed as 'ethnic minority members' raise issues around concepts of 'ethnicity', 'culture' and how the operationalisation of these terms in policy and practice leads to ethnic minority marginalisation from mainstream HIV prevention and harm minimisation. In this chapter I explore some of these issues, arguing that minority ethnic drug users are a highly heterogeneous group. Their experiences and responses vary, both between and across groups officially defined as 'ethnic minorities'. This chapter seeks to avoid 'tribalising' those from particular cultural 'groups': a black or Cypriot drug user is a drug user, to paraphrase Max Gluckman loosely. It also seeks to avoid reducing culture to ethnic identity: Cypriot drug users do not do what they do simply because they are Cypriot.

This chapter will argue that drug-related harm and its reduction cannot be understood without reference to wider issues of power and its conceptualisation. I regard 'culture' as created in complex interaction that is structurally rooted and contingent, and will argue that the concepts of culture and power are not separable.

Power is examined as something that is exercised rather than possessed; it is productive of knowledge, and also of policy, practice and resource allocation. The chapter will investigate the capacity of HIV prevention, harm minimisation and drug treatment to attract or repel Cypriots and other minority ethnic drug users and wider populations. It will examine aspects of the broader social, cultural and political context of risk reduction initiatives and will explore how marginalisation from services operates. The chapter will examine if and how effective mainstream intervention can be achieved when resources and symbolic imagery are controlled by others.

Data discussed here have been collected in North London between 1991 and 1996 for two inter-disciplinary studies. The first research project partially focused on Greek and Turkish Cypriot populations and investigated issues pertaining to mainstream HIV and drug service purchase and provision. The second study is based on interviews with 150 dependent heroin and/or crack cocaine users, 60 per cent of whom were women. The majority of the latter (60 per cent) had no current contact with harm minimisation or drug treatment services and 63.3 per cent injected at the time of the interview. Informants represented the 'ethnic' and 'cultural' diversity of the area and approximately half of them were from minority ethnic 'groups' (Abdulrahim *et al.* 1994, 1996).

THE BACKGROUND OF HIV-RELATED POLICY, PRACTICE AND RESEARCH

In Britain, the HIV epidemic amongst injecting drug users anticipated in the mid-1980s has been, to a large extent, averted (Stimson 1994a, 1994b, 1995). The low and stable rates may be partially explained by genetic variations in susceptibility and viral strain, sampling bias and the dynamics of the injecting population. There is, however, much evidence that low prevalence rates are also the result of behavioural changes amongst the target group and of the wide range of prevention initiatives available (Stimson and Hunter 1996; see also Des Jarlais and Friedman 1996). Factors identified as instrumental to the success of British interventions included the quick response of policy-makers and the presence of a comprehensive range of services aimed at drug users (Stimson and Hunter 1996). However, the current epidemic levels of hepatitis C infection reveal continued high-risk injecting practices. Resources need to continue to be directed at drug users so that rates of HIV infection remain low.

Injecting drug users were not alone in demonstrating that they are willing and able to make behavioural changes, and in demonstrating the effectiveness of behavioural change at the community level. Although gay men continue to be affected by HIV and AIDS, the mobilisation of British gay men and their adoption of safer sex practices undoubtedly curtailed the surge of the HIV epidemic. Despite the expectation that rates of infection through homosexual intercourse are set to continue and rise (Public Health Laboratory Service 1990), research in the early 1990s showed an 'alarmingly low level' of HIV prevention work targeting gay or bisexual men (King *et al.* 1992: 1). More recently, activists have been calling for the 're-gaying' of AIDS to ensure that statutory and voluntary resources are targeted at them (Weeks *et al.* 1996).

HIV has been the catalyst of the proliferation of research on sexual and injecting practices. Although a small body of pre-AIDS knowledge does exist, the dearth of even basic descriptive information meant, for example, that HIV prevention was not able to learn from the lessons of the earlier hepatitis B epidemic (Strang *et al.* 1992: 344).

Frankenberg (1992) argues that social scientists working on HIV often used theoretical tools similar to a flawed concept adopted in earlier decades for the understanding of issues of 'race' and 'ethnicity' in social work and medicine. The much criticised notion of 'ethnic non-compliance' was based on the perception that people were unhealthy because they did not comply with advice given by professionals, and that their 'culture' prevented them from doing so. Within HIV-related research, a similar notion was extended to cover indigenous groups. Researchers were often expected to 'discover' homogeneous 'cultures' and 'communities' of gay men and drug users, and by so doing change their behaviour. Research and practice often reified these 'cultures' or 'subcultures' and promoted ideas such as that the sharing of injecting equipment is a 'cultural' bonding mechanism. Implicit in this notion was the belief that the 'culture' or 'sub-culture' itself creates risk (Frankenberg 1992).

Notions that the homosexual or drug dependent 'other' 'is' behaving, and 'must' behave, in certain ways raise issues of power and control. It has been argued by Quimby (1992) that HIV has forced social scientists to view the concepts of power and culture as inseparable. According to this view, power should be viewed as a part of social life, giving rise to notions of cultural legitimacy and illegitimacy and shaping meanings of, and reactions to, normality and deviance. The notion of 'cultures' or 'subcultures' as immoral, illicit or illegal has been applied to politically marginal or powerless groups, such as gay men or drug 'addicts', and reflects aspects of labelling by dominant groups (Quimby 1992: 166). Research can, thus, create and reproduce a social reality that excludes people from resources. Sophie Day (1990) investigates the contemporary cliché of research that female sex workers insist on condom use, and how this may divert resources away from appropriate interventions.

Over the span of the epidemic many simplistic notions have been challenged and resisted. People affected by HIV were able to read the texts produced by researchers and practitioners and tested or contested their characterisations. They also drew attention to the dangers of generalisations which may further stereotype, exoticise and marginalise groups of people. Gay activists in particular called for a type of indigenisation of theory and for the need to reformulate research questions with the aim of engendering empowerment over health and lifestyle. Issues raised in this context are relevant to the study of 'ethnic minority drug users' and the design of services aiming to meet their needs. Significant advances have been made with regard to knowledge and understanding of both injecting and sexual practice. Sociology has been invaluable in providing in-depth information and understanding. Studies have shown how different people may give different meanings to sexual or drug using behaviours, and have investigated differences based on ethnicity, sexuality, gender, and so forth. The need to avoid resorting to new orthodoxies is emphasised by Barbour (1993), who urges us to remain alert to the differences that exist within groups. Research has shown how failure to do so can lead to cultural stereotyping (Kline *et al.* 1992: 455); the obscuring of differences in safer sex practices amongst gay men belonging to different age groups (Hart *et al.* 1992); or the failure to recognise the differences between the needs of gay men and bisexual men who do not identify themselves as part of the gay community (Bloor 1995).

STUDYING ETHNIC MINORITY DRUG USERS: POWER AND CULTURE

Despite a wide body of knowledge on illicit drug users in Britain, little systematic research has been carried out amongst those from minority ethnic 'groups' (exceptions include Mirza *et al.* 1991; Awiah *et al.* 1992; Daniel 1992; Abdulrahim *et al.* 1994; Klee & Owolabi 1993; Perera *et al.* 1993; Johnson and Carroll 1995). The report of the Task Force to Review Services for Drug Misusers looked at drug service provision and identified a number of factors to explain their possible under-utilisation of services. These included the fact that they may be less aware of services, concerns about confidentiality and anonymity, and the fact that the social risks of disclosing drug use may be seen as more significant than the personal risks associated with drug use. The tendency of drug treatment agencies to adopt simplistic views of ethnic minorities and of ways of addressing their needs was also emphasised (Task Force to Review Services for Drug Misusers 1996: 89).

An early 1990s review of generic HIV primary prevention initiatives aimed at minority ethnic populations in general also showed a dependence on rudimentary notions of minority ethnic 'culture' (Abdulrahim 1991). These mirrored the discourse that has come to dominate the representation, descriptive as well as polit-ical, of people singled out as 'ethnic minorities'. This equates ethnic categories to social groups under the name of 'community' and identifies each community with its own reified 'culture' (Baumann 1996: 188). Minority ethnic populations in general were frequently placed by HIV prevention in the nebulous category of 'hard to reach'. In the name of cultural sensitivity many groups of people were reified as essentially 'traditional' and cultures as 'immutable', especially around issues of sexual behaviour, sexuality and gendered relations of power. HIV preven-tion generally viewed people as passive carriers of exotic cultural baggage rather than active agents of culture. Too much was too often ascribed to this reified 'culture' without taking into account the socio-economic and political conditions that contribute to alleged cultural patterns. This frequently contributed to a simplistic analysis of the powerful behavioural, social and political forces that construct people's understanding of HIV and AIDS. Service providers' task was conceptualised as reaching people in spite of their culture (Abdulrahim 1991).

The present research on the access of drug users to services in North London also showed that harm minimisation policy and practice often stereotyped minority ethnic 'cultures' as generating the problem. This frequently resulted in cultural stereotyping and led to the creation and reproduction of social boundaries and the increased marginalisation of people from mainstream resources. By focusing on the reified cultures of minority ethnic drug users, harm minimisation policy and practice failed to identify how the cultures and most mundane practices of institutions, organisations and bureaucratic structures can exclude people from services/resources. The structural constraints which impede innovative and equitable strategic service development were overlooked. In order to rectify this omission, we need to examine institutional arrangements and their operation so as to identify the mechanisms via which discrimination or marginalisation occurs. There is no doubt that the kind of 'ethnic absolutism' identified by Gilroy (1987) has been integral to much service delivery, and that the emphasis on ethnic or cultural specificity has become an important feature in rationalising the failure to achieve equity.

However, as argued by Baumann (1996: 11), the concepts of 'culture' or 'community' may hold relevance and meaning for social actors despite being deconstructed in an academic context. Informants in the present research mobilised these notions of culture as received heritage to identify their sense of exclusion or marginalisation from mainstream harm reduction initiatives. They essentialised majority society and culture and held reductionist views of its members, thus alluding to the influence of ethnocentric assumptions in shaping harm minimisation interventions. They also manipulated notions such as 'mentality' as an 'artifact used in the construction of difference' (Herzfeldt 1997: 70), in this case based on 'culture' or 'ethnicity' to allude to wider political issues of public service delivery. For example, one said:

> A lot of the establishment that are like this [community drug service], they are actually run by white people or English people, not like by ethnics. . . . because, an English person can never really understand the mentality of a Jamaican and the mentality of a lot of other people, 'cos they're English, and that's just the way it is. . . .
>
> (Jamaican dependent drug user)

In recent years, dominant notions of 'culture' and 'community' have also been enmeshed in the politics of the public funding of social welfare and health care. Partially at least, they form part of what Stolcke (1994) referred to as the 'new rhetoric of exclusion'. These concepts allude to differential access to the public domain and raise questions about the exercise of power. Like 'culture', 'power' has been deconstructed as a universally valid and applicable concept whilst structural contingencies continue to shape both our lives and our experience of them. Respondents in the present study did not engage in a discourse about 'power', as such. However, they knew very well what 'power' was – in the sense of structural constraints and social barriers – and experienced and reacted to it from a position of disadvantage. Their reactions and interpretations of their relationship to drug agencies forced analysis to look at 'power' and 'culture' as inseparable. They were aware of the role of power in their interaction with drug services and were conscious of its different causes and manifestations, such as those emanating from colour racism, those emanating from the ethnocentric nature of mainstream service purchase and provision, and those emanating from the wider historical and contemporary context of minority/majority power relations. They were aware that contact with harm minimisation and HIV prevention initiatives cannot be dissociated from the complex social and political contexts within which relationships occur. Informants thus wanted analysis to incorporate the fact that notions central to HIV prevention and harm minimisation have to be located in wider contexts of perceived and/or objective powerlessness or marginalisation. Although their discourse differed from that of the social researcher, it echoed Schneider's definition that 'Social relations of race, class and gender are hierarchically organised, resting on and resulting in inequalities of social and political power over labour, resources and services' (Schneider 1992: 21).

Informants also forced analysis to view them as social actors, not exclusively and passively 'locked into an ideational predestination' (Herzfeldt 1997: 29; also see Fardon 1985: 6), and to explore issues of independent action and agency in drug service (non-)utilisation. Drug users, regardless of 'ethnicity', are often reluctant to use services because HIV prevention and harm minimisation are viewed as power–knowledge relations that participate in social control. The analysis of service non-utilisation by minority ethnic drug users also reveals the role of agency.

This non-utilisation has to be viewed, at times, as a positive act and as a form of resistance to imposed and stigmatising cultural and community identities and should be analysed as existing within a wider collective processes of self-determination. The chapter will also show how, at other times, resistance to mainstream initiatives is part of a wider project of the social construction of culture, community and continuance. HIV and drug use are sometimes constructed as conditions of 'Otherness' in order both to forge cultural and moral separateness from the majority society and to counteract domination by the 'culture' of the majority.

HIV AND THE CONSTRUCTION OF 'OTHERNESS'

Mainstream HIV prevention has often ignored the diversity of its target population. A North London survey of two thousand young people aged 13 to 18 years showed that those from affluent social classes had better levels of knowledge of HIV prevention than others; those from the majority white society had more than their peers from minority ethnic 'groups'. Partially at least, these statistically significant differences revealed a cultural and class bias of the school-based interventions and their ineptitude at making HIV equally relevant to all young people (Abdulrahim *et al.* 1994). Of course, many other elements determine young people and adults' responsiveness to prevention campaigns, and their willingness or ability to act upon information. Despite mass prevention campaigns and an increased awareness of the 'non-discriminatory' nature of the virus, there is no doubt that HIV and AIDS remain for the bulk of adult British society conditions of 'Otherness'. HIV continues to be associated with homosexual men, injecting drug users and sub-Saharan Africans, and these continue to define HIV as a metaphor for 'Otherness'.

Research carried out amongst Greek and Turkish Cypriot adults revealed that these same factors also created and reproduced HIV as a condition of 'Otherness'. HIV is constructed as a marker of separateness, and as a condition of the white English majority, specifically because it is perceived as a condition of gay men, injecting drug users, promiscuous women and sex workers. It is a condition of 'Otherness' precisely because expressions of ethnic identity require that individuals do not engage in perceived high-HIV risk activities, that is, are heterosexual and drug-free. A blind eye is often turned to their existence in the societies of origin. HIV is perceived as an indigenous English phenomenon, produced by a permissive society; it is merely further evidence of the moral decadence of the host society. This was summed up by a Cypriot respondent:

> As far as [London] Cypriots are concerned there is no one in Cyprus that's got AIDS. It comes from America and England and dirty countries, know what I mean, because we do class ourselves as a little better than the English.
>
> (Greek Cypriot heroin user)

As a result, many deny that AIDS affects them, because they believe themselves to be 'protected by their culture'. Cypriots are not alone in holding this belief. A study conducted in London, for example, found that many Chinese people thought that a combination of their conservative attitudes, social pressures and self-discipline made them believe that they are less at risk from AIDS. This meant that they did not see a need to change their behaviour (Ethnic Response and Communication Research Council 1988). The present research amongst Cypriots also revealed that as high-risk HIV behaviours are generally constructed as the behaviours of the 'Other', HIV is turned into a signifier of the potential 'corruption' of young people and women by the dominant society and culture and of the moral disorder resulting from migration and contact with the host culture and society. Generic drugs and HIV prevention messages are thus often seen as being devised for the 'Other' and do not affect them, because they have their own forms of regulation. Effective HIV and drug prevention are thus perceived by many as primarily a process of resisting aspects of the dominant culture and of teaching their children to do so. They are part of a wider project of constructing community and continuity.

THE POLITICAL CONTEXT OF DRUG USE, HARM MINIMISATION AND HIV

There is, of course, no denying that some Cypriots engage in high-risk behaviours, despite prevailing taboos around addiction and drug use, same-gender sex, extra-marital sex and commercial sex, and despite taboos around injecting, held even by many heroin users. Over the years, drug agencies in North London have seen a slow but steady trickle of Cypriot drug users, but professionals believe that only a minority are accessing their services, or using needle exchange facilities. It has also been noted by drug professionals and Cypriot drug users alike that contact with agencies is often sought at times of crisis; users thus miss out on the opportunity to reduce drug-related harm at earlier stages of their careers. Cypriot heroin users said for example:

> . . . Greeks would rather go out and buy them [sterile needles] and say I'm diabetic or something.
>
> (Cypriot heroin user)

> . . . like the Cypriot guys, the Cypriots that I know, they knew about the needle exchange but they never use it.
>
> (Cypriot heroin user)

> People come to the programme when they are in the last state. I mean you have to be very desperate.
>
> (Turkish Cypriot heroin user)

Barriers to the utilisation of harm minimisation and drug treatment agencies have been identified by all drug users, regardless of culture or ethnicity. They included waiting lists for methadone prescriptions, expected levels of compliance, ignorance of services' working practices, fear of social services involvement with children. Informants also confirmed that drug users – regardless of their ethnicity – were often suspicious of drug services and described them as instruments of social control and as extensions of the 'system', the 'authorities' or 'officialdom'. Whilst the fear of the breach of confidentiality was identified as an obstacle to service utilisation by all drug users, minority ethnic drug users were significantly more concerned about this issue than were their peers from the majority white society (Abdulrahim et al. 1994; see also Klee and Owolabi, 1993). Many believed that their minority status made them particularly vulnerable to potential breaches of confidentiality and anonymity, and they feared the exchange of information between drug services and other statutory agencies. Informants mentioned areas where perceived or objective differentiation or discrimination operated. Black informants mentioned, for example, issues of colour racism, control and policing:

> I don't know what the fear is, but with black people there's some kind of fear of telling the authorities [interestingly referring to GPs as well as drug services] about things that you do, that are actually illegal.
>
> (African-Caribbean crack user)

Others mentioned their fear of breach of confidentiality concerning their foreign national and/or refugee status. Alluding to his fear of deportation, the highest risk of all, an Iranian asylum seeker said:

> Not in every sense I don't trust them [drug agency]. . . . I mean I don't trust that if the Home Office [Immigration Department] really needed information they wouldn't really give it to them, definitely.
>
> (Iranian heroin user)

Other areas of differentiation identified centred on a more abstract sense of exclusion and on the wider historical and contemporary context of minority/majority relations and wider issues of power and marginalisation. For example:

> Many [Cypriots] don't use drug projects because they don't trust the system, this is it, really, they don't trust the system. [The English are more likely to do so because] the difference is that the English are in their community you know, it's their own society.
>
> (Greek Cypriot heroin user)

The political context of drug use, HIV prevention and harm minimisation cannot be ignored and should be taken into account in the design of interventions aimed at both drug users and the general population. Many Turkish and Kurdish people in Britain feared that drugs awareness initiatives aimed at the non-drug using population will reinforce stereotypes of Turkish and Kurdish men as heroin traffickers. A Turkish drugs worker who suggested to a community organisation the possibility of providing a drugs education session was accused of being a 'traitor'. This reaction can be explained by reference to the concern to project to the majority society the image of a minority ethnic 'community' that does not distinguish itself by anything problematic or stigmatising and which may, in turn, bring additional discrimination. With regard to other areas of social and health care, community organisations representing 'ethnic minorities' are actively seeking to be placed on the agenda of policymakers, but, in the case of drugs and HIV, such organisations wish to render both themselves and those whom they represent invisible. Similarly, resistance by many African-Caribbeans to mainstream drugs awareness messages, and especially crack cocaine, cannot be regarded in isolation from racist stereotypes, especially of the black man. In a process not unlike one that took place in the US, the 'crack addict' in Britain was also for many years portrayed as a black man, the worst urban nightmare, and the (black) 'crack house' has been turned into a metaphor of high-risk sexual behaviour. Within the black communities in Britain, the war on crack was also often perceived to be a 'selective battle against black men' as it had been in the US (see Quimby 1992).

Research in North London clearly shows that political considerations and the fear of unwillingly participating in the promotion of racist stereotypes sometimes influenced drug users' decisions about whether or not to establish contact with drug services, even at times when they acknowledged a need for these services. Often, simple and mundane drug agency practices reinforced these fears and acted as disincentives to service utilisation, especially if the rationale of these practices was not explained to the clients. Fearing that ethnic monitoring data will be manipulated to create and reproduce the symbolic link between black people and drug use, a crack user said:

> For example they [drug agency] have a register out there and you're supposed to sign your name down and you're supposed to say whether you're white or you're black. But a lot of black people they wouldn't like to see their name going down as black because they're thinking, 'What everyone is going to be saying, they are going to collate these figures and saying: look how many blacks are drug addicts!' and that type of thing, so they're very wary of that kind of thing.
>
> (Afro-Caribbean crack user)

Whether the fears held by many minority ethnic drug users are real or imaginary is not what is at issue here. What cannot be ignored is the wider political context of 'minority' status and the fact that the drug user's ability to reduce the risk of HIV and other drug-related harm is partially located in wider contexts of perceived and/or objective powerlessness or discrimination. Such fears also exemplify how people believe that their ability to minimise drug-related harm is limited because of feelings of powerlessness to change other aspects of their lives and those of wider social bodies. They show the need to develop a wider under-standing of what constitutes drug-related harm, HIV prevention and harm minimisation to individuals and wider communities.

'CULTURAL' APPROPRIATENESS AND SERVICE RESPONSIVENESS

To a large extent, HIV prevention in Britain has taken account of the fact that high-risk injecting or sexual behaviours are the outcome of a multiplicity of complex individual, social and practical factors. However, despite long-standing public acknowledgement of the need to respond appropriately to the cultural/ethnic diversity of local communities, mainstream policy and practice are based on the assumption that the dominant culture is neutral. What is often ignored is the obvious: that mainstream professionals work within their own values and norms, and constantly use these for comparison. Harm minimisation and drug treatment practice are generally presented as being a-cultural or universal. What is also ignored is that the meaning and social reality of drug use and HIV are negotiated and constructed within the cultural contexts in which they are placed. Professionals and indigenous drug users from 'white mainstream society' neither share the same experiences nor do they negotiate the culture of harm minimisation from the same premise. Their structural position is very different. However, a dynamic understanding of culture should not obscure the symbolic importance of culture, experienced as a reified heritage. Nor should it imply that differences do not exist, but these should be understood and incorporated in service provision.

To a large extent, drug using Cypriot informants perceived drug use, drug-related harm and its reduction as inherently cultural matters. When asked about the effectiveness, efficacy and acceptability of mainstream services, they often located problems in what they believed to be mainstream professionals' ignorance of the social construction of illicit drug use and drug-related harm amongst Cypriots. Like young recreational users also interviewed, drug-dependent adults placed drug use firmly within the Eastern Mediterranean shame/honour paradigm, created and reproduced in North London. This ideology underpins conformity to central moral principles; underlies every aspect of social and economic life (Delaney 1986: 35); and views drug use as a source of shame. The shame/honour paradigm and its notions of 'reputation' and 'respectability' operate to prevent the use of drugs. However, they also result in keeping existing drug use deliberately hidden (Abdulrahim et al. 1994).

Cypriot informants were aware that the shame/honour ideology could hinder contact with prevention and care services, thus potentially making drug use more hazardous (Abdulrahim et al. 1994). They believed that the social risks of disclosing drug use may often be seen as more significant than the personal risks associated with drug use. However, drug-dependent Cypriots also believed that the practice of mainstream agencies often worked against persuading them to adopt the interventions. They located obstacles in the most mundane of drug service practices, as well as in more complex structural factors. Drug services were, for example, often unable to provide the level and type of confidentiality required by Cypriots and therefore posed a social risk; the particular location of an agency was identified as a deterrent, as it could maximise the risk of drug use being made public:

> . . . look around here [drug agency], there's Greek factories right, when I walk in here they know it's a drug place right, if somebody sees me, they know I'm coming here because of my drug problem. It takes a lot of guts to walk into this place, it's embarrassing you know. People know what it's [the agency], for. And let's face it, [name of area given here], it's full of Greeks here you know, it's difficult for people [Greek Cypriot drug users] to come . . . so if they decide to come off the gear [heroin], they don't decide to come here, they buy methadone on the black market, because of course it's easier than coming here.
>
> (Greek Cypriot heroin user)

Informants also believed that professionals' ignorance of family models other than their own often compromised the effectiveness of interventions. In particular, they mentioned the inability of professionals to grasp the fact that the shame associated with drug use operates within the fluid boundaries that exist between self and family and between individual and collective identity. The stigma carried by a Cypriot drug user involves his/her immediate family. Informants often located problems in what can crudely be described as the inter- action of the culture of the mainstream professional, a culture of guilt, and that of a Cypriot client, a culture of shame. Like those quoted below, others also confirmed their belief that mainstream professionals often found the 'shame' phenomenon difficult, or impossible, to interpret:

> They [mainstream drug workers] haven't a clue . . . like when you start to telling them about shame and things like that they say to you, 'Don't blame yourself.' They don't understand that you're bringing the whole family down. I mean, if I talk to my drug worker about it she wouldn't understand that, she'll go, 'Don't be silly, they're putting pressure on you.' But it's me putting pressure on my family, it's not them putting pressure on me. . . . I put shame to my family you know. . . .
>
> (Greek Cypriot heroin user)

> I tried to make my drug worker and probation officer know my problem, they don't understand it, they just think I'm blaming myself. . . . I've tried to explain it all, they think I've got psychological problems . . . they can't under- stand what I'm trying to put to them. . . . I have a problem but I don't think that they'll be able to help me with that.
>
> (Greek Cypriot heroin user)

The disregard of the role of the family by professionals is by no means universal: on the contrary, many were particularly conscious of its central position – espe- cially as family members often did establish contact with specialist drug agencies. However, research also shows that professionals frequently held simplistic inter- pretations of the Cypriot family, similar to the view of the reified 'Asian' family, prevalent in social and health care. Professionals reified communities as essen- tially 'close-knit' and interpreted the kinship group as a comprehensive welfare and support system which is able and willing to fulfil all the needs of an indi- vidual. A drugs professional said:

> . . . I feel personally that if they've [Cypriot drug users] got a problem, they've got their aunts or their uncles that they can talk to. They solve it within the family. I think that when they actually do come to us, it's gotten out of control and the parent, the uncle, brother whatever will arrive with them. . . . They've got more of a family unit.
>
> (Mainstream drug worker)

Professionals often construed Cypriot family involvement as disruptive and as essentially detrimental to the drug treatment or support process and to the long- term benefit of the individual drug user. It was also viewed as operating against many of the tenets of harm minimisation and drug treatment ideology, such as confidentiality or the non-directive nature of counselling. Mainstream drug workers said for example:

. . . their family members tend to want to get involved. They want you to take ultimate control: [they say,] 'Look here he is, do something.' And because the whole family does tend to get involved, that can get very chaotic.

Mother would phone up [the drug agency], brother would phone up, aunts, sisters, uncles would phone up! Obviously because of confidentiality, you can't just give out information.

Undoubtedly, the need to protect the confidentiality of drug agency clients is paramount. However, what professionals often ignore is that people may hold different interpretations of problems and ways of dealing with difficulties. Drug and harm minimisation workers may draw on culturally defined notions of problems as personalised and private, and disregard Cypriot notions of problems as concerns of a wider group of people. They may thus diminish the opportunity to tap a strong resource for prevention and support in the culture. This is not unique to Cypriots. Research on HIV and drug use amongst black women in the US has also suggested that an insensitivity to cultural values such as the extended family may be a major barrier to a responsive delivery of alcohol and drug services, and that prevention and treatment initiatives must include families (Taha-Cisse, 1991: 56). It is, of course, important not to generalise as many Cypriot drug users clearly rejected any type of family involvement or support, while others were denied it, sometimes in the extreme form of ostracisation. However, many were likely to look to their families as a source of strength, protection and help from drug-related harm. A Cypriot woman said about her release from prison, for example:

. . . and if I didn't have my family to go home to, I would have got nicked [imprisoned] again within a week, or done something really stupid. But I had my family behind me, because some girls haven't. Because if you're down on your luck and you can't go back to your family, where can you go? You'll end up going to your junkie friends and that will only get you to yet deeper trouble.

(Greek Cypriot heroin user)

Ethnocentric assumptions made by mainstream professionals were also identified as limiting the effectiveness of interventions as well as reducing the benefits of support. Cypriot informants mentioned, for example, the frequent advice given to them to focus on their needs as individuals and not on family pressures. They often believed that solutions proposed indirectly encouraged them to adopt irrelevant mainstream cultural notions of what constitutes family involvement: support is thus ineffective and solutions proposed out of reach. One said, for example:

I mean up to this day my family give me hard times. . . . S [drug worker] and M [probation officer] say, 'Tell her [mother] to back off you know, it's your business, you're a big woman.' I can't do it to my mum. I can't tell her, 'Look, mind your own business.' An English girl could do that but I couldn't.

(Greek Cypriot heroin user)

Moreover, there is a need to look at drug users' own choices in accepting the parameters of their culture. Professional advice and support is often viewed as being ultimately based on particular cultural notions of self, other and family not shared by Cypriots and not necessarily wanted by them. It is viewed as based on a majority culture, reified as uniformly reinforcing the individual and his/her selfish need, as opposed to a Cypriot culture, often perceived as morally superior because of its emphasis on reciprocity and sharing. Informants often complained bitterly about pressures placed on them by their own families, but generally situated them as part of a wider cultural package worth preserving. Non-compliance to professional advice is part of the process of resisting domination by the reified culture of the majority society. It is part of the wider process of forging cultural and moral boundaries and of the social construction of community. This was summed up by an informant who said:

> [About family involvement:] That's the way we [Cypriots] are, we cannot change it, and I don't want to change it, I don't want to become like an English person you know. I don't really like the way their families sort of spread around and don't really care about each other. I like the way my family care about me you know, even though it gets on my nerves sometimes, I do like it.
>
> (Greek Cypriot heroin user)

CONCLUSION

This chapter has explored the access of minority ethnic populations to HIV prevention, harm minimisation and drug treatment, and the effectiveness of initiatives in meeting their needs. I have argued that many of these initiatives are participating in the creation and reproduction of marginalisation, whereby populations constructed as 'ethnic minority' are excluded from resources available to prevent the spread of HIV. In 1993 Perera *et al.* called for the need to empower communities to 'reassess outdated and possibly high-risk culturally-specific beliefs' – such as the myth that injecting is a 'white' or 'English' phenomenon.. This remains true today.

HIV prevention and harm minimisation interventions exist within, but do not effectively respond to, ever broader contexts – themselves dependent on diverse senses of history, order, structure and power – within which 'ethnic minorities' are constructed. Marginalisation cannot be understood in isolation from the legacy of social barriers that affect persons of minority status in British society, and from the historical and current differences of power in a minority/majority context.

I have shown how ethnic minority drug users, on the one hand, and agents of harm minimisation policy and services, on the other, operate with different notions and interpretations of the term 'culture'.

Notions and labels such as 'hard to reach' create and operationalise a social reality that marginalises people and denies them resources. They place the blame on minority ethnic populations and their reified cultures, and obscure the complex and diverse range of factors that undermine service utilisation and effectiveness. Harm minimisation policy and practice ignore the possibility of minority ethnic populations having a say in shaping public culture, but view development as adding a little 'ethnic' or 'culturally sensitive' bit on the side. They therefore conceal the need to look at how organisations and bureaucratic structures exclude people from services, and how service access/effectiveness is undermined by people's lack of control over resources and symbolic imagery.

Notions of 'culture', reified as heritage, were mobilised to identify informants' sense of exclusion from, and views on effectiveness of, mainstream interventions. Services ignored the social context of drug-related harm and were deemed ineffective and inappropriate. Moreover, views of mainstream support as ethnocentric raise questions about the politics of public funding, and the labelling of minority ethnic groups by bureaucratic machineries. The issue is not simply about the cosmetics of communication, however, but about structural dynamics and tangible outcomes. Concerns such as these should not be considered as a footnote, a 'by the way' fact. They are major determinants of social reality, should be placed in conjunction with other factors at the centre of analysis and should be analysed as reflecting the wider structural constraints that undermine service access and/or impede effective service responsiveness.

ACKNOWLEDGEMENT

Research funded by North East Thames Regional Health Authority/HIV/AIDS Unit.

REFERENCES

Abdulrahim, D. (1991) *Working with Diversity: HIV Prevention and Black and Minority Ethnic Communities*, London: North East/North West Thames Regional Health Authorities.

Abdulrahim, D., White, D., Phillips, K., Boyd, G., Nicholson, J. and Elliott, J. (1994) *Ethnicity and Drug Use: Towards the Design of Community Interventions* (4 vols), London: North East Thames Regional Health Authority.

Abdulrahim, D., White, D., Phillips, K. and Boyd, G. (1996) *HIV Infection Control: Drug Use and Health Care for Women in a Multi-Ethnic Setting* (A Report to Funding Body).

Awiah, J., Butt, S. and Dorn, N. (1992) *Race, Gender and Drug Services*, ISDD Research Monograph 6, London: Institute for the Study of Drug Dependence.

Barbour, R.S. (1993) 'HIV/AIDS and medical sociology in the nineties', in M. Haralambous (ed.) *Developments in Sociology*, Vol 9, Ormskirk: Causeway.

Baumann, G. (1996) *Contesting Culture: Discourses of Identity in Multi-Ethnic Britain*, Cambridge: Cambridge University Press.

Bloor, M. (1995) *The Sociology of HIV Transmission*, London: Sage.

Daniel, T. (1992) *Drug Agencies, Ethnic Minorities and Problem Drug Use*, London: Centre for Research on Drugs and Health Behaviour, Executive Summary.

Day, S. (1990) 'Anthropological perspectives in sexually transmitted diseases', in

N. Job-Spira, B. Spencer, J.P. Moatti and E. Bouvet (eds) *Santé Publique et Maladies à Transmission Sexuelle*, Paris: John Libbey, Eurotext.

Delaney, C. (1986) 'Seeds of honour, fields of shame', in D. Gilmore (ed.) *Shame and Honour and the Unity of the Mediterranean*, Washington, DC: American Anthropological Association Publications 22.

Des Jarlais, D. and Friedman, S. (1996) 'HIV epidemiology and interventions among injecting drug users', *International Journal of STD and AIDS*, 7 (S.2): 57–61.

Ethnic Response and Communication Research Council (1988) *Qualitative Research on Attitudes to AIDS and AIDS Publicity among Ethnic Minorities in the UK: The Chinese*, Leamington Spa: Report no. 3.

Fardon, R. (1985) 'Introduction: a sense of relevance', in R. Fardon (ed.) *Power and Knowledge: Anthropological and Sociological Approaches*, Edinburgh: Scottish Academic Press.

Frankenberg, R. (1992) 'What identity's at risk? Anthropologists and AIDS', *Anthropology in Action*, 12: 6–9.

Gilroy, P. (1987) *There Ain't No Black in the Union Jack*, London: Hutchinson.

Hart, G., Boulton, M., Fitzpatrick, R., McLean, J. and Dawson, J. (1992) 'Relapse to unsafe sexual behaviour amongst gay men: a critique of recent behavioural HIV/AIDS research', *Sociology of Health and Illness*, 14 (2): 216–32.

Herzfeldt, M. (1997) *Cultural Intimacy: Social Poetics in the Nation-State*, New York and London: Routledge.

Johnson, M. and Carroll, M. (1995) *Dealing with Diversity: Good Practice in Drug Prevention Work with Racially and Culturally Diverse Communities*, London: Home Office Drugs Prevention Initiative, Paper 5.

King, E., Rooney, M. and Scott, P. (1992) *HIV Prevention for Gay Men: A Summary of Initiatives in the UK*, London: North West Thames Regional Health Authority.

Klee, H. and Owolabi, O. (1993) *A Study of Drug Use among Afro-Caribbeans in Central Manchester*, Manchester University: A report prepared for the Department of Health.

Kline, A., Kline, E. and Oken, E. (1992) 'Minority women and sexual choice in the age of AIDS', *Social Sciences and Medicine*, 34(4): 447–57.

Mirza, H., Pearson, G. and Phillips, S. (1991) *Drugs, People and Services in Lewisham*, London: London University Monograph, Goldsmith's College.

Perera, J., Power, R. and Gibson, N. (1993) *Accessing the Needs of Black Drug Users in North Westminster*, London: Centre for Research on Drugs and Health Behaviours with the Hungerford Drug Project.

Public Health Laboratory Service (1990) 'AIDS in England and Wales to end 1993: projections using data to end September 1989', *Communicable Disease Report* (The Day Report).

Quimby, E. (1992) 'Anthropological witnessing for African Americans: power, responsibility and choice in the age of AIDS', in G. Herdt and S. Lindenbaum (eds) *The Time of AIDS: Social Analysis, Theory and Method*, Newbury Park, CA: Sage.

Schneider, B. (1992) 'AIDS and class, gender and race relations', in J. Huber and B. Schneider (eds) *The Social Context of AIDS*, Newbury Park, CA: Sage.

Stimson, G.V. (1994a) 'Minimising harm from drug use', in J. Strang and M. Gossop (eds) *Responding to Drug Misuse: The British System*, Oxford: Oxford University Press.

—— (1994b) 'Reconstruction of sub-regional diffusion of HIV infection among injecting drug users in South East Asia: implications for early intervention', *AIDS*, 8: 1630–2.

—— (1995) 'AIDS and drug injecting in the United Kingdom 1987–1993: the policy response and the prevention of the epidemic', *Social Science and Medicine*, 41(5): 699–716.

Stimson, G. and Donoghoe, M. (1996) 'Health promotion and the facilitation of individual change: the case of syringe distribution and exchange', in T. Rhodes and

R. Hartnoll (eds) *AIDS, Drugs and Prevention: Perspectives on Individual and Community Action*, London and New York: Routledge.

Stimson, G. and Hunter, G. (1996) 'Interventions with drug injectors in the UK: trends in risk behaviour and HIV prevalence', *International Journal of STDs and AIDS*, 7 (suppl.2): 52–6.

Stolcke, V. (1994) 'Europe: new boundaries, new rhetoric of exclusion', paper presented at the European Forum, European University Institute, Florence; quoted in S. Vertovec (1996) 'Multiculturalism and public incorporation', *Ethnic and Racial Studies*, 19(1): 49–69.

Strang, J., Stimson, G. and Des Jarlais, D. (1992) 'What is AIDS doing to the drug research agenda?', *British Journal of Addiction*, 87: 343–6.

Taha-Cisse, A. (1991) 'Issues for African-American women', in P. Roth (ed.) *Alcohol and Drugs are Women's Issues*, Vol. 1, New Jersey and London: Women's Action Alliance/Scarecrow Press.

Task Force to Review Services for Drug Misusers (1996) *Report of an Independent Review of Drug Treatment Services in England*, London: Department of Health.

Weeks, J., Aggleton, P., McKevitt, C., Parkinson, K. and Taylor-Laybourn, A. (1996) 'Community responses to HIV and AIDS: the "de-gaying" and "re-gaying" of AIDS', in J. Weeks and J. Holland (eds) *Sexual Cultures: Communities, Values and Intimacy*, London: British Sociological Association/Macmillan.

Chapter 4

Policing boundaries

Linking the theory and experience of psychotherapy in HIV/AIDS research

Philip Gatter

INTRODUCTION

Psychotherapy is now (at least in the West) a dominant discourse through which the self is refracted and interrogated. Telling psychotherapeutic stories is kin to telling sexual stories, most obviously in the apprehension and confession of the sexual self. However, there are more compelling reasons to apply Plummer's framework in *Telling Sexual Stories* (1995) to psychotherapy. Psychotherapy involves the unfolding of a personal narrative between a client and therapist. As Rose (1989) argues, psychotherapy is one of the 'professions of the self' which provides a grammar for discussing problems of living. It is also a social construct in terms of the process that leads the client to the therapist in the first place, and because accounts of why certain kinds of individuals have socially recognisable selves with attendant psychosocial problems are generated through public debates. As critical social scientists, following Foucault, we might wish to ask whether psychotherapy, in making subjects aware of themselves, is not also producing the subjectivities of which it speaks (Silverman 1990: 208).

HIV and AIDS have created a niche, in which psychotherapy and related forms of counselling take on a new significance. AIDS is potentially life-threatening, and also stigmatises with associations of the socially and sexually unacceptable. It has psychosocial implications for the individual. Being tested for HIV antibodies, and experience of 'seropositivity', were seen from early in the epidemic as necessitating appropriate counselling and psychotherapeutic inter-vention. David Silverman describes well how genito-urinary medicine (GUM) lost its Cinderella status because of AIDS, and the associated professional rivalry between primary care (GPs), doctors and health advisers in GUM clinics, and social workers working for local authorities, as to who was best positioned and qualified to provide HIV counselling.

Social scientists have made a strong contribution with such empirical accounts of the institutionalisation of HIV/AIDS. Others with more interest in theory have been preoccupied with psychotherapy as a model of human subjectivity. The lived experience of psychotherapy and its connection with institutional contexts, in other words psychotherapy as discourse, has received less attention.

This chapter addresses this gap and outlines its consequences in terms of both political and theoretical aspects of the research role.

The research described here involved participant observation and an experience of psychotherapy for me as the researcher. Within an interpretevist framework, I aim, firstly, to examine my own subjectivity as implicated in the generation of any account of the relationship between subjects and institutional context. The second aim is to explore critically the reflexive dimensions of social research on HIV and AIDS. Thirdly, I aim to demonstrate the need for social theory which illuminates the relationship between the subjective and the collective.

Some research topics will have more emotional impact on the researcher than will others. The exact nature of this impact varies with the evolution of each research project and the biography of each researcher (Jill Bourne, Chapter 6), together with the methodological and political approach to the study and the relationships it engenders. However, collective reactions to the theme of research in important respects both shape our experience of research and provide the language for its articulation. Methodological texts are emerging on researching sensitive topics (for example, Renzetti and Lee 1993), AIDS having recently emerged as a prominent example. Extensive literature also exists on *why* AIDS creates such societal shockwaves: its association of death with stigmatised sexuality and illness (for example, Sontag 1988; Patton 1990); ideas of moral contagion (Watney 1987); a body blow to the science born of the Enlightenment (the virus is always one step ahead of the opposition). What is notably lacking, in both sociology and anthropology, is an adequate *theoretical* account of the links between the subjectivity of the researcher and the field of research. This has been due largely to a rejection of questions which are regarded as psychological in orientation. Cousins, in agreement with Born and Moore, detects a considerable *rapprochement* here between anthropology and psychoanalysis, at the expense of psychology. Both disciplines are interested in the cultural unconscious; both are concerned with 'a point where unconscious categories and the category of collective thinking are synonymous', divorced from psychologistic reasoning (Cousins 1989: 85). Relevant literature spans several disciplines, none of which locates and theorises the point where this 'synonymy' occurs.

The acquisition of personality and psychological disposition are treated by anthropologists and sociologists as if they were anterior to culture, and, thus, properly the domain of methodologically individualistic science. Anthropologists say they are not interested in the acquisition of individuality, but in such questions as 'what constitutes the idea of individuality in a given cultural context'. As Henrietta Moore argues in *A Passion for Difference* (1994: ch. 2), such a position is question-begging since it leaves untheorised any link between individual and group self-consciousness; hence the new interest in reviewing Freud as a possible key to understanding simultaneously the development of individual and collectivity without *a priori* falling into the trap of methodological individualism versus methodological collectivism. Likewise, Antony Cohen (1994: ch. 1) has explored the idea of self-consciousness in a way which transcends the limitations inherent in symbolic interactionism, the analytic frame which has tended to dominate questions of self in sociology and anthropology. His complaint is that within symbolic interactionism the self becomes a cipher, a mere contingency, bearing no relation to a real person's sense of self. Cohen, though taking respondents' accounts of selfhood seriously, nevertheless follows in the anthropological and sociological tradition of being chiefly interested in the self as symbolic construct.

Within sociology and anthropology, the past twenty years have seen a great expansion in interest in theories of mind and the subject; specifically Freudian, Lacanian and (to a lesser degree) Kleinian psychoanalysis (Hollitscher 1970; Wallace 1983; Manson, 1988; Obeyesekere, 1990; Born 1994; Heald and Deluz 1994). This interest has been heavily theoretical, with psychoanalysis providing a heuristic and hermeneutic device for exploring the subjectification and encultura-tion of the individual. Some sociologists have also looked more generally at psychoanalysis and psychotherapy as social phenomena (see Edelson, 1970; Weinstein 1973; Roman and Trice, 1974; Smith, 1982). However, within the social sciences little attention has been given to their therapeutic aspects, nor have psychoanalysis and psychotherapy been examined as discourses of mental health.

Anthropologists have written much about the differing paradigms of cause and effect which underlie indigenous aetiologies of illness (meaning illness in its widest sense) and cure. The African literature covers innumerable examples of divination and healing involving spirit entities (see, for example, Evans-Pritchard 1937, or, more recently, Peek 1991). Closer to home, Ursula Sharma (1992) has reviewed the recent explosion in interest in the so-called complementary thera-pies in Britain (Sharma, 1992). In contrast, psychotherapy has been little explored. Moore (1994: 55) sees this as an effect of a primary focus, at least in anthropology, on cultural difference at the expense of exploring other forms and processes of difference.

Antony Clare, as a psychiatrist, has explored the semantic dimension of psychotherapeutic claims to therapeutic value (Clare and Thompson, 1981: 8): part of the problem in comparing psychotherapies with the drug treatments central to psychiatric practice is that notions of treatment and cure are constructed very differently by the two discourses. None the less, Clare tends toward viewing many of the new psychotherapies as very idiosyncratic in their claims to effectiveness, and in this sense is conventionally psychiatric.

Anthropologists and interpretive sociologists might have some distaste for the positivistic interests of psychiatry, but the dynamic aspects of psychotherapy should be of interest to us since, like Marxism, psychoanalysis claims to be both a theory of the subject and a programme for potential change. The two aims are dialectically linked, so one might justifiably consider psychoanalysis *as praxis* to qualify as discourse in a Foucauldian sense.

SETTING THE SCENE

The analysis offered in this chapter is prompted by what was initially an emotional reaction to a set of events in which my professional and personal concerns intersected with psychotherapy in a particular context: therapy as a professional support mechanism in a voluntary sector HIV/AIDS social care organisation in Britain. The emotional reaction is crystallised in a letter I wrote to the newsletter of an HIV/AIDS voluntary organisation offering support to current and ex-injecting drugs users. At the time of publication I withheld my identity.

> Dear Mainliners,
> Following the recent controversy over Cass Mann's *Deadly Counsels* (but unconnected with it), I have an experience to share with your readers which has both disturbed and angered me.
> I work in a research post, and spend much of my time interviewing people living with HIV about how the virus has affected their lives. As personal support, I receive counselling privately from a therapist who works also for a high-profile, highly respected HIV/AIDS voluntary organisation.
> In a recent session, the subject of criticism of HIV service providers by HIV service users arose incidentally. The therapist then probed further, inviting me, I felt, to repeat *specific* complaints against *named* staff of another HIV/AIDS voluntary organisation. He then *explained* that when people living with a potentially life threatening condition make complaints against service providers, these are usually exaggerated and are *really* a misdirected expression of anger.
> I have two points to make:
>
> 1 I did not take the bait. I felt I was being led toward a breach of confidentiality; that the counselling relationship was being abused by the therapist.
> 2 I accept that psychotherapy has given valid insight into how anger becomes (or fails to be) expressed. However, to say that complaints against professionals by service users are all about anger can be nothing more than a gross generalisation. But a greater cause for concern is that such claims *could* be used to political ends: to place counsellors and other HIV service providers above criticism and beyond accountability.
>
> Yours in shock
>
> (Letter in Mainliners 1992)

Before explaining the circumstances of the particular research project in which my reaction arose, some definitional issues surrounding psychotherapy and counselling need to be explored in order to understand the organisational and ideological underpinnings of psychotherapy as practice.

PSYCHOTHERAPY

Defining counselling and psychotherapy, and the relationship between them, is not possible independent of context. Their lexical and practical connections are inextricable.

In modern practice, psychotherapy is most broadly defined as the treatment of disorders by psychological (as distinct from medical) methods (see Liddell 1983: 19). More precisely, the British Psychological Society has defined psychotherapy as

> Informed and planful application of techniques derived from established psychological principles, by persons qualified through training and experience to understand these principles and to apply those techniques with the intention of assisting individuals to modify such personal characteristics as feelings, values, attitudes and behaviours which are judged *by the therapist* to be maladaptive or maladjustive.
>
> (British Psychological Society, Division of Clinical Psychology 1979: 6; emphasis added)

However, within psychotherapy there is a diverse spectrum of theory, practice and practitioners, not least because what constitutes 'disorder' is left unspecified. At one end of the spectrum are those Freudians and neo-Freudians who work with psychodynamic models concerning the personality as a whole. At the other are those behavioural therapists who aim to induce behaviour change through diagnosing and responding to specific presenting symptoms (echoing a medical model of intervention).

To practise as a member of the British Psychoanalytic Association requires four years' training, including a period in analysis for the analyst, and now costs tens of thousands of pounds. Members of this élite will work in private practice, as do others who train in neo-Freudian psychodynamic therapies. Their clients tend to be metropolitan middle-class people who can afford the fees (typically upwards of £30 per hour), have an interest in holistic approaches to health, and a dislike of drug-based therapy. Psychodynamic therapies are also practised by a range of psychiatrists and clinical psychologists.[1] However, the greater proportion of clinical psychologists in Britain use behavioural techniques, though some employ a mixture of methods, even with a single client.

In Britain and elsewhere there is considerable overlap between professions, institutions and clients, despite the gatekeeping efforts of various interest groups. Many of the HIV positive men interviewed in our research encountered clinical psychologists either after an inpatient stay in hospital or as part of ongoing monitoring and care in a GUM clinic. Since the kind of psychotherapy received depends largely on the training and aptitudes of the individual therapist, comparison of these HIV positive men's experiences was limited due to lack of information on their therapists.

COUNSELLING

Counselling is an even more equivocal term than is psychotherapy, in terms both of the range of practices it covers, and of who qualifies as a practitioner. The difference between counselling and psychotherapy is most often expressed in terms of time-scale and purpose. Counselling is usually aimed at identifying a specific problem and enabling a client to reduce anxiety in relation to that problem (such as an HIV diagnosis). Psychotherapy tends to be a lengthier process (notably this is so for psychoanalysis) which explores in greater depth the psychological attributes of an individual. Counselling is available in a wider set of environments than is psychotherapy, and a broader sample of the population will receive counselling at some point in their lives than receive psychotherapy.

Many counsellors are also trained psychotherapists, and there is a tendency for literature in this field to use the terms counselling and psychotherapy as if they were interchangeable or simply to differentiate them as 'related fields' (for example, Burck *et al.* 1973; Kahn *et al.* 1975). However, counselling is much less professionalised than psychotherapy, and it is possible for anyone in Britain to describe him- or herself as a counsellor, regardless of qualifications.[2] Counselling is a contested arena. Taking counselling as applied to HIV and AIDS alone, a national survey in 1990 had to devote an entire chapter to 'The search for an agreed meaning of the term "HIV counselling"'. The survey found that differences in meaning arose due to (a) different professional traditions, (b) differences between job title and role, and (c) a belief that 'counselling' had become a devalued and unhelpful term. GPs saw themselves as offering counselling, whereas members of the British Association for Counselling saw this as an unwarrantable appropriation of the term.

The 1990 empirical study illustrated ambiguities in the definition of counselling, over the relatively narrow field of HIV and AIDS. Nevertheless, some attempt was made to synthesise a core definition, drawing on established professional definitions of counselling. In the terms of the British Association for Counselling, the main professional body in Britain, counselling is

> the skilled and principled use of relationships which develop self-knowledge, emotional acceptance and growth, and personal resources. The overall aim is to live more fully and satisfyingly. Counselling may be concerned with addressing and resolving specific problems, making decisions, coping with crises, working through feelings and inner conflict, or improving relationships with others.
>
> The counsellor's role is to facilitate the client's work in ways that respect the client's values, personal resources, and capacity for self-determination.
>
> (British Association for Counselling 1990)

This definition is perilously close to that quoted earlier for psychotherapy. I am not attempting here to resolve definitional problems, but rather to illustrate the difficulties of attempting an institutional analysis starting from the rubrics of either counselling or psychotherapy.

COUNSELLING AND THERAPY IN AN HIV/AIDS ORGANISATION

Definitional problems surrounding counselling and psychotherapy are important when turning to their application within an HIV/AIDS organisation. The activities of professionals must, in some sense, be linked to how they define their role. I will argue, however, that this is not a simple relationship. In an institutional context, professional practices can have effects beyond those intended. In this particular case, the unintended consequences were beyond the professional grasp of therapists due to lack of adequate theory.

Since definitions are problematic, an argument can be made for using inductive research techniques to arrive at an understanding of counselling and psychotherapy in context, which will then produce an interpretation stronger in its account of praxis than of theory. The data reported here were gathered during the evaluation of an HIV/AIDS voluntary sector social care organisation, and arose from participant observation, interviews, and the therapeutic relationship between the author and a psychotherapist working with the organisation. This psychotherapist was trained in the psychodynamic tradition, strongly influenced by Adler. He described his work as both psychotherapy and counselling and, where support to in-house staff was concerned, 'supervision'. The analysis presented here relates to a particular form and context of psychotherapy, but I aim to raise issues relevant to the interrogation of other forms of psychotherapy and other contexts.

Within the organisation which was evaluated (referred to here as 'The Centre') there were a number of definable interest groups operating, some of which were overlapping.

In this general milieu counselling and psychotherapy were present in two main ways. Firstly, counselling was offered as a confidential service to people infected and affected[3] by HIV, bookable at The Centre reception. Three counsellors were available, with expertise in different areas (such as stress and depression, relationships and bereavement) who could be consulted on an individual basis, or with a partner or group.

Secondly, psychotherapists/counsellors were involved in the training programmes for The Centre volunteers, in the areas of Listening Skills and Death, Dying and Bereavement. Listening Skills was aimed at equipping volunteers with some rudimentary counselling skills, to facilitate empathic interaction with Centre users. The Death, Dying and Bereavement training was to help volunteers operate effectively in an environment in which mortality was an issue, in the senses both of working with those facing their own deaths, and coping with the loss of others (which all within the organisation might expect to experience). The work of Elizabeth Kubler-Ross featured prominently in this area of training (for example, Kubler-Ross 1970, 1982).

The counsellors and psychotherapists at The Centre generally organised their time between working through organisations (whether HIV-dedicated or not) and offering private consultations. It was thus common for those who wanted (and could afford) extra input from a counsellor or psychotherapist to become the private clients of the professionals operating through The Centre, or be referred by them elsewhere in their professional networks. This was the case for some volunteers, some staff members, some service users and myself.

Experiences of counselling and psychotherapy among service users were subjects of the evaluation research and counselling also informed my own experience of The Centre. I wish to analyse these two sets of 'data' together. I will begin with the rationale for my seeking counselling and an account of the experience, followed by the stories told by other subjects. A deliberate shift of style is made here, to speaking in a subjective tone. Such a shift is encouraged by psychotherapeutic discourse, and in returning to a more analytic frame I will argue this is an aspect of the (potential) insidiousness of psychotherapy and counselling, whereby an uncritical focus on the 'subjective' leaves unnoticed the political implications and effects of therapy.

THE AUTHOR'S TALE

Having previously studied processes of rural development in Zambia, evaluating an inner city HIV day centre in Britain represented a new set of challenges and opportunities to me. A Zambian village held its own predicaments: malaria; social and cultural alienation; midnight trips to the pit latrine; a high incidence of disease and death, especially in the rainy season. Yet the alienation perversely had the positive effect of enforcing some emotional distance between ethnographer and informants. This was not to be the case in the evaluation of The Centre.

I had applied for the post of researcher on the evaluation to gain experience of research in a British context and, as a gay man, out of a personal wish to make a contribution in the field of HIV and AIDS. The component of the evaluation which was to be my chief responsibility was the Direct Impact Study, by which was meant an assessment of the impact of the services offered by The Centre on its clientele.[4] This was to involve in-depth interviewing of a cohort of seventy-five service users (and potential service users), to which I appended participant observation within The Centre, to generate richer contextualising material in which to locate individual responses at interview. I decided to train as a volunteer as well, which would allow me to make a practical contribution to The Centre whilst integrating me for the purposes of research.

Volunteer training made me aware of the likely personal impact of involvement with the organisation. The start of interviewing sharpened this awareness. In interview, respondents discussed the history of their experience of HIV, which could be distressing both for them and for me. Though labelled as research interviews, these encounters could feel more like therapy sessions. As the research could not alleviate the problems which interviewees aired, interviews could leave me feeling both distressed and powerless. These feelings were enhanced by my identification with my respondents, many of whom were gay men. This form of identification and involvement had never been present in my Zambian field experience.

I approached a psychotherapist who had been involved in the volunteer training about supervision/counselling to help alleviate some of the anxiety I was experiencing. We agreed to work together, and began weekly private consultations.

Analytically, the focus of our sessions soon became consideration of ego boundaries. We identified a problem lying in my occupation of several different roles within The Centre, the boundaries between which were not always clear to those I interacted with, nor, more importantly (from a psychotherapeutic perspective), to me. This problem of ego boundaries took various forms, but was present both in face-to-face interviews and in the group context of The Centre. Thus, it was important for me to distinguish my own problems from those presented by my respondents, so that I could leave interviews without feeling any burden of responsibility and with a clearer idea of the limits of my role as a researcher, and making explicit to respondents the limits of my responsibilities. I was also encouraged to be more candid about my activities within The Centre, lessening the opportunity for confusion over my role, which could lead to mistrust (a potential impediment to the research).[5]

These sessions undoubtedly equipped me to deal better with the emotional impact of the interviewing process, and to develop a greater sense of purpose and clarity during participant observation. Interviews became less exhausting, and participant observation more structured around roles within The Centre. I note, however, that the relationship between myself and the therapist was not examined or discussed – from either a professional or a personal perspective. Thus, the therapist invited me to break confidence and I lacked an authoritative position from which to challenge him.

At the start of the evaluation no contingency (in the sense of resources) had been made in the research plan to offer the kind of support to researchers which I subsequently demanded. Implicitly, the evaluation was grounded in the positivist assumption that researchers are external to the object of investigation, and that evaluation by implication is a disinterested process. Existential aspects of the research had been underplayed, if not ignored. This was in stark contrast to the position held by the management of The Centre, which was that all workers involved in HIV/AIDS organisations should have access to supervision and (if necessary) counselling as a condition of their employment. Although postmodernist and feminist social science holds that research is necessarily a reflexive process in which subject and object positions are themselves products of interaction and interpretation, this is essentially a theoretical concern. Neither positivist evaluators nor interpretive social scientists have considered in detail the importance of the psychodynamic aspects of research. I will go on to demonstrate that this has implications beyond the welfare of the researcher and that this limits the contribution which social science might make.

RESPONDENTS' VOICES

My interviewees in the Direct Impact Study had encountered counselling or psychotherapy in a number of different contexts. Nearly all of them had received pre- and post-test counselling when they had tested positive for HIV antibodies. There were a few, significant, exceptions. These were individuals who had been tested in the mid-1980s, at a time when procedures had not been definitively and consistently scripted for all institutions offering HIV testing in Britain. Such individuals felt, in retrospect, that the personal crisis of diagnosis had been worsened by a lack of appropriate support, delaying (perhaps for years) their ability to approach HIV/AIDS organisations for services. In the worst cases, the HIV test had allegedly been made without the consent or knowledge of the interviewee, drastically increasing the trauma occasioned by the test result.

Subsequent experience of counselling and psychotherapy depended on the network of referral between services, determined both by the individual respondent and professional service providers. Many of the gay men interviewed had discovered their positive HIV status through attendance at a GUM clinic. In this context they would be referred to a clinical psychologist if a definite psychological need were identified by a clinician, or a health adviser for general emotional support in the context of health advice. Similarly, women diagnosed through antenatal testing might initially receive counselling in a clinical setting. Emotional support would also be available via social workers, either in specialist HIV-support teams attached to hospitals, or through referral to local authorities. None of the interviewees had experienced psychotherapy directly via a clinical setting. This might be expected, given the historical dominance of psychiatry as discourse of mental health in post-war Britain, and the relatively minor role of psychotherapy in state health care (as compared with the American situation; see Clare and Thompson 1981: 23).

After initial contact with counselling in a clinical setting, interviewees were commonly referred to voluntary sector organisations such as the Terrence Higgins Trust, Positively Women and The Centre, where a much greater variety of counselling and psychotherapy was available.

A striking feature of our data is that the experiences of counselling and therapy as reported are similar regardless of their institutional or definitional contexts.

I felt that she'd got a lot out of me basically, that we talked, a lot that came out was quite good because it made me understand a few things, and it made me realise that we all need to talk. And also it showed me why, you know, I'm getting so wound up all the time. She said, she could see everything I was saying. And I felt, oh gosh, you know, I talk to you about this and that, and I feel as if I've got it off my chest.

(Gay man, with reference to a clinical psychologist in a GUM clinic)

I went for counselling, which really helped me a lot. I saw a woman there who

was very good. I knew my main problem was denial. I knew I had, I knew
that it was AIDS. I didn't really want to discuss it. I wouldn't talk, and my
partner understood and didn't push me, then one day one of my very dear,
very close friends found out he was HIV. And I was talking to him on the
phone about it. And he was so together with like chatting about it and how he
felt and how did I feel and all that. And I came off the phone and I thought
God I should be more like him. You've got to talk about it, you've got to
discuss it, you know. So I went for counselling.

(Gay man, discussing counselling in a voluntary organisation)

There were negative as well as positive experiences, again not readily associable
with kinds of organisation or intervention:

There was no point, I had a specific legal matter to sort out. For general information they're fine. But once you've been through it once, that's all you need.

(Gay man, with reference to a clinical psychologist)

She seemed to me to be inexperienced and very, very tired. We didn't develop
a rapport. It felt more like a befriending session and what I needed was
specific counselling to do with bereavement.

(Gay man, with previous counselling experience, on a counsellor
in a voluntary sector organisation)

The benefits, in the sense of emotional support, which interviewees obtained
through HIV-related services were weakly related to professionally defined areas
of competence. Indeed, some respondents felt that just sitting in the drop-in area
of The Centre and talking with other service users provided all the social and
emotional support they needed. Others were organised into confidential support
groups facilitated by a social worker. Yet others felt that one-to-one sessions with
professional counsellors were what most benefited them. All such observations
were made from a perspective of personal tastes and aptitudes, in the context of
a history of referrals between organisations, not in terms of needs as defined by
professionals.

PSYCHOTHERAPY AS DISCOURSE

The descriptions offered so far have all been in terms of personal experiences of
counselling and therapy as directed at the problems of individuals.
Psychotherapy and counselling rest on theories of formation of the subject and
self-consciousness. It is easy therefore to imagine the operations of
psychotherapy as being solely on the individual psyche, and therapists often
speak as if this were the case.

The crisis outlined in my letter earlier in this chapter was experienced initially
as a jolt in my relationship with an individual psychotherapist. On reflection it
leads into a questioning of the wider discursive role of counselling and therapy.
What effects do counselling and psychotherapy have on the culture, politics, and

activities of organisations – effects which are separable from their direct therapeutic role with clients, but are nevertheless linked to the ethos of counselling
and psychotherapy?

In the context of the relationship between therapist and therapised, all interactions between people are conceptualised by the therapist in an ego-focused
manner. Thus, if one describes a problematic relationship with another individual in a therapy session, the focus is always on how one's own emotional states
arise within the relationship. The therapist does not encourage interpretation of
the absent third party's motivations, emotions and thoughts. Psychotherapy
therefore treats all dyadic relationships from a monodic perspective (and it could
not do otherwise except, perhaps, in the context of couples' counselling) and
assumes emotion as authentic and ontologically prior to reason and intellect.

Inevitably, organisations which seek to be relatively informal and to some
extent user-led in their services (such as many voluntary sector HIV/AIDS
organisations in Britain) are likely to experience some tensions and difficulty in
mediating between the interests of different groups involved in the organisation.
This theme was prominent in our evaluation of The Centre. The organisation
set out to be participatory and had to balance the needs and demands of a
diverse client base against the necessity not only of maintaining coherent
management structures and procedures but also of meeting the demands of a
funding environment driven by government policy in the direction of the quasi-
market (see NCVO 1989; NHS Management Executive 1991; Bebbington et al.
1992; Feldman 1995). My interviews recorded a number of problems as well as
benefits which service users perceived in the organisations which served them.
The perspective adopted within the research was to treat these perceptions as
valid, aside from the question of their reasonableness, since they evidently were
integral to the relationship between service organisation and service user.

In contrast to the perspective adopted by the evaluation on users' complaints,
the position advanced by my psychotherapist can be construed as a highly selective reading of events. His contention that the response of HIV positive people
to organisations which serve them is founded on and identical with their
emotional experience of HIV amounts to a denial of agency; persons become
mere ciphers of emotion.

There is, I would argue, a paradox at the heart of the therapeutic perspective
(as outlined above) when considered in one institutional context. Whilst the therapeutic relationship is constructed by therapists as one in which the therapised
realise self-awareness in a manner which is never coerced by the therapist, at an
institutional level the theoretical insights of therapy can lead to generalisations
about emotional states of people as members of prescriptively defined groups.
Psychological propensities may be attributed in a way which a psychotherapist
would never allow a client to do in a one-to-one therapeutic relationship.

In caring organisations which deal with personal, emotional issues,
psychotherapists and counsellors are attributed expert status in defining the characteristics of subject populations. Their expertise is valuable to the organisation

in aiding sensitivity to its clients' problems and understanding the emotional impact of working with them. But simultaneously it may act as a silencing mechanism. If HIV positive people are treated as ciphers of their emotions (emotions which can be accurately predicted), then their dissatisfactions with an organisation may be construed as emotionally contingent, as *essentially* being an expression of anger over HIV status. In the particular context I encountered, the psychotherapeutic perspective effectively discounted certain voices before they could enter into dialogue. And interestingly, it was never suggested that the *positive* things my respondents reported about The Centre were products of emotional disturbance. An HIV positive status is unarguably a cause of fear and anxiety, and the anger this may entail can spill over in unexpected places. But this is not a constant factor for all people who are HIV positive; nor does it preclude problems and dissatisfactions which anyone, regardless of HIV status, might experience with an organisation.

My claims here are necessarily limited. I do not have evidence that a particular psychotherapist directly influenced the attitudes of an organisation to its clients. Rather, as an evaluator I was presented by him with, and strongly urged to adopt, a framework for interpreting and making value judgements of statements made by interviewees which conflicted with the interpretational framework I expected to use as a professional anthropologist. Had I adopted the suggested framework, the findings of the evaluation would have been distorted towards treating service users as 'patients' in relation to the service providers as 'agents'. The findings of the evaluation have subsequently been used by The Centre in policy and service development, so there was at least a potential for this distortion to have limited effects on the organisation, with the researcher acting as catalyst.

A transcript of one of my service user interviews would be interpreted quite differently by a social scientist and a psychotherapist. The crux of my argument is that it would be naive to treat these interpretations straightforwardly as different, yet equivalent, readings. In the context of evaluation research which is intended to influence the policies and activities of an organisation, each reading may hold quite distinctive implications for the world beyond the text itself.

CONCLUSIONS

From a social scientist's perspective, a gap exists in the literature between method and theory which might fruitfully provide an account of the researcher as subject in the research process. A link needs to be made between ethnography (meaning both participant observation and writing) and theories of the subject. This chapter has presented a limited empirical case as a starting point for discussion. I have tried to examine the relationship of psychotherapeutic and interpretive social science discourses in the context of evaluation research. An important dimension of the role of the researcher here is the relative inclusiveness of the anthropological/sociological discourse. This inclusiveness (the interpretation and presentation of multiple perspectives) has a tendency to problematise the claims to authority and exclusivity of other professional discourses. This might provide a better nuanced account of an organisation, yet we run the risk of marginalising the researcher during fieldwork, and in reaction to what he or she might later write. Our evaluation revealed that the contexts in which service users of The Centre experienced support through what might, in the widest sense, be labelled counselling and psychotherapy were very diverse. A great deal of the benefit associated with "talking about things" at The Centre arose in the context of service users informally talking to each other, or in facilitated groups. This suggests an interesting (though provocative) question: Who needs psychotherapists and counsellors?

There are specific contexts in which professional counselling and therapy are indispensable, especially for someone in extreme distress. Yet psychotherapy, amongst other things, is a professionalising discourse which claims authority in defining how we are emotional beings.

There are parallels here with how medicine claimed dominion over the body, and psychiatry over the mind, in the nineteenth century. We can now be therapised as well as medicalised. However, there seem to be important differences in the discursive capabilities of psychotherapy and psychiatry. In the work of Foucault, and other historians of medicine and science, we see how changes in the interpretation of madness and its institutionalisation arise with the birth of psychiatry (Foucault 1967, 1985; Bynum et al. 1985a, 1985b, 1988). In his later work Foucault related this process to a wider set of discourses governing the body, with a particular interest in sexuality. The development of the concept of discourse as a regimen of power/knowledge existing historically through human subjects and their institutions is suggestive of why psychoanalysis and psychotherapy have a particular status among discourses which theorise the subject (Foucault, 1979, 1986, 1990). Psychiatry is integral to a wider (and, since the nineteenth century, hegemonic) biomedical discourse which claims authority in describing and administering to mind and body. It has its grounding in biologically deterministic natural science, and relies on logico-deductive reasoning in developing its theories and therapies. Psychoanalysis and its offspring rest on a different set of premises, making them theoretically interesting to interpretive social scientists, and empirically dubious to psychiatry. Psychoanalysis mediates between biological and cultural determinist positions by associating sexuality with the unconscious, a psychic realm through which biology and socialisation mediate. As an unfalsifiable project, psychoanalysis has tended to be marginalised by psychiatry. At the same time, 'the talking cure' does not claim expert status for its practitioners in the same way as psychiatry. The problems, outlined earlier, with definitions of psychotherapy and counselling are connected with the fact that practioners allow that we are all, to some degree, amateur counsellors and psychotherapists: the psychotherapist constructs his or her role as facilitation rather than pedagogy.

The 'need' for therapy is always contingent, and what counts as therapy, as well as the gatekeeping mechanisms of the profession, are much more fluid than for psychiatry. Under these conditions, I suggest, psychotherapy and counselling cannot assume the status of dominant discourse which psychiatry can.

There are specific circumstances, though, under which psychotherapy can become a relatively powerful discourse. Voluntary sector HIV/AIDS organisations in Britain are not direct employers of psychiatrists. Their professional culture also tends to be one which fosters alternative and holistic approaches to well-being, particularly through offering complementary therapies. Counselling and psychotherapy have established a niche in this context, forming part of a culture which runs parallel to, but in contrast with, a biomedical culture centred on allopathic drug treatments.[6] Under conditions where tensions may arise between those running and those using such organisations, psychotherapy can participate in legitimising the ascendancy of the views of the former. My major contention has been that there is a problematic division between the theoretical and therapeutic dimensions of psychotherapy. While therapeutic practice claims to engage only with individual egos, its theoretical underpinnings lead to pronouncements on collective egos and ego states. The two positions are in tension and, as I have argued, this tension can have implications outside the discourse of psychotherapy.

The requirement of reflexivity leads me finally to a questioning of the role of the discourse of research in the case described, and the researcher as subject in this discourse. Issues of displacement and representation need addressing. My letter was my response to a situation as I perceived and felt it during fieldwork. What I have written here is a reinterpretation of those events in a more analytic mode and with the benefit of hindsight. I have, in effect, challenged the authority and representations of psychotherapy, and, to borrow crudely from a popular image, taken the side of the inmates against the asylum. This is a political act, and a common one in the annals of anthropology, which has traditionally sought to represent the underdog against authority. In all fairness, one should also address the question of the grounds on which interpretive social scientists justify *their* generalisations. Given the lack of claim to authority in exploring matters of emotion which we make for ourselves, by what authority can we seek to argue with psychotherapists? Is there not a danger here of reactively objectifying therapists at the expense of their clients?

Second, what is written here is a displacement from the original context. I have discussed my interpretation of the interests of the social actors involved at the time, but addressed these issues to an academic audience (even accepting some of the *dramatis personae* might read this book). The issue of responsibility must be faced: supposing my interpretations are correct, is writing this piece a dereliction of duty in that it is directed (as a psychotherapist might say) somewhere safe and comfortable? My excuse, such as it is, is that my original letter did raise the issues with a group of people living with HIV and AIDS, albeit anonymously. The possibility remains, however, that any catharsis I have achieved here should better have been gained by directly addressing my concerns to the particular psychotherapist involved, and not writing anything.[7]

NOTES

The empirical research described in this chapter was part of a larger evaluation, funded by the Department of Health, and conducted jointly with Rayah Feldman at South Bank University and Andrew Bebbington and Pat Warren of the Personal Social Services Research Unit, University of Kent, between 1989 and 1992.

1   Conventionally, a distinction between psychiatrists and clinical psychologists is that the former tend to work with a pathological model in which their concern is mental illness, whereas the latter take a broader, psychological approach. In practice, severe psychological disorders which might be identified as psychoses are referred by clinical psychologists and GPs to psychiatrists. Despite the medical orientation of psychiatry, a sizeable group of psychiatrists in Britain practise psychodynamic therapies in addition to using drug therapies.

2   The same applies to the use of the general term 'therapist', though psychotherapists as such try harder to guard the boundaries of their profession.

3   HIV/AIDS organisations in Britain conventionally use the term 'affected' by HIV to refer to anyone who, though not HIV positive themselves, is considerably affected by it through being a carer, partner, relative, and so on, of someone who is. Services are generally made available by voluntary organisations to both the infected and affected.

4   The subject of what constitutes the impact of a service (and, by implication, what is meant by quality of life) is worth a book in its own right. Anthropologists and other interpretive social scientists are increasingly contributing to debates over the simplifying and positivistic tendencies of much evaluation research.

5   Boundaries in an institutional professional sense are explored in greater detail by Katie Deverell in her chapter.

6   Voluntary sector HIV/AIDS organisations (with the exception of some marginal ones) do not discourage the use of allopathic medicine, but it is not their role to provide clinical care.

7   After the research reported here, I consulted a second psychotherapist under a different set of circumstances. I discussed the concerns I have expressed in this chapter and, from a therapeutic point of view, she was of the opionion that it was ill advised, if not unprofessional, for the first therapist to have agreed to work with me, given his close involvement with the organisation and people I was researching. Psychotherapy holds that the therapeutic relationship should be one in which the therapist is a disinterested third party.

REFERENCES

Bebbington, A., Feldman, R., Gatter, P. and Warren, P. (1992) *Evaluation of the Landmark: Final Report*, Canterbury: PSSRU, University of Kent, Discussion Paper 901/2.

Born, G. (1994). Unpublished paper, Medical Anthropology Seminar, University College London, Spring.

British Association for Counselling (1990) *Definitions of Counselling: Project Information Sheet*, Rugby: BAC.

British Psychological Society, Division of Clinical Psychology (1979) *Report of a Working Party on the Definition of Psychological Therapies*, Leicester: BPS.

Burck, H.D., Cottingham, H.F. and Reardon, R.C. (1973) *Counselling and Accountability: Methods and Critique*, New York: Pergamon Press.

Bynum, W.F., Porter, R. and Shepherd, M. (1985a) *The Anatomy of Madness: Essays in the History of Psychiatry Vol. 1: People and Ideas*, London: Tavistock.

Bynum, W.F., Porter, R. and Shepherd, M. (1985b) *The Anatomy of Madness: Essays in the History of Psychiatry Vol. 2: Institutions and Society*, London: Tavistock.

Bynum, W.F., Porter, R. and Shepherd, M. (1988) *The Anatomy of Madness: Essays in the History of Psychiatry Vol. 3: The Asylum and its Psychiatry*, London: Routledge.

Clare, A.W. and Thompson, S. (1981) *Let's Talk about Me: A Critical Examination of the New Psychotherapies*, London: British Broadcasting Corporation.

Cohen, A.P. (1994) *Self-Consciousness*, London: Routledge.

Cousins, M. (1989) 'In the midst of psychoanalysis: Lévi-Strauss on Mauss', *New Formations*, 7: 77–87.

Edelson, M. (1970) *Sociotherapy and Psychotherapy*, Chicago: University of Chicago Press.

Evans-Pritchard, E.E. (1937) *Witchcraft, Oracles and Magic among the Azande*, London: Oxford University Press.

Feldman, R. (1995) 'User empowerment: contradictions between self-help and service delivery in AIDS Service Voluntary Organisations', unpublished paper.

Foucault, M. (1967) *Madness and Civilization: A History of Insanity in the Age of Reason*, London: Tavistock.

—— (1979) *The History of Sexuality Vol. 1: An Introduction*, London: Allen Lane.

—— (1985) *The Birth of the Clinic: An Archaeology of Medical Perception*, London: Routledge.

—— (1986) *The History of Sexuality Vol. 2: The Use of Pleasure*, Harmondsworth: Viking/Penguin.

—— (1990) *The History of Sexuality Vol. 3: The Care of the Self*, Harmondsworth: Penguin.

Heald, S. and Deluz, A. (eds) (1994) *Anthropology and Psychoanalysis: An Encounter through Culture*, London: Routledge.

Hollitscher, W. (1970) *Sigmund Freud, an Introduction: A Presentation of his Theory, and a Discussion of the Relationship between Psychoanalysis and Sociology*, Freeport, NY: Books for Libraries Press.

Kahn, T.C., Cameron, J.T. and Giffen, M.B. (1975) *Methods and Evaluation in Clinical and Counselling Psychology*, New York: Pergamon Press.

Kubler-Ross, E. (1970) *On Death and Dying*, London: Tavistock.

—— (1982) *Living with Death and Dying*, London: Souvenir Press.

Liddell, A. (ed.) (1983) *The Practice of Clinical Psychology in Britain*, Chichester: Wiley.

Mainliners (1992) *Newsletter of Mainliners Ltd*, an agency working with and for people affected by drugs and HIV, London, no. 20, March.

Manson, W.C. (1988) *The Psychodynamics of Culture: Abram Kardiner and Neo-Freudian Anthropology*, New York: Greenwood Press.

Moore, H. (1994) *A Passion for Difference*, Oxford: Polity Press.

NCVO (1989) *Contracting: In or Out?*, guidance notes on contracting for voluntary groups, London: NCVO.

NHS Management Executive (1991) *NHS Reforms: The First Six Months*, London: HMSO.

Obeyesekere, G. (1990) *The Work of Culture: Symbolic Transformation, Psychoanalysis and Anthropology*, Chicago: University of Chicago Press.

Patton, C. (1990) *Inventing AIDS*, London: Routledge.

Peek, P.M. (ed.) (1991) *African Divination Systems: Ways of Knowing*, Bloomington: Indiana University Press.

Plummer, K. (1995) *Telling Sexual Stories: Power, Change and Social Worlds*, London: Routledge.

Renzetti, C.M. and Lee, R.M. (eds) (1993) *Researching Sensitive Topics*, London: Sage.

Roman, P.M. and Trice, H.M. (eds) (1974) *The Sociology of Psychotherapy*, New York: J. Aronson.

Rose, N. (1989) *Governing the Soul: Technologies of Human Subjectivity*, London: Routledge.

Sharma, U. (1992) *Complementary Medicine Today: Practitioners and Patients* (1st edn), London: Routledge.

Silverman, D. (1990) 'The social organisation of HIV counselling', in P. Aggleton, P. Davies and G. Hart (eds) *AIDS: Individual, Cultural and Policy Dimensions*, London: Falmer Press.

Smith, A. (1982) *The Relational Self: Ethics and Therapy from a Black Church Perspective*, Nashville: Abingdon.

Sontag, S. (1988) *AIDS and Its Metaphors*, New York: Farrar, Straus & Giroux.

Wallace, E.R. (1983) *Freud and Anthropology: A History and Reappraisal*, New York: International Universities Press.

Watney, S. (1987) *Policing Desire: Pornography, AIDS and the Media*, London: Methuen.

Weinstein, F. (1973) *Sociology: An Essay on the Interpretation of Historical Data and the Phenomenon of Collective Behaviour*, Baltimore: Johns Hopkins University Press.

Part II

Boundaries and identities

Chapter 5

It's a family affair
On public and private accounts of HIV/AIDS

Hugh Masters

INTRODUCTION

Derek was 35 when he died of AIDS in Milestone House. He was one of the first patients to die in the newly opened hospice. Derek had been infected with HIV whilst injecting drugs with his two younger sisters, both of whom subsequently contracted the virus. Derek had four children, ranging from 6 to 17 years of age, two with his present partner, two from a previous marriage.[1] Two weeks before his death Derek married his partner, with his children at his bedside, in the hospice. He was by this time very weak and barely had the strength to speak the vows to the hospice chaplain. His children, apart from the eldest, who lived with his ex-wife and rarely visited, were at Derek's bedside for long periods during the final weeks of his life, and Milestone House became their home during this period. They ate, played and were naughty with the staff, who daily took them to and brought them back from school. Derek's wife never left his bedside in case he should die without her there. After many discussions with the staff and several weeks after being told that 'there was nothing else the doctors could do', Derek, when he had the strength, stopped telling his children that he was 'going to get well' and spoke to them about his illness and impending death. They all cried and repeatedly promised to be good to their mum/step-mum after he died.

Derek's death was like many at Milestone House: he was comatose during his final week, his breathing became increasingly difficult and distressing; it was not 'a very easy death'. The family reacted as many have since, swinging from sadness and tears to becoming increasingly frustrated and angry at what they saw as his inability to 'let go'; they often pleaded with staff to 'do something'. The funeral was attended by Derek's immediate family; his wife's family refused to attend. His youngest daughter was kept away from the funeral, despite her father's prior wish for her to be there. His wife and children found it hard to leave Milestone House after 'living' there for almost two months, but eventually the staff managed to persuade them to return home and restart their lives. The two families no longer have any contact; in his ex-wife's family HIV and AIDS are never spoken about now. Derek's father, a widower, no longer has any contact with his grandchildren; since that time he has attended the funerals of his two daughters, who also leave behind three children under 12.

I was a charge nurse at Milestone House during the time of Derek's death. I had been involved in planning for the opening of the hospice, but, as I think the above scenario shows, the number of issues that caring for young families raised was staggering and consequently we were overwhelmed. Of the first 100 patients admitted, 60 were parents, who had a total of 105 dependent children. The children were often resident in the hospice during the whole of their parent's stay; many were single parents who were unable or reluctant to arrange alternative care. As part of the staff response, a 'children and families planning group' was established. I searched the literature and contacted other services for any previous experience of this type of provision. This yielded nothing that specifically addressed parents and children affected by HIV. There were not even any estimates of the number of children in Lothian with an HIV positive parent to gauge how many parents we were likely to admit, although the Lothian AIDS Forum had recently begun to express concern about services for children and parents. It quickly became clear that the service offered at Milestone House was essentially new and that there was a gap in knowledge around the impact of HIV on affected children and families.

I contacted Lothian Health Board's AIDS team and participated in producing a report which estimated that there were potentially 500 children living with an HIV positive parent in Lothian (Duncan 1992). Useful though this estimate was, it could not offer any insights that might lead to an understanding of the problems and issues that the families faced, or were likely to face in the future. As a consequence I applied for, and was awarded, a two-year fellowship by the Scottish Office to carry out a qualitative study which would investigate, in-depth, families affected by HIV. Twenty families in Lothian where one or both parents were HIV positive were studied over an eighteen-month period; multiple contacts including repeat in-depth semi-structured interviews were conducted both with parents and with members of the extended family (Masters 1997).

This chapter describes the process by which I entered the research field and charts my journey from nurse to ethnographer. I played out this change of roles to one audience, who, in turn, changed roles from 'clients/patients' to 'research respondents' in their relationship to me. The blurring of roles and relationships which ensued was at times extremely difficult to handle, particularly as it intersected with my own biography in specific ways. However, I will go on to suggest that the uncertainty was also productive in that it created a space for the construction of accounts outside of a standard repertoire of public HIV narratives.

HIV/AIDS is an emotive research topic. I found the impact of HIV even more so because of the absence of a public and therefore emotionally 'safe' language by which to articulate often painful experience (see also Clive Foster, Chapter 9). The research interacted with events in my own and my respondents' lives and consequently affected all of us in various ways. These issues are the subject of much debate in qualitative methodology and in particular in relation to HIV research (see Lee 1993; Sieber 1993). I will discuss the impact of the research on the respondents and the researcher and the effects this had on data generated. I will also discuss ethical issues around the dissemination of findings.

NURSE, RESEARCHER, ETHNOGRAPHER, RESIDENT, PATIENT, RESPONDENT: CHANGING AND ADJUSTING TO NEW ROLES AND RELATIONSHIPS

Through my work in a variety of inpatient and community-based HIV services, I had 'nursed' many of the respondents, who were therefore to some extent aware of my personal circumstances, social class and educational background. In addition I already had information about the respondents' past and present circumstances and therefore they were less able to put on a 'best face' or 'stick to the relative security offered by public accounts' (Cornwell 1984: 15). Some ethnographers, such as Taylor (1993), advocate conscious attempts to change vocabulary and accent in order to establish rapport with respondents. In my case, I consider that this would have immediately been seen to be false. In any case, I remain unconvinced of the wisdom and benefits of making these changes as a matter of course as respondents are likely to be more sophisticated and tolerant of the researcher's identity and foibles than the sort of approach advocated by Taylor suggests.

What *was* different was my change of role from nurse to researcher and the associated change in the relationship between the respondents and myself. The individuals were no longer patients or clients but research subjects or respondents. The research 'setting' (here 'setting' means both the change in role of researcher and researched *and* change of physical location from inpatient unit to respondents' homes and communities) was to a large extent unfamiliar to the respondents and myself. A period of adjustment was necessary as this relationship changed from a therapeutic focus to a research focus. Various researchers have discussed the benefits of participation by respondents (Oakley 1981; Finch 1984; Olesen 1994). It can be argued that interviewing brings an element of catharsis and therefore *is* therapeutic (see Jill Bourne, Chapter 6, for example), but this is secondary to the main purpose of the relationship, which is to gather data (see Holland *et al.* 1994 for a discussion of the distinction between interviewing and counselling).

My nursing experience had taught me that parents will only begin to discuss HIV, death and child care issues when a high degree of trust has developed. This 'delay' in discussing delicate issues has also been described by Silverman and Perakyla (1990). I now had to build this trust on a different ground than the nurse–client relationship in which I had previously operated. This task involved the resolution of complex role conflicts and made me face issues around the effect of the subjectivity of the researcher. It also forced me to consider ethical questions.

THE RESEARCHER AS 'INSIDER': SHIFTING BOUNDARIES

The debate surrounding the influences on the research process of being a 'known' researcher, and of conducting research in 'your own setting' (Schwartz and Jacobs 1979; Lipson 1984, 1992), are ongoing in qualitative methodology. Lipson (1984) argues that there are potential benefits in being a known researcher, including ease of access, prior knowledge of some relevant research questions and an enhanced capacity to elicit in-depth data. Overall, I feel that there were definite benefits to being 'known': the data gathered were genuinely 'in-depth' and the existing trust and rapport overcame some of the problems of public accounts. There was a level of co-operation and agreement to participate that I feel that an 'outsider' would not have been able to achieve. The downside of having experience of the research setting is that the researcher may not see the things that are routine or obvious (Strauss and Corbin 1990).

The boundaries between 'insiders' and 'outsiders' are, however, a matter of definition and shift according to context. Although I was neither an HIV positive parent nor a researcher conducting research in my own work setting I was an 'insider' in the sense that I knew all except one of the parents before the start of the study. The issue of subjectivity in the researcher is therefore pertinent. Undoubtedly the value of having worked in the HIV field for a number of years meant that I already had ideas about the questions that would be addressed from the 'inside' view of professionals working with families affected by HIV. Indeed the whole study came about as a result of my experience of nursing the parents and identifying the gap in both clinical provision and research on families affected by HIV. To research these issues, however, I had to establish an analytical position outside of these views. I had to detach myself from my nursing role and renegotiate the relationship with my former clients. This involved redrawing boundaries of involvements and detachment, a task which went far beyond a mere intellectual realignment of my position.

THE RESEARCHER AS EX-NURSE AND CARE PROVIDER

The nurse–patient relationship has been extensively studied (Benner and Wrubel 1989; May 1990, 1992; Morse 1991, 1992). However, as Morse notes, the difficulties encountered when the relationship between nurse and patient becomes over-involved have not been well described. HIV, particularly when allied to palliative care, has brought this issue to the fore. Barbour (1993), in a study of staff tensions and conflicts in HIV/AIDS work, found that concerns of over-involvement and burnout were common in those involved in HIV-related work. The factors identified by research studies as being particularly stressful were the youth of patients, 'bereavement overload', dementia (Ross and Seeger, 1988) and working with marginalised groups such as drug users and the difficulties that their demands can make on workers (Bulkin et al. 1988).

After years of working with people with HIV and drug users in a variety of settings, I was very aware (almost obsessively) about the need to set limits on the amount of personal involvement and to seek help when problems of this nature arose. My experience of individuals who do not follow these basic rules is an early, often painful, exit from the HIV field. Maintaining an individual's independence and discouraging over-reliance on 'helping agencies' and professionals is central to the role of nurses. This runs contrary to the concept of reciprocity in research relationships, where some researchers consciously seek to help, for example by running errands, either in order to compensate for the respondents' participation or as a token of good faith (Mitchell 1993). Working with drug users had also made me aware of the need to maintain boundaries and cautious about being 'suckered' (Berk and Adams, 1970) by, for example, offering loans of money or transport. Memories of my early days as a community drugs nurse were still fresh in my mind: on one occasion I offered to take a drug user to various locations to 'pick up clothes and giros'. After several stops I had the dawning realisation that I was in fact acting as his driver whilst he dealt drugs. The debate surrounding the practical and ethical wisdom of providing goods and services to respondents is ongoing (Lee 1993: 138).

Lipson describes how 'being a psychotherapist affected my interviewing style . . . it was almost too easy to probe into emotionally sensitive areas' (Lipson 1984: 350). For me, as a nurse rather than a psychotherapist, there were similar issues. Respondents were unsure of my change of role and there were three instances where families appealed to me directly to help in their attempts to get their children back into their care. Two families asked me to assist in talking to their children about their HIV status. I had to avoid trying 'to find solutions', either short-term or long-term, and to learn to listen to people's problems without trying to steer them towards problem-solving and 'therapeutic' outcomes. As I will go on to describe, just listening and probing did not sit comfortably at first – as Morse (1991) suggests, nurses are particularly bad at 'doing nothing' Perhaps what is important here is that I was constantly aware of these possible pitfalls and their impact on the data generated throughout the research process. However, research interacts with other parts of life in unexpected ways and it is impossible to completely anticipate one's reactions and plan for all possible events.

THE INTERACTION OF PUBLIC, PRIVATE AND PROFESSIONAL ROLES

Strauss and Corbin (1990) coined the term 'theoretical sensitivity' to refer to previous experience of the field. They define it as 'a personal quality of the researcher . . . one can come to the research situation with varying degrees of sensitivity depending upon previous reading and experience with or relevant to an area' (Strauss and Corbin 1990: 41). Professional *and* personal experience are important sources of 'theoretical sensitivity'. I have raised issues around my professional experience as a nurse. Some details of my family circumstances are also pertinent. I am an age peer of the respondents, and, like them, I have children under the age of 10. Personal experience of loss and illness of family members during the study period also impacted on the progress and completion of the study.

I do not intend to go into a discussion of my own background, assumptions and priorities, but some detail is needed to describe the interaction of my personal circumstances with those of the respondents. There is also an issue around the degree to which this should be articulated by the researcher. Lofland and Lofland write that an excess of self-reflexivity can lead to reports being viewed as 'narcissistic and exhibitionist, and simply dismissed as uninteresting' (Lofland and Lofland 1995: 14). Burton (1978: 167) argues that it is in reality impossible for the researcher to be aware of all their assumptions and characteristics that may impact on the research, and quotes Johnson (1976), who is similarly sceptical of attempts by researchers to 'let the reader know that they cried twice, made love fifteen times and changed their socks once a week while in the field'. However, it should be acknowledged that in qualitative *and* quantitative studies the researcher's own perspectives and characteristics will to some extent affect the priorities given to certain topics and to the collection of data (Pavis 1993).

As a nurse, the intention is to make the relationship with patients therapeutic. May notes that for nurses 'there is not only a direct and intimate connection between "work" and "relationships", but for all practical purposes the two are indivisible' (May 1992: 598). The problems I encountered were twofold. Firstly, I lost this 'therapeutic' role and the merely listening and observer role was difficult initially; there was a feeling of helplessness and guilt. These persistent feelings of 'guilt' are also common to naturalistic observers (Bluebond-Langner 1978; Wilkins 1993) and the sense of being a 'data mugger' (Lofland and Lofland 1995) was very real. Secondly, after working in a close-knit team setting with other nurses and professionals, I felt isolated and yearned for the support that such a setting affords. Frequent meetings with my supervisors were necessary to discuss these issues, although ultimately I was guilty of not paying enough heed to the emotional difficulties I was experiencing.

The situation was compounded by two unexpected deaths within my close family, one just before the study began and one during the study. A third member of my close family was diagnosed with cancer during the study. After the death of two respondents to whom I felt particularly close and whose families and children I had known over a number of years, it became very difficult for me to carry on the research. As Lee (1993) has commented, the lone researcher is particularly vulnerable to emotional difficulties when respondents die. The problem of over-identification was all too apparent at that stage. I was the same age as many of the respondents and like them also had young children.

There was also a great expectation from the HIV field for some feedback from the research and many requests for talks, workshops and seminars, my positive response to which added to the pressure. This may have been an attempt on my part to regain a therapeutic role or to assuage some of the 'guilt'. I also gave interviews to a national newspaper and to television and radio current affairs programmes.

Ultimately I was overwhelmed by the feeling that my life was dominated by death and that I was surrounded by dying and ill people. I found it increasingly difficult to spend both my working and private life thinking about death and dying. It became impossible for me to lift anything written about terminal illness or the death of parents, and it was at this stage that the research was put on the back burner after the fieldwork had been completed. It was only after carrying through a conscious decision to spend a year away from the HIV field that I felt able to return to write up the study.

My experiences changed my thinking as a researcher and of the research process in two ways. Firstly, I initially shared the view expressed above by Burton (1978) and also by Rosaldo, who warns against the 'frequent violation by essays laced with trendy amalgams of continental philosophy and autobiographical snippets' (Rosaldo 1989: 7). However, personal experience can be used to great analytical and theoretical gain and Rosaldo eloquently describes how the death of a partner was instrumental in gaining greater theoretical insight during a study of loss and grief. He also details this in a critical analysis of anthropological method. Secondly, my tradition (or profession) was nursing, where the teaching, as described earlier, warns against over-involvement, divulging personal information and the use of self. Nursing has to a large degree used quantitative nursing and medical research as the source of knowledge (Benner and Wrubel 1989; Morse 1992; Tilley 1995). However, as Rosaldo states, 'Such terms as "objectivity", "neutrality", "impartiality" refer to subject positions once endowed with great institutional authority, but they are arguably neither more nor less valid than those of more engaged, yet equally perceptive, knowledgeable actors' (Rosaldo 1989: 21). Therefore, through the research process I learnt to worry less about truth and objectivity, and to embrace 'the truths of case studies that are embedded in local contexts, shaped by local interests, and colored by local perceptions' (Rosaldo 1989: 21). My own experiences enhanced my perceptiveness and analytical engagement, but only once I could give them the space to do so.

THE IMPACT OF THE RESEARCH ON THE RESPONDENTS: PUBLIC AND PRIVATE ACCOUNTS

HIV research has been directed at a small 'captive' population. Although rarely explicitly stated, there is a general feeling among researchers that the HIV population is perhaps over-researched (Blaxter 1994) and that to some extent many of this group have now become weary of research involvement. Consequently, perhaps, many studies are now conducted on a small group of subjects who *are* still willing to be involved in research. I was keen not to impose any additional burdens on those already seriously ill or facing high levels of stress in their lives (Zich and Temoshok 1986). However, from previous experience and my initial review of the literature, I was satisfied that this was a new and important area to study. Indeed many of the respondents stated that it was the subject matter of this study that persuaded them to take part; they felt that the issues surrounding HIV and families needed to be addressed.

In order to gain an overview of the respondents' previous and current research involvement, I included a question in the second interview schedule that asked respondents to identify and list the studies with which they had been involved and their attitude to research in the HIV field. The respondents divided into two groups in relation to this. The first group had always been wary of joining in research, but felt that if a study was going to be of benefit to themselves or others they might agree to participate. However, they recounted that they often felt treated as 'guinea pigs' and that they 'never heard the results' of any study they had been involved with. Consequently most were not involved in research and two was the maximum number of studies in which any one respondent had participated. The reasons they gave for agreeing to this study were the perceived salience of the research topic and the fact that I was already known to them.

The second group reported that they were happy to join in any study that might be of benefit to themselves or others with HIV. Some respondents agreed to involvement in studies if they felt it might be of benefit to a researcher's studies or career. The maximum number of studies that any respondent was able to identify having been involved with was four. However, although adult respondents may have been willing to consider their own participation in research, they were all very protective of their children being involved in research. Some even withdrew their children from the follow-up study of children born to positive mothers (European Collaborative Study 1992; Mok 1993). Again the term 'guinea pig' was used to describe how they felt about the role of their children in research, as the following quote illustrates:

HM: The visits to the hospital, you've stopped that now or stopping . . . ?
G: I've stopped that now, because I just felt they wanted to use him as a guinea pig, there's no reason for them to see him now, he's clear he'll not convert now and he's perfectly healthy.
HM: Have they said that to you?
G: Oh aye, [the doctor] said it's just a formality type thing to keep them up on their research, but there's no way he's going to convert now he's perfectly well.

Respondents' knowledge about different types of research and research methods varied and the basis upon which they made decisions regarding participation in research was not always clear. They often appeared to have difficulty in identifying *what* a research study was, or what researchers did. This uncertainty was particularly marked when they described qualitative or community-based studies. In this study respondents would often ask in mid-interview, 'When are we going to start?' or 'What is it you're after?' As Becker states, 'If research participants are unfamiliar with social research they may feel uncomfortable with the "abstract, relativist, generalising" approach of the social scientist' (Becker 1964; quoted in Lee 1993: 190). Studies associated with drug trials and clinical procedures (discussed in more detail by Neil Small, Chapter 8) were usually what respondents appeared to be able to identify as research.

HM: Have you had people sort of asking you to join in this piece of research or that study?

L: No, but I wouldnae mind daeing that because I believe that you need our help tae find oot, I dinnae mind as long as I can tolerate the drug, I really dinnae mind because it's the only way they're gonnae find oot.

In addition to research projects, many of the respondents were in touch with a number of services. All had a GP and all but two attended the infectious diseases hospital for regular check-ups. Many used community nursing, social work-supported accommodation services and a range of other statutory and non-statutory agencies. The maximum number of agencies that an individual was in touch with was nine and the minimum was three.

The respondents were thus used to talking about themselves to a variety of people and they were not always entirely clear about the exact purpose of the tales they were asked to tell. They report sometimes feeling that 'they could give their story asleep'. They may have become adept at telling professionals what they want to hear and hiding difficult or problematic issues. Bloor similarly notes that many rent boys were able to give fluent accounts of their drift into prostitution and that 'such practised accounts confound attempts by interviewers to pursue biographical topics like the possible association between childhood abuse and a subsequent prostitution career' (Bloor 1995: 93).

Some topics were clearly outside of these standard and well rehearsed autobiographies, however. When probing did take place on difficult issues raised by myself it was obvious that the respondents were no longer on 'auto-pilot'. The less comfortable respondents felt with a particular topic, the less likely they were to introduce it into the interview. Disclosure, reproductive choices, and death and dying were rarely raised spontaneously by respondents. Discussion on the future care of children was always instigated by myself. The responses around these issues were obviously unrehearsed and painful to talk about.

The issue of 'disclosure' or how children learn about their parents' HIV status illustrates this point. The research process was particularly important in this area, as to some extent it both constituted, created and reflected the process of disclosure. The topic normally surfaced when discussing general areas such as school or using HIV services. The interview schedule contained the question: 'What do the children know about your health at the moment?' Here prompting was often necessary to elicit what the respondents *suspected* the children knew. In several cases it appeared that the interview made respondents give this serious consideration for the first time. Many were surprised on reflection that the children were showing signs of knowing more than they had been told. The interviews uncovered the important processual nature of disclosure and also got behind the static categories of telling, not telling, knowing, not knowing. Here, a mother sums up many of these issues when she describes how her daughter, who has been told nothing of the mother's HIV infection, has begun to think about her mother dying. The mother is also surprised, on reflection, to realise that her daughter 'knows more than she is letting on':

B: I've just told her I'm no well and that I just go into hospital sometimes for a rest and that's all I've told her, but she said 'mum, when you die will you leave me something that I can cuddle into that will remember me of you?' and then another time she says 'I'll make you a picture and I'll make you a kite, ken so's it will come away up to heaven', but certainly I havenae said anything to her about when I die or anything like that, as far as she is aware, from what I have told her I'm just no well and that's that.

HM: Do you think she maybe suspects or is guessing?

B: Aye, I think so . . . I think so . . . maybe she kens a little bit more than she's actually letting on, I never actually gave it a thought, her kenning more than she really does, but now that you've said it, aye I think she does.

I was often asked by the respondents how other families were generally dealing with talking to the children about HIV, illness and death. I was also asked by the parents in two families if I would be involved in telling the children about the parents' HIV status. Our in-depth discussions about these issues may have interacted with difficulties respondents had in adapting to my change of roles from nurse to researcher. I discussed my involvement with the study supervisors and we felt it was not appropriate for me to become involved in *directly* helping the parents with disclosure, both in order not to compromise the research relationship and due to the need for long-term follow-up which I would be unable to provide. This was communicated to the parents, who accepted the need to seek assistance from the services that they were in contact with.

In summary, I felt that being a researcher known to the research participants allowed sensitive and difficult issues to be addressed by the respondent in a more relaxed manner than they would perhaps have done to a stranger. Only rarely did respondents relate information that I knew to be factually incorrect (for similar findings on research with drug users see Taylor 1993).

The personal effect on the respondents can, of course, only be partially assessed through comments either made by the respondents themselves during visits and interviews, or by partners and extended family. 'Denial', or, less critically, not wishing to address issues at this particular stage, was a common feature in the study group. Therefore I was often asking respondents to consider areas that they either consciously avoided or were as yet unprepared to look at. This was particularly the case when the discussion moved to issues around their children. To discuss telling children about HIV and death, as well as planning future care, was to acknowledge the terminal nature of HIV infection.

There were two instances where the research was reported as having direct consequences for the respondents. However, in neither case was research participation a decisive factor in what turned out to be important life events. One male respondent felt that my interview with his female partner had been 'the last straw', as his partner had left the relationship shortly afterwards:

HM: When was this then Brian?

B: She has been away for about three months, and one of the final things that done it, remember when she was talking to you about certain things? Between that and other things, it is the first time that she has looked at realities in four years man, ken what I mean?

I was the only person apart from her partner to whom she had disclosed her HIV status. He felt that she was already on the verge of ending the relationship, but that during the interview she had for the first time addressed issues about becoming HIV positive and living with the virus and this had deepened her antipathy towards him. A similar picture emerged from his partner. She did indeed 'blame' him for 'infecting' her, and whilst acknowledging the impact of the interview, she felt she had by then decided to leave the relationship.

A second male respondent, who at the time of the initial interview had recently separated from his wife and children, felt that discussing the future of his children had put him on a 'real downer'; he started to use street drugs heavily and consequently received two short prison terms. His partner agreed that it *was* the first time he had 'faced up' to these issues, but his drug use had started before the interview and indeed was the reason for her asking him to leave the relationship.

The above are two extreme examples of 'the impact' perceived by respondents. More generally, although respondents were often distressed by some of the issues we raised in the interviews, they ultimately expressed that they had valued the opportunity to explore these with someone other than their families and the professionals with whom they were in contact. The respondents who were HIV negative reported that although they did attend HIV services with their partner, they felt that the services were very much for their partner. These respondents seemed to find the interviews of particular value.

DISCLOSURE AND DISSEMINATION

Lack of emotional distance and the difficulty of publishing unflattering or critical accounts of the respondents where a prior relationship exists constitute a considerable challenge for the researcher (Lipson 1984; Lee 1993). The problems around disclosure and dissemination of this type of study are issues that have concerned me all through the study process. Lee (1993) notes that a number of writers warn against an overly 'sentimental' approach to publication and that researchers need to be aware of the possible harms to respondents by publication. These harms need to be assessed rather than simply assumed, and need to be weighed against gains to the wider community of making the information available. The potential harm to respondents from disclosure of their HIV positive status or drug use is, of course, of great importance. Although many of the respondents are known within their communities as being HIV positive, there are others whose status is still not widely known and one respondent's status was only known by the partner and myself. The children of many of the respondents are not fully aware of their parents' diagnosis, and the impact and stigma that could follow any disclosure should not be underestimated.

Some disguise was therefore necessary, but anonymising the data was far from easy (as Cathy Stark, Chapter 12 also discovered). The original transcripts were not initially anonymised as this was too confusing. As Lee states, 'removing real names from field material can prove problematic . . . retaining real identities aids navigation through the material and prevents confusion' (Lee 1993: 180). Some disguising of the respondents and their families is possible, such as using pseudonyms for all the individuals within the study. This practice of using pseudonyms and disguising the research site and other details is now widespread in social science research. However, this has been challenged by Colvard (1967, quoted by Lee 1993), who feels that the onus is on the researcher to demonstrate that the need for pseudonyms is essential. A more wide-ranging consideration is that altering too many details can distort the data. Disguising research in readily identifiable cities is also difficult (Punch 1994). This is particularly true given the known pattern of HIV infection in Edinburgh, which is unique in the UK. Indeed given that one of the main findings from the study was how local differences affect the issues that people face, disguise would be undesirable. However, individual locations within Edinburgh were not given in the text and neither was the exact time period when interviewing and follow up took place.

Previous studies have changed males to females, ages, number of children and family structures. However, to alter any of these characteristics would have distorted the central findings in this study, which addressed: gender; the relationships of both parents and carers; and the length of time respondents had been infected with the virus. The age of the children is also crucial in the decision-making process of the respondents. Hence, although some changes were made, many of the details were as described. A series of profiles of the families were initially written but were not included as it proved impossible to find a balance between changes that preserved both anonymity *and* the unique characteristics of the individual families. Additionally, the respondents' pseudonyms were not used in the body text in order to focus on themes from parents and families collectively rather than on individual families. The length of time between fieldwork and publication also helped to disguise the events. The issue of confidentiality was discussed with respondents and it was made clear that no real names would be used in publications.

Self-censorship has been used in previous studies to protect both respondents and researchers. This can range from not publishing at all, publishing only in certain forms or omitting specific items of sensitive information, Adler and Adler (1993) argue that, when work is self-censored, the wider social science community is 'duped, deceived or misled'. The type of self-censorship envisaged by this researcher as regards this study was that it would only be written in the original format for the purposes of an academic thesis. Complete confidentiality or complete safety from inadvertent disclosure of identification still cannot be guaranteed as the thesis is still 'a public document lodged in a library and open to all' (Wallace 1977: 159, quoted in Punch 1994). However, publishing as a thesis is less visible than other forms such as journal articles or books (Adler and Adler 1993). Not to make the thesis available for viewing by placing a restrictive order seemed a betrayal and exploitation of the respondents' time and involvement in the study and this was not pursued. I decided that any subsequent publication in a more visible medium would necessitate less of an emphasis on individual circumstances and more on the general findings of this study. This seemed the only practical way to overcome at least some of the pitfalls of inadvertent disclosure of the identity of the respondents. In interpreting the findings and writing up the research I tried to follow the advice of Sieber, which is 'to design ethically and culturally sensitive research and to interpret the findings tactfully and judiciously with concern for the research participants, the gatekeepers and society' (Sieber 1993: 184).

CONCLUSION

It seems almost *de rigueur* to end any qualitative or ethnographic study of drug users with statements of how normal and indistinguishable the drug users were from people in general; how unthreatened and accepted the researchers felt doing the fieldwork; how co-operative the respondents were; and how sad the researchers were to be leaving the field. Perhaps this is an over-reaction to the bad press that drug users (particularly as parents) have traditionally received. Although I share some of these sentiments, I also want to avoid some of the clichés and 'romanticism' often seen in HIV research. My overriding impression is that the pattern and scale of infection within such an already disadvantaged group generates a unique complex of difficult circumstances. Yet, some of the remarkable routes that the families were navigating through these circumstances, including contemplating their own premature death, were truly remarkable. As to the other clichés: the respondents were co-operative (on the whole); I did feel safe (on the whole); and I did enjoy carrying out the research (on the whole).

In this paper I have documented the processes involved in conducting research about the impact of HIV in families in a particular city. I have described how my background as a nurse impacted on the research process and the difficulties I faced in changing from a nurse to a researcher. I have also suggested that the change of roles ultimately helped me gain a valuable perspective on ways in which people with HIV manage their family relationships. More crucially, it has given me a unique perspective on the role of research in the construction of knowledge. Coming to research as an 'outsider' has thus helped me consider the research enterprise itself. Whilst trying to steer clear of excessive personal revelation, I hope I have demonstrated the importance of serious reflection regarding research and its relationships.

NOTE

1   The composite family described here is built from the circumstances of several families, but accurately portrays the range of issues that any one family faces. Throughout
this chapter all identifying names and places have been changed. The only exception
is Milestone House, as it would prove difficult to disguise the only AIDS hospice in
Scotland; however, in common with other HIV services, all references to the hospice
in the respondents' quotes have been removed. Other characteristics, such as age,
gender and family composition, have also been changed where this does not conflict
with the findings from the study.

REFERENCES

Adler, P. and Adler, P. (1993) 'Ethical issues in self-censorship: ethnographic research on
sensitive topics', in C. Renzetti and R. Lee (eds), *Researching Sensitive Topics*, London: Sage.
Barbour, R. (1993) '"I don't sleep with my patients – Do you sleep with yours?": Dealing
with staff tensions and conflict in AIDS-related work', in P. Aggleton, P. Davies and
G. Hart (eds), *AIDS: Facing the Second Decade*, London: Falmer.
Becker, H. (1964) 'Problems in the publication of field studies', in A. Vidich, S. Bensman
and M. Stein (eds) *Reflections on Community Studies*, Chicago: Aldine.
Benner, P. and Wrubel, J. (1989) *The Primacy of Caring: Stress and Coping in Health and Illness*,
Menlo Park, CA: Addison-Wesley.
Berk, R. and Adams, J. (1970) 'Establishing rapport with deviant groups', *Social Problems*,
34: 102–17.
Blaxter, M. (1994) 'Towards the mainstreaming of HIV research', in M. Boulton (ed.)
Challenge and Innovation: Methodological Advances in Social Research on HIV/AIDS, London:
Taylor & Francis.
Bloor, M. (1995) *The Sociology of HIV Transmission*, London: Sage.
Bluebond-Langner, M. (1978) *The Private Worlds of Dying Children*, Princeton, NJ: Princeton
University Press.
Bulkin, W., Brown, L., Fraoli, D., Giannattasio, E., McGuire, G., Tyler, P. and Friedland,
G. (1988) 'Hospice care of the intravenous drug user AIDs patient in a skilled nurse
facility', *Journal of Acquired Immune Deficiency Syndromes*, 1(4): 375–80.
Burton, F. (1978) *The Politics of Legitimacy: Struggles in a Belfast Community*, London:
Routledge & Kegan Paul.
Colvard, R. (1967) 'Interaction and identification in reporting field research: a critical
reconsideration of protective procedures', in G. Sjoberg (ed.) *Ethics, Politics and Social
Research*, London: Routledge & Kegan Paul.
Cornwell, J. (1984) *Hard Earned Lives*, London: Tavistock.
Duncan, B. (1992) How Many Children Live At Home with HIV Positive Parents in
Lothian?, unpublished dissertation, Department of Public Health Sciences, University
of Edinburgh.
European Collaborative Study (1992) 'Risk factors for mother-to-child transmission of
HIV-1', *Lancet*, 339: 1007–12.
Finch, J. (1984) '"It's great to have someone to talk to": ethics and politics of interviewing
women', in C. Bell and H. Roberts (eds) *Social Researching: Politics, Problems, Practice*,
London: Routledge & Kegan Paul.
Holland, J., Ramazanoglu, C., Scott, S., Sharpe, S. and Thompson, R. (1994)
'Methodological issues in researching young women', in M. Boulton (ed.) *Challenge and
Innovation: Methodological Advances in Social Research on HIV/AIDS*, London: Taylor &
Francis.
Johnson, J. (1976) *Doing Fieldwork*, New York: Wiley.

Lee, R. (1993) *Doing Research on Sensitive Topics*, London: Sage.

Lipson, J. (1984) 'Combining researcher, clinical and personal roles: enrichment or confusion?', *Human Organisation*, 43(4): 348–52.

—— (1992) 'The use of self in ethnographic research', in J. Morse, and J. Johnson (eds) *Qualitative Health Research*, Newbury Park, CA: Sage.

Lofland, J. and Lofland, L. (1995) *Analyzing Social Settings: A Guide to Qualitative Observation and Analysis* (3rd edn), Belmont, CA: Wadsworth Publications.

Masters, H. (1997) Parents, Human Immunodeficiency Virus and Drug Use: A Qualitative Study of Families Living in Lothian, unpublished M.Phil. thesis, University of Edinburgh.

May, C. (1990) 'Research on nurse–patient relationships: problems of theory, problems of practice', *Journal of Advanced Nursing*, 15: 307–15.

—— (1992) 'Individual care? Power and subjectivity in therapeutic relationships', *Sociology*, 26(4): 589–602.

Mitchell, R. (1993) *Secrecy and Fieldwork: Qualitative Research Methods*, Monograph 29, Newbury Park, CA: Sage.

Mok, J. (1993) 'HIV seropositive babies: implications for planning for the future', in D. Batty (ed.) *HIV Infection and Children in Need*, London: British Agencies for Adoption and Fostering.

Morse, J. (1991) 'Understanding the illness experience', in J. Morse (ed.) *The Illness Experience: Dimensions of Suffering*, Newbury Park, CA: Sage.

—— (1992) 'Negotiating commitment and involvement in the nurse–patient relationship', in J. Morse and J. Johnson (eds) *Qualitative Health Research*, Newbury Park, CA: Sage.

Oakley, A. (1981) 'Interviewing women: a contradiction in terms', in H. Roberts (ed.) *Doing Feminist Research*, London: Routledge & Kegan Paul.

Olesen, V. (1994) 'Feminisms and models of qualitative research', in N.K. Denzin and Y.S. Lincoln (eds), *Handbook of Qualitative Research*, Thousand Oaks, CA: Sage.

Pavis, S. (1993) Expressed Emotion and Supported Accommodation for Sufferers of Severe Mental Illness: An Ethnographic Study of Four Community Based Houses, unpublished Ph.D. thesis, University of Edinburgh.

Punch, M. (1994) 'Politics and ethics in qualitative research', in N.K. Denzin and Y.S. Lincoln (eds) *Handbook of Qualitative Research*, Thousand Oaks, CA: Sage.

Rosaldo, R. (1989) *Culture and Truth: The Remaking of Social Analysis*, London: Routledge.

Ross, M. and Seeger, V. (1988) 'Determinants of reported burnout in health professionals associated with the care of patients with AIDS', *AIDS*, 2: 395–7.

Schwartz, H. and Jacobs, J. (1979) *Qualitative Sociology: A Method to the Madness*, New York: Free Press.

Sieber, J. (1993) 'The ethics and politics of sensitive research', in C. Renzetti. and R. Lee (eds) *Researching Sensitive Topics*, Newbury Park, CA: Sage.

Silverman, D. and Perakyla, A. (1990) 'AIDS counselling: the interactional organisation of talk about "delicate" issues', *Sociology of Health and Illness*, 12(3): 43–54.

Strauss, A. and Corbin, J. (1990) *Basics of Qualitative Research*, Newbury Park, CA: Sage.

Taylor, A. (1993) *Women Drug Users: An Ethnography of a Female Injecting Community*, Oxford: Clarendon Press.

Tilley, S. (1995) *Negotiating Realities: Making Sense of Interaction Between Patients Diagnosed As Neurotic and Nurses*, Aldershot: Avebury.

Wallace, R. (1977) 'The moral career of a research sociologist', in C. Bell and H. Newby (eds) *Doing Sociological Research*, London: Allen & Unwin.

Wilkins, R. (1993) 'Taking it personally: a note on emotion and autobiography', *Sociology*, 27(1): 93–100.

Zich, J. and Temoshok, L. (1986) 'Applied methodology: a primer on the pitfalls and opportunities in AIDS research', in F. Douglas and T. Johnson (eds) *The Social Dimension of AIDS*, New York: Praeger.

Chapter 6

Researchers experience emotions too

Jill Bourne

INTRODUCTION

> Traditionally, little attention has been paid to the place of emotions in research. Recently, this has begun to change, and a focus on researcher's self-reflexivity and the power of emotion in the research process has emerged.
>
> (Gilbert 1996: 2)

Rose Barbour and Guro Huby first approached me after I had presented a paper on my research into carers of people with HIV and AIDS. They asked whether I might be interested in contributing to this collection and put several questions to me about the emotional impact on me of carrying out the research. Up until that time no one had asked about my reactions to the distressing stories which I was eliciting from my respondents. My subsequent conversations and reading brought the realisation that I was not alone in experiencing emotional reactions to and involvement in the research project.

The Fourth International Social Science Methodology Conference (Essex '96) identified the issue of emotions in fieldwork as an important aspect of the process of the research process. A stream was dedicated to this: 'The Emotional Nature of Qualitative Research', through which these issues could be addressed. For many of the participants at the conference it was the first time they had been able to discuss these issues with like-minded academics and researchers. Much scholastic work never discusses the emotional dimension or impact which the research has or had on the researchers, and most methods chapters are bereft of discussion on this subject. For this neglected area to be admitted into the academic world both through the conference and through this book is a tribute to those who have 'gone public'.

I contend that, for those who research the emotions of others, the privilege and the pain (Walsh 1992) encountered in doing research can be more intense than had been envisaged. As researchers, we attempt to tread a fine line in seeking both to keep an interpretive distance from those we are studying and to attempt to understand issues from their point of view (Corbin and Strauss, 1988). Those researching what have been termed 'sensitive topics' (Lee, 1993), are expected to remain emotionally detached during the whole of the research process, including the analysis, writing up and reporting of findings as well as during the period of data collection.

The research arena of HIV and AIDS is a highly emotive one, with emotional implications for both researched and researcher. Lutz and White (1986) have explored the relationship between researcher and informant, arguing that both parties come to the relationship with cultural and personal knowledge which will lead to assumptions about the self and about emotions. This knowledge is bound up in the personal biography of the researcher and inevitably colours his/her reaction to the descriptions and expressions of emotional trauma which are elicited and encountered in the course of the research process. Issues of emotional disclosure in the personal, private and public sphere are addressed here from the perspective of the researcher. I base my description on the experience of conducting some twenty-six in-depth interviews with family members of persons with HIV and AIDS.

This chapter offers an examination of the manifold emotions exhibited and expressed in the research setting, and also during the stages of analysis and writing up. This includes the emotions expressed and displayed by both respondents, and researcher. It is an exploration of the times when the personal and private emotional world of the researcher meets the public world of research: a situation which forces a juxtaposition of 'researcher' and 'self'. It offers a view from a researcher's perspective, given via personal biography and experiences related from interviews, fieldnotes and a diary written during the research process. I suggest that the emotions of the researcher cannot be ignored when offering an explication of emotions in analysis of data. For as Kleinman and Copp (1993) argue: 'we can learn a good deal more from the field by treating our feelings as aids to analysis rather than hindrances' (Kleinman and Copp 1993: viii).

RESEARCHING EMOTIONS

> In listening to these stories, I felt both pain and privilege. By inviting people to share their story, a researcher is asking to hear the raw truth.
>
> (Walsh 1992: 10)

All but one of the people interviewed told stories of their experiences of being a family of a person with HIV or AIDS. The vast majority of their stories were those of sadness and grief; indeed, when reading the transcripts from the interviews the emotional change in them leaps off the page and hits the reader in the face. Grief is everywhere, on almost every page, in all of the stories and at times in every paragraph. The data appear almost consumed by the emotions which are contained within them, as the respondents have poured out their version of events. Although we can, of course, never be certain that the data collected are the 'raw truth', we must accept that they are the truth which the respondents wish us to perceive.

In the interview setting there were portrayals of negative feelings which respondents experienced but were unwilling or unable to display to the person with HIV/AIDS and other family members. Feelings expressed to the researcher were thus often contrary to the more positive ones that the respondents acknowledged they displayed to others, which were a display of what have been termed 'feigned feelings' (Hochschild 1983: 83). Hochschild describes these as feelings which are perceived to be appropriate in a given situation, rather than those considered 'genuine' or 'true' but concealed, and not displayed to some significant others.

A kaleidoscope of emotions is experienced during the course of a research project by both respondent and researcher, including laughter and tears, happiness and grief, love and anger, longing and fear. During the course of a single interview the range of emotions expressed and experienced may slip and merge one with another: some of them intense; others carefree. Sad memories may loom like black clouds overshadowing the proceedings, or happy memories may be recalled, with treasured moments brought back to life. For many of the respondents, especially where the research is of a sensitive nature, these are intensely personal feelings, private emotions which are expressed in the public arena of the interview setting. However, during the interview at least, the personal emotion of the researcher remains suppressed and controlled.

I argue that emotions can be seen to exist in three arenas: the public (where emotions are played out to a general audience); the private (where emotions are displayed in the presence of significant others); and the personal (where emotions are seen as controlled by the self, deeply internalised, and not for public or private display). My central argument is that feelings which are displayed in public – and in private with significant others – may not be those which either researcher or researched is consciously acknowledging at that time, but those which they wish others to see. Their 'real' or personal feelings are not displayed in these situations, but only in personal moments when the individual is alone. These personal feelings become 'secrets' and the keeping of these 'secrets' becomes a constant burden (Voysey 1975), as 'personal' feelings have to be suppressed, controlled and hidden.

My typology of 'arenas' follows from a culturally specific view of 'emotions'. 'Emotions' are not simply given psychological entities, but are also social constructs. In the context of the academic setting in which my doctoral thesis was conceived and carried out, it was respondents' emotions which were viewed as 'data', whilst the researcher's emotions were viewed as being external and incidental to the research enterprise in hand. Marshall and Rossman (1995) have pointed out that autobiography – and, hence, experience and emotion – frequently plays an important role in the selection of research topics and in the formulation of research questions. However, such admissions are not acknowledged as part of the conventions of academic presentations, which require that our topics be seen as emerging from the literature and gaps therein, and that our research questions be seen as engaging with theoretical rather than personal debates. This construction of 'emotion' as irrelevant profoundly affected my experience of the research and the way in which I engaged with the tasks involved. By contrast, I will argue here for a view of 'emotion' as integral to understanding both the research process, in general, and researcher–researched relationships, in particular. Such a focus on 'emotion' as a 'significant' rather than 'trivial' (Rosaline Barbour and Guro Huby, Chapter 1) aspect of the research enterprise will, hopefully, provide support and reassurance for individual researchers as they encounter the prevailing 'conspiracy of silence' surrounding this taboo topic, and will also allow for the collection of richer data and the production of more subtle analyses. Wilkins looks at her own emotional responses in the field and argues that examining these 'can foster a sophisticated sensibility in the research setting and enhance sociological understanding' (Wilkins 1993: 93). Thus, according to Wilkins, instead of being regarded as a weakness or 'shortcoming', emotions can be viewed as an 'academic resource'.

DISPLAYING EMOTIONS

With respect to display rules, it has been well established that human males, in particular, require ceremonial permission in order to express their feelings (Hochschild 1983: 68). This certainly appeared to be the case for the heterosexual men who took part in my research study. Embarrassment at any outward display of emotion was often evident, and they all appeared to be slightly ill at ease, sitting quite stiffly and frequently not offering elaboration with regard to the emotional issues raised. Their discomfort was also apparent in their recounting of their behaviour in other situations.

One respondent, Ian, described his embarrassment at his emotional reaction to the news when he was told that his brother had AIDS:

That keeps flashing back in my mind thinking about that, how upset I was in front of everyone as well which I know was embarrassing me at the time.

Huw, another brother in this family, described his reaction to the news:

Em . . . well . . . I think it took a while for it to sink in, you know. Like I mean my eldest brother, he broke down straight there and then like, but you know I was a bit upset. Because of where I worked I'm there by myself and you know it's er, I think you know a bit more time to think you know, and that's when I–I got upset about it.

Whilst Ian was embarrassed by what he saw as his emotional outburst, Huw was unwilling to display his emotions in public. This held true in front of his family and even his own wife. He described how he waited until he was alone for any emotional release, when the reality of the situation came to the fore. Huw's wife was present during the interview, being in the main a silent observer. However, she interjected at this stage with her own opinion on the issue of Huw's emotional display. She said that since hearing of his brother's illness, Huw had become much more withdrawn emotionally – even from her. This control and suppression of emotion remained in the interview setting, where both men appeared to keep their feelings in check.

In contrast, most of the homosexual men who took part in this research freely expressed their feelings and emotions with partners, close female friends, and with the researcher in the interview setting. One respondent, Jeff, talked about the importance of having someone to talk to about his feelings. He described how their house was always full of other gay male friends as the end drew near for his partner:

> There was always someone here that, if you wanted to cry, you could have a cry on somebody's shoulder and vice versa; there was no embarrassment about it.

It would appear that for Jeff at least there was no need for ceremonial permission to express his feelings.

The issue of grief loomed large in this particular research project, and grief was an emotion which emanated at every interview. Whilst I had expected from the outset that this would have some impact on me, I had underestimated the effects on both myself and the respondent, and the intensity of the feelings which might emerge. For one respondent many of the feelings which he had kept suppressed and controlled, not only during his partner's illness, but also after his death, became externalised in the interview setting. This was especially true in relation to the grief which he appeared still to be experiencing.

> Grief is a funny thing it er . . . keeps the world out. Keeps the world away from you, and you cope quite well even though you . . . you're grieving, things aren't really all that you think, problems can be kept out . . . and problems can be kept out, you pull this cloak around yourself like putting the bed clothes over your head and it's OK. The problem is that the world is a very cruel place in a sense and it doesn't let me grieve for very long.
>
> (John)

John felt that he was not allowed to grieve for what he perceived to be the proper length of time for his partner. As a same-sex partner, he was not accorded the same degree of emotional involvement as a spouse would be. In the eyes of society he has lost what he said others referred to as 'just a friend'. John's experience of having to constrain his expression of grief offers a parallel with my own situation as a researcher.

The display of emotion is constrained by what is expected in a given situation and our anticipation and understanding of others' reactions. The emotions of researcher and respondent are each determined by the expectations and assumptions of the other. Whilst the researcher is expected to elicit information from respondents about their personal and private feelings s/he is expected, at the same time, to keep her/his own emotions under control: only certain researcher emotions are considered appropriate in an interview or fieldwork setting and these do not include distress, anger or grief. Writers such as Oakley (1981) have challenged this uneven view of the research encounter, pointing out that, particularly where we engage with respondents with whom we share vital characteristics of gender or experience, we become involved in reciprocities which involve us, as researchers, in exchanging some information about ourselves. This process has been referred to by anthropologists as part of the process of humanising the researcher and enabling rapport with respondents to be established. However, most accounts are concerned with the 'trading' of snippets of information about the more mundane aspects of our personal lives and stop short of addressing issues to do with the exchange of emotional dialogue or displays of emotion.

For all of my interviewees, initial reaction to the news of the diagnosis was one of extreme distress (Lippman *et al.* 1993): for HIV they read AIDS, and AIDS they equated with imminent death. As such they grieved from the moment they became aware of the seropositive status of their loved one. This was a traumatised grief in which the researcher could become embroiled. This was especially the case where the respondents had been unable to externalise or share these very intense emotions with anyone else. In such situations, the researcher became privy to privileged information and, thus, a keeper of the 'secrets' of others.

Whilst all of my interviews contained a degree of emotional intensity that had an impact on me, some were more intense than others. For the majority of people I interviewed there were some negative feelings which they had not discussed with anyone prior to being interviewed. In these cases a torrent of emotional outpouring ensued during the interview. Respondents were encouraged and allowed to talk about their feelings in relation to their situation, thus granting ceremonial permission to display emotion. There was no requirement for them to hold back their emotion out of respect for someone else's feelings; consequently, the floodgates opened. At times the feelings expressed were quite evidently distressing for the respondent to discuss, and indeed for the researcher to hear.

One particular instance occurred when interviewing a woman whose son had died from an AIDS-related illness. The impact on me of her expressions of grief gathered intensity, and I was forced to control and suppress an internal resurgence of almost overwhelming grief. After leaving the room, emotion poured out of me through tears which had been kept in check during the interview. This was perhaps the most dramatic case of my own emotions surfacing through exposure to respondents' narratives – emotions which I assumed I had 'dealt with' many years before. On several occasions it took immense willpower and professional detachment to retain the degree of emotional neutrality expected and required in the research setting. I frequently left an interview feeling emotionally drained and shaken. I would get into my car and drive a short distance before stopping. It often took some time for me to control my emotions sufficiently to be able to drive back to my office or home.

It would be foolish to ignore such sentiments; as reflexive sentient beings we cannot be immune to the emotions of others. To fail to address such issues can also have a profound impact on the analytic rigour of our research. Wilkins argues that our emotional responses may aid 'a sophisticated sensibility' in two ways: firstly, an awareness of our own feelings can have a 'sensitising, cognitive function which alerts us to the meanings and behaviours of others'; secondly, they have an important 'interpretive function' acting as 'a medium through which intuitive insight and inchoate knowledge arise' (Wilkins 1993: 96).

Okely argues:

> The anthropologist-writer draws also on the totality of the experience, parts of which may not, cannot, be cerebrally written down at the time. It is recorded in memory, body and all the senses. Ideas and themes have worked through the whole being through the experience of fieldwork. They have gestated in dreams and the subconscious in both sleep and in waking hours, away from the field, at the anthropologist's desk, in libraries and in dialogue with the people on return visits.
>
> (Okely, 1994: 21)

My reactions were, in part, due to the emotional intensity of the stories that had been narrated, but sometimes interviews reawakened emotional issues of my own. Personal responses are not, of course, synonymous with empathic understanding, but I would agree with Wilkins (1993), who reports being similarly affected by personal issues which arose during fieldwork, that they may allow the researcher to tap a rich vein which may provide important insights. 'An analytic exploration is achieved through grasping the behaviour emotionally and then working with and beyond that to sociological insight' (Wilkins 1993: 97). I would argue here that only someone able to execute extreme emotional detachment could have been untouched by the narratives encountered and, further, that such a detachment would have detracted from the analysis of the data collected. As Wilkins (1993) argues, 'if we are to extend beyond ourselves into sociological understanding it remains important to appreciate the ways in which we are socially and emotionally constituted, both to the advantage and detriment of the research' (Wilkins 1993: 98).

In eliciting powerful responses, researchers assume considerable responsibility. When interviewing another member of a respondent's (John's) family, the extent of the emotional effect, for John, of taking part in the research became apparent. He had telephoned this family member to ask if she would be willing to talk to me, and told her that he had cried for about an hour after I had left. In a similar vein, Hugh Masters (Chapter 5) talks about the perceived impact of one of his research interviews on a relationship which was terminated shortly afterwards – and which was described by the other partner as being 'one of the final things' which precipitated his partner's decision to leave. The impact, for respondents, of being interviewed (or, even, of taking part in a research project) is not always given the consideration it merits – particularly when our contact with respondents is a 'one-off' event and we, as researchers, have little opportunity (or, perhaps, inclination) to engage in follow-up discussions.

The comments from John's relative caused me some concern and made me realise the enormity of the responsibility I had undertaken in asking people to discuss issues of such sensitivity. There came the realisation that, as researchers, we are not engaged in isolated incidents; research is not conducted in a vacuum. Rather, the experiences and emotions which we encourage our respondents to divulge can have a more profound impact than we envisage on all the interactants involved. Even when functioning as researchers we are changed to some degree, however minuscule, by those with whom we come into contact, and they by us. In our efforts as social scientists to gain insights into the world of others, we sometimes forget that no matter how skilful and careful we are – or believe we have been – we sometimes can (and do) inadvertently cause distress to the respondents themselves. Conversely, we can also have a positive effect (as Neil Small, Chapter 8, points out, with regard to the potentially therapeutic effect of taking part in research inter- views). For John and my other respondents, taking part in the research gave them space – or even ceremonial permission – to talk about and make sense of their 'reality'. Especially for those who had talked to no one else about their experiences as carers, the interview situation could be said to have had a cathartic effect, not unlike Murray Parkes' (1972) 'quiet catharsis of comprehension'.

All of the respondents who participated in my research study displayed – at some point – emotions corresponding to each of the three categories outlined in the typology of emotional display which I have outlined. However, heterosexual men, in particular, more frequently reported refraining from exhibiting their emotions either in public or in private. As a researcher I found myself in the same situation. I had to suppress and control my emotions both in the interview setting and when discussing the research with members of my own professional peer group, whom I believed to attach little significance to the topic of emotions in the research process.

THE AURA OF CONFIDENCE

We behave as we are expected to behave given the context in which we are situ- ated. We show commitment to the other by concealing 'true' and 'genuine' emotions and entering into a false consciousness with them. Thus, family members of persons with HIV and AIDS are fulfilling their commitment to the patient as they see it. This is achieved by pretending that everything is all right, whereas, in reality, they are concerned about their ability to continue to give the emotional support they perceive the patient will require for a considerable time. All the key family members, that is, those who were closest emotionally to the patient, talked about 'maintaining an aura of confidence' or donning 'a mask' in order to hide their real feelings, and to portray only those that they perceived the person with HIV wished to see. Throughout this time they were suppressing what one respondent, Carrie, termed her 'silent scream'.

I get, you know, it hurts, I get a pain in my chest, and I think Ohh if I could give one of them [a scream she expelled outside the hospital when she first

heard of the diagnosis]. Because I can remember that scream so vividly. . . .
But I can't.

It's like a pain which won't ever go away, a pain inside that I can't let out. I
don't tell anyone about it, I just keep it to myself.

She described her anguish in terms of physical symptoms as she attempted to
conceal her emotional turmoil. One of the other respondents, John, recounted
how he attempted to project an aura of confidence in an attempt to ensure that
his partner had confidence in his ability to continue to deal with the situation.

He kept asking me will you be able to cope, you know when it really gets bad,
and er . . . and that was obviously of concern to him because if I couldn't
cope he was going to be in one hell of a mess. And, er . . . so I was continually
trying to give him the confidence that I could cope, to maintain this aura of
confidence.

Researchers also have to don their own 'aura of confidence' and keep their own
version of a 'silent scream' controlled and suppressed, whilst their internal state
may be in turmoil. They are required to keep this controlled state not only in the
research setting, but also in interaction with their professional significant others.
For the researcher, it is the commitment to produce an analytical scientific piece
of research work which is the prime directive; work which can be demonstrated
to have been undertaken and produced with visible neutrality and competence.
The issue of the emotional impact of the research on the researcher has, until
now, been given little credence in the 'scientific' world. The portrayal of
emotional aspects connected to a research project in any public arena could be
said to be both discouraged and, some may argue, unethical.

Sharing the confidences of those whom we research raises important ethical
issues (see Cathy Stark, Chapter 12, for a discussion about the difficulties in
operationalising the concept in a situation characterised by low prevalence of
HIV/AIDS). Confidentiality – at least within the context of one-to-one interviews – is negotiated with individuals, but, by virtue of our data gathering, we
become keepers of 'secrets' and private feelings of an anonymised group or
collectivity. We also thus assume responsibility with respect to divulging these
'aggregated secrets' in public arenas – indeed, the feeding back of anonymised
findings to policy-makers or service planners may form part of our negotiated
research bargains with respondents. As Rosaline Barbour (Chapter 11) points
out, deciding which aspects of respondents' 'secrets' to present is far from
straightforward. The need to address this issue and make decisions which are
often irrevocable can place the researcher under immense pressure, and could be
said to be another form of 'the constant burden' which Voysey (1975) identifies
in relation to carers. Parallels can also be drawn here with counsellors, who can
become burdened with their clients' troubles and problems – indeed, at times,
this was exactly how it seemed. This burden affected me personally, but it also
impinged on my work; and, in particular, on the analysis of data.

For some family members in my study, the requirement of maintaining an 'aura of confidence' culminated, at times, in a detachment from the reality of the situation. This was manifested in withdrawal into themselves, and one respondent described how this ended with a psychiatric assessment. An equivalent denial of reality can also occur for the researcher; not only withdrawal from the fieldwork itself, but also from the process of data analysis and even that of writing up.

Analysis and writing up tend to be time-consuming and somewhat lonely pursuits – even where the topic involved is less emotive than the one under discussion here. As researchers, we are all familiar with the difficulty in resigning ourselves to what we know, from past experience, will be a task which dominates our lives for several months. However, my reluctance to embark on each successive stage of analysis and the delaying tactics which I employed exceeded 'normal' bounds.

Rereading transcripts brings the interview back to life, and with it the emotions encountered – both positive and negative. Listening to the tapes themselves can lead to more detailed recall, as one hears tones of voice and significant silences, and remembers body language and tears. The emotions involved can be exacerbated during analysis and writing up, unless these are externalised in some way.

It was at this stage that I used fieldnotes and a research diary as a form of therapeutic writing as I attempted to come to terms with the emotions – both those emanating from the research and those from my own personal biography which had been exposed by my fieldwork. However, I found little guidance in the literature with respect to ways of integrating such emotional 'off-loading' into my emergent theoretical analyses.

THE ROLE OF SUPPORT

It has been established that emotional support is important for informal carers of persons with HIV and AIDS (Green 1992, 1993; McCann and Wadsworth 1992). A lack of support results in what has been termed 'emotional exile' (Giacquinta 1989), which the key family members of this particular research experienced most acutely as they kept their own emotional turmoil locked away, hidden out of sight from significant others.

Arguably, lone researchers, in this particular instance a doctoral student, may also experience this 'emotional exile', and lack of emotional support. For a researcher ceremonial permission to display his/her feelings is rarely offered. Indeed, it could be argued that little support of an emotional nature is available, and this is especially true for research students. This may partly be because of their reluctance to admit to significant others that they are becoming emotionally embroiled and drained by the research they are undertaking. More importantly, as trainee researchers, we are taught and encouraged to perceive our research as 'data'. Data are often portrayed in the abstract, to be interpreted and analysed, with no room for emotional entanglement.

Before beginning fieldwork I talked to a female researcher who had been engaged in research in a similar field to the one I was about to enter. She explained how emotionally draining she had found her interviews, and that she had used the services of a counsellor to off-load. It was suggested that I might wish to consider making similar arrangements for off-loading some of the more distressing aspects which might affect me. However, as we sometimes do when offered sound advice, I believed that I would not need to consider such an arrangement. In retrospect I wish that I had heeded her advice more closely.

As the research undertaken has identified differences between homosexual and heterosexual males in relation to their displays of emotion, it is open for discussion whether or not heterosexual male researchers are reluctant to discuss this aspect of their work. Certainly discussions with a male colleague working in a similar field of inquiry, with male researchers at the 1996 International Social Science Methodology Conference, and at a post-graduate course funded by the European Union on qualitative research would suggest that male researchers may also feel burdened by the emotional discharge of their respondents. However, given the well-documented difficulties which men may experience with regard to the expression of feelings, it may well be that male researchers face a double burden.

My own experiences suggest that a support group for researchers engaged in sensitive or potentially emotionally draining research may be a worthwhile consideration. This is especially true where the researcher is a research student, with the implications of an imbalance in the power relationship between researcher and project director or supervisor.

Although support groups can be extremely valuable in therapeutic terms, there is a danger that they will be conceptualised as separate from the processes of analysis and theorising, thereby 'ghettoising' discussion of the emotional impact of research. However, it is possible and potentially illuminating to combine support and theorising. Green *et al.* (1993) report how a group of four women AIDS researchers, who began meeting in order to provide support for each other, used these meetings as an opportunity to develop an analysis of sexual harassment in research settings. An alternative reading of this account, however, might suggest that the outcome in the form of a published paper testi-fies to the academic community's discomfort with the notion of support and underlines its tendency to intellectualise feelings.

CONCLUSION

During my research there were times when it felt as if the whole research process entailed being swallowed up and subsumed by the emotions which emanated both from the data and from my reaction to them. As researchers we have to keep our emotions controlled and suppressed in the fieldwork setting, for, as Shaffir *et al.* remark:

The intensity of the fieldwork process is typically accompanied by a psychological anxiety resulting in a continuous presentation and management of self when in the presence of those studied.

(Shaffir *et al.* 1980: 4)

Emotional knowledge is negotiated and constructed through relationships, in this case between the respondent and researcher and their respective significant others. Emotions are important ingredients in the construction of social reality. The researcher is not immune to the emotions which emanate from their research, nor to the distressing topics under discussion. As Holland *et al.* point out:

Awareness of our own humanity should never be far away. We cannot simply separate our sociology from our own fears and losses; from our own concepts of danger and deviance; from our own sexuality and our own deaths.

(Holland *et al.* 1990: 515)

Nor indeed should our sociology be separated from a recognition of our own emotions.

The use of fieldnotes and research diary as a means to externalise feelings can be extremely effective, and, as data themselves, can be used to achieve self-reflexivity in data analysis (see Gilbert and Schmid, 1995; Gilbert, 1996). Corbin and Strauss contend that

The researcher's problem is to be both theoretically and interactionally sensitive, to walk a fine line between keeping interpretive distance from the people they are studying and at the same time seeing things as they do insofar as that is possible.

(Corbin and Strauss 1988: 1)

The separation of 'emotion' from 'data' in research leads to a juxtaposition between the emotions of the researcher and the researched. Hence another 'fine line' is added: that of remaining emotionally detached throughout the whole research process (as access is negotiated, as the data are collected, as they are analysed, written up and reported), whilst addressing the need to express the emotional impact which the research is having on the researcher.

Research involving people in distressing situations throws into particularly sharp focus the practical limitations of our professional remit to maintain emotional detachment. However, there is also the danger of pursuing reflexivity too far (see, for example, Tierney 1995) and giving vent to our own emotions to the detriment of formulating potentially more sophisticated analyses. Hugh Masters says:

My own experiences enhanced my perceptiveness and analytical engagement, *but only once I could give them the space to do so.*

(Masters, Chapter 5; my emphasis)

It is essential that we allocate the space to consider the full implications and potential of our own emotional reactions as a resource in our academic endeavour. An adequate allocation demands that we give space to our emotions in terms of the time dedicated to consideration of this aspect of our work; in terms of the importance attached to the topic; and in terms of allowing ourselves the opportunity to revisit our data and our own reactions from the vantage point afforded by the passage of time.

It has been argued that, for some respondents, participating in a research project can be seen as an emancipatory experience, whereby taking part enables them to come to a clearer understanding of the reality of their situation. Arguably this chapter has afforded the same scenario for me, as I have been able, for the first time, to externalise and reflect upon the emotional impact upon me of my research project; for, without doubt, in this instance, the researcher experienced emotions too.

REFERENCES

Corbin, J. and Strauss, A. (1988) *Unending Work and Care: Managing Chronic Illness at Home*, London: Jossey-Bass.
Giacquinta, B. (1989) 'Researching the effects of AIDS on families', *American Journal of Health Care*, May/June: 31–6.
Gilbert, K.R. (1996) 'Indirect exposure to emotions in qualitative research: issues relating to teaching students and training staff', paper presented at Essex '96, the Fourth International Social Science Methodology Conference, University of Essex, 1–3 July.
Gilbert, K.R. and Schmid, K. (1995) 'Bringing our emotions out of the closet: acknowledging the place of emotion in qualitative research', *Qualitative Family Research*, 8(2): 4–6.
Green, G. (1992) 'A review of the literature on social support and health with special reference to HIV', *Medical Research Council Working Paper*, No. 34.
—— (1993) 'Social support and HIV: a review of the literature', *AIDS Care*, 5(1): 87–104.
Green, G., Barbour, R.S., Barnard, M. and Kitzinger J. (1993) 'Who wears the trousers? Sexual harrassment in research settings', *Women's Studies International Forum*, 16(6): 627–37.
Hochschild, A. (1983) *The Managed Heart: The Commercialisation of Human Feeling*, Berkley: University of California Press.
Holland, J., Ramazanoghi, C. and Stott, S. (1990) 'AIDS: from panic stations to power relations: sociological perspectives and problems', *Sociology*, 25(3): 499–518.
Kleinman, S. and Copp, A (1993) *Emotions and Fieldwork*, Thousand Oaks, CA: Sage.
Lee, R. (1993) *Doing Research on Sensitive Topics*, London: Sage.
Lippman, S., James, W. and Freirson, R. (1993) 'AIDS and the family: implications for counselling', *AIDS Care*, 5(1): 71–8.
Lutz, C. and White, G. (1986) 'The anthropology of emotions', *American Review of Anthropology*, Summer: 405–36.
McCann, K. and Wadsworth, E. (1992) 'The role of informal carers in supporting gay men who have HIV related illness: what do they do and what are their needs?', *AIDS Care*, 4(1): 25–34
Marshall, C. and Rossman, G.B. (1995) *Designing Qualitative Research*, London: Sage.
Murray Parkes, C. (1972) *Bereavement: Studies of Grief in Adult Life*, New York: International Universities Press.

Oakley, A. (1981) 'Interviewing women: a contradiction in terms', In H. Roberts (ed.) *Doing Feminist Research*, London: Routledge & Kegan Paul.

Okely, J. (1994) 'Thinking thorough fieldwork', in A. Bryman and R.G. Burgess (eds) *Analyzing Qualitative Data*, London: Routledge.

Shaffir, W., Stebbins, R. and Turowetz, A. (1980) *Fieldwork Experience: Qualitative Approaches to Social Research*, New York: St Martins Press.

Tierney, W.G. (1995) '(Re)presentation and voice', *Qualitative Inquiry*, 1(4): 379–90.

Voysey, M. (1975) 'Impression management by parents with disabled children', *Journal of Health and Social Behaviour*, 13(1): 80–9

Walsh, M.E. (1992) *Moving to Nowhere: Children's Stories of Homelessness*, New York: Auburn House.

Wilkins, R. (1993) 'Taking it personally: a note on emotion and autobiography', *Sociology*, 27(1): 93–100.

Chapter 7

Fact-finder, fag hag, fellow and funambulist

Research as a balancing act

Katie Deverell

INTRODUCTION

This chapter is based on my experiences as the evaluation fieldworker for the community development and HIV prevention initiative MESMAC (men who have sex with men – action in the community). Funded by the Health Education Authority (HEA), it comprised a national structure and four local projects each housed in a host organisation in a different city in England. The projects had their own distinctive briefs but all worked with men who have sex with men in relation to HIV, safer sex and other health needs. This was done through a range of methods including outreach, group work, work on the commercial gay scene, one-to-one work and work with existing organisations.[1]

Evaluation was built into MESMAC from the start and designed to cover all its aspects: national and local structures; the detailed work of the projects; their impact on project users; the role of funders, managers and co-ordinators; and the national training programme for workers. Its design was firmly rooted in the illuminative paradigm (Stenhouse 1975; Aggleton and Moody 1992), which meant that we acted as partners, facilitating the overall evaluation process in collaboration with project members. As evaluators, Alan Prout and I played both a formative and summative role. We were expected to provide feedback to participants during the course of the initiative in order to improve and develop the work, and we were also expected to make judgements at the end.

The evaluation[2] involved the use of both quantitative and qualitative methods but drew heavily on the ethnographic fieldwork tradition, utilising participant observation and interviews. The use of such methods, our collaborative approach and the fact that the evaluation lasted for three years led to the development of relatively in-depth and long-term research relationships. These obviously changed over time and were influenced by different perceptions and understandings both of our roles and of the purpose of the evaluation.

My role in the project and ways in which I was identified changed over time and over different contexts. At times, I was strongly identified with the traditional research role, as the following description shows:

Someone with a measure of objectivity, who questions motives and has an overview. Asks questions others wouldn't ask which makes us think about what we've done.

(Project worker)

However, I was also variously seen as: a 'checker upper'; advice giver; source of knowledge, information and support; trainer; colleague; honorary gay man; and friend.

It seems that in part such differing identifications related to my different formative and summative evaluation roles.[3] Being seen as the friendly, useful adviser fitted my formative role of using evaluation to help develop the work and train others in evaluation; while the more questioning, checking up identifications related to my summative role as an external evaluator who would make judgements on the work. These diverse roles and identifications highlight the tensions involved in an evaluation which tried to balance a critical distance and an outside view with supportive and sympathetic engagement.

There is a complex relationship between research practice and processes of identification. In this chapter I explore some of the ways in which I was identified, or saw myself (fact-finder, fag hag, fellow and funambulist) and show how these affected my relationship with research participants. As Narayan notes in her account of being a 'native anthropologist', our relationships are not always straightforward:

... we might more profitably view each anthropologist in terms of shifting identifications amid a field of interpenetrating communities and power relations. The loci along which we are aligned with or set apart from those whom we study are multiple and in flux.

(Narayan 1993: 671)

I will discuss my different identifications in the context of crucial tasks I had to negotiate in the course of the evaluation, namely gaining access and credibility, maintaining neutrality and confidentiality, analysis and writing. I also describe how wider frames of reference all played a part in the way researchers and participants viewed both the evaluation and the role of the evaluator/researcher. Thus, the organisation's need for specific kinds of evaluation outputs, social and cultural ideas about gender and sexuality, personal values, and the politics of HIV work all impacted on the construction and negotiation of identities within the evaluation.

'YOU'RE ALL RIGHT YOU ARE': CREDIBILTY, IDENTITY AND ACCESS

At the beginning of the project we were seen by the workers as part of the funding body (HEA) and thus associated with hierarchy and power. This meant that gaining access and credibility involved overcoming initial fears that the evaluation was there to provide surveillance. On an early site visit I was asked: 'Where do your loyalties lie in relation to the HEA?' Around the same time, on another site visit, jokes were made about the vicious evaluator making people scared! They asked, 'Was I going to put in the report that [this project site] spend their money on lunches [for visitors to the project]?'

Although we were clear about our distinct role ourselves, we had to communicate to other project members that we were not part of the HEA but independent. Therefore, we spent a lot of time drawing up guidelines and explaining that we were evaluating all levels of the project and not there to feed back information direct to funders.

In common with other researchers, initially a lot of my time 'in the field' was spent building up relationships and gaining some kind of trust. Particularly at the start of the work, I felt I was being tested to discover whether I was truly committed or just doing the work for a 'quick buck'. This is indicated in the following quote from a worker, discussing the sexuality of the evaluators:

> It would not have made much difference if the evaluators had been gay men. [It] may have added something but it's not been a problem because of the evaluators' attitudes. . . . *[It] would have been an issue if we had felt you were just involved for research purposes, but because it seems you are committed to the project it's OK.* You seem to have been sensitive to a lot of the issues and understood and empathised with things that have been said. [I] know lots of gay men who could have made a mess of it.
>
> (Emphasis added)

Having been involved in the HIV field for some time, part of my credibility and acceptance as a researcher came from the personal and political motivation for doing the work which I shared with many of the workers. This emphasis on personal commitment was a predominant theme in the HIV field at the time and those 'not truly committed to the cause' were often looked down upon or mistrusted. Indeed trust seemed to be built on assumptions about personal values, commitment to HIV, knowledge of gay slang and gay communities. A few years before I had worked for six months as a full-time unpaid volunteer at the Terrence Higgins Trust (THT – Britain's largest HIV charity) and I am sure this was seen as evidence of my long-term personal, political and practical commitment to HIV-related work. In other words, I was identified as 'one of us', despite my different role.

The importance of previous experience, interest and motivation in doing a particular piece of research has probably been brought to the fore in HIV research because of the culture of personal commitment and distrust of professionals that has often seemed to exist.[4] This situation meant that it was my past experience, shared values and personal commitment which gave me credibility. For example, at a project training weekend, held shortly after I had taken up my post, there was much heated discussion about the issue of equal opportunities. Over lunch a project worker talked to me about what I thought of the issue.

After hearing my response he patted my hand, looked me in the eyes and said: 'You're all right, you are,' before walking off. At this point I felt I had passed some invisible test of credibility.

The fact that participants observe researchers and make assumptions as to their identifications and motivations (Shaffir, 1991) inevitably limits the extent to which researchers can control and play around with their identity. This has implications for the research outcome. In terms of MESMAC, the ways in which we were identified were tightly bound up with the access that people were willing to give us. These understandings affected both what we were told and also what it seemed appropriate for us to do. Gaining access and credibility was a continual process which involved negotiated definitions and understandings of our role and relationships. To appear credible to so many different people we had to continually reflect on our role. As the project progressed, fears that the evaluation would be used to check up on people declined. Indeed, project members were very forthcoming about their work and gave us complete access to any materials we asked for. For example, one worker responded to my request for information with: 'There's the filing cabinet!' Nevertheless, continual thought had to be given to ensuring that good access and credibility were maintained. This was particularly important when we began to collect information from project users, at which point new issues of access arose.

My past experience and commitment to HIV work was not just important for gaining credibility but also motivated me as a researcher. This obviously brought the potential for boundary blurring as my work was driven by political and emotional agendas as well as a desire to undertake good quality research. As noted in the introduction to this collection, the urgency of the epidemic and the small and networked nature of the HIV field has led to close relationships between many researchers, practitioners and service users. At times our shared aims took on more importance than our distinct roles. This sense of common purpose may create bonds absent in other research and also raises particular issues around both personal/professional and disciplinary boundaries.

In the next section I look more closely at some of the boundaries I had to negotiate within the evaluation and draw out how these were related to understandings of my role.

NEGOTIATING BOUNDARIES

As many researchers have pointed out, fieldwork is often a lonely occupation where one is never fully involved and therefore plays a marginal role. In addition the work itself is stressful, as Baum notes:

> . . . a community health researcher faces the task of walking a tightrope between three often conflicting worlds: the immediacy of service delivery, the complex politics of the health bureaucracy, and Ivory Tower academe. The researcher must develop a good sense of balance. This will often be as

essential to the success of a particular research enterprise as the actual design
and implementation of the investigation.

(Baum 1988: 260)

Being somewhat outside the project, but keen to maintain good relations with
everyone in it, we felt in a particularly difficult position at times of tension
between different groups. At such times differences between various project
constituents would be clearly marked. It was hard for us to maintain trust with
everyone and still appear credible. In these instances tightrope walking became a
familiar occupation. Our marginal role was often symbolised spatially in whole
project meetings. Having no constituency to which we belonged, we tried to mix
with all members and this sometimes involved literally being in the middle! At
times of tension and mistrust whom we were seen to spend time with had big
implications. For example, if I sat and had lunch with the co-ordinators I would
receive half-joking comments from workers such as: 'I see you are siding with the
enemy again.' On the other hand, I was sometimes accused of being too close to
the workers. As I wrote in my Project Diary:

> Felt attacked by [co-ordinator] who said: 'Why do you go to clubs with the workers?' I think
> they [co-ordinators] feel I'm too involved with them. I think the ethnographic tradition is
> different from training and managing, etc. where it seems more emphasis is placed on creating
> and sustaining boundaries. When I explained that there was an opportunity to build rela-
> tionships, follow up issues, talk, see how conflicts were resolved, etc. in a social setting, they
> said they thought people would be horrified if they thought I was evaluating them then.

For me, good fieldwork involved building up trusting relationships and
immersing myself as fully as possible in the project.[5] Indeed, developing good
quality relationships with regular communication has been highlighted by others
as essential in doing good ethnographic research (Gans 1968: 303; Baum 1988:
261; Aggleton et al. 1992: 16). For this reason my ideas about appropriate
personal and professional boundaries were often different to those of other
project constituents. Although I would not actively take notes or specifically use
material gathered in social situations, I believe that my participation here helped
to build relationships and develop a greater understanding of the political
context and pressures of the work. In this way it enriched the data collection.
Interestingly, the co-ordinators did not have the same concerns about my
spending time with them. For example, I was invited to accompany them on
shopping trips or sit with them during training weekends. I also socialised with
them at meals or in the bar after project events.

Although I tried to ensure that I spent time with all project constituents, my
behaviour was not always perceived this way by others. Many project members
were concerned if I did not spend all my time with them. This often revealed a
great deal about the concerns and power dynamics within the project and this
was useful for the research. However, on a personal level it was hard to find an
optimum balance of interaction across participants and to decide where to place

boundaries. This meant that the role of fieldworker was often lonely and uncomfortable. However, as tensions between project constituents died down, so did comments about whom I spent time with. In addition, by carving out a role which was to some extent accepted by all, I managed to communicate the sense of balance which Baum highlights as important.

Other boundaries which had to be negotiated concerned the sharing of information about myself and others within the project. I often felt under pressure to talk to others about what people had said in confidential interviews. Although it was made clear from the start that we would not reveal such information, this did not stop people from asking us. Often this occurred in the form of a general question, but occasionally it was more direct, for example: 'What has X been saying to you?' This could prove frustrating and difficult, as this extract from my diary shows:

> *[A co-ordinator] talked about showing his interview to others and asked about how other people's interviews had gone, 'Had they said the same things?' I wish they wouldn't. It's hard [for me] as they obviously tell each other loads of things anyway but if I say what they've said it breaks confidentiality. I said that 'factually they seemed very similar'.*

When I avoided, or could not answer, people's questions because it would break confidentiality, I sometimes felt dishonest. This was particularly the case when I became friendly with people in the project.

As a friend I would also want to talk about my own frustrations with work, but given my role this did not seem appropriate. However, the fact that I knew so much about some people's thoughts, experiences and feelings and they knew so little of mine made relationships feel unbalanced. In order to maintain good working relationships and credibility I felt it was sometimes necessary to give my opinion or talk about how I felt. Judging when to reveal personal information was never easy, particularly as a decision usually had to be made on the spot. For example:

> *[Worker X] asked me how I felt, said I'd seemed down at the weekend. Said he thought my job must be awful, he feels distanced but I'm even more removed . . . wasn't sure if I should talk to him about it or not, in the end I said a bit. Maybe it was not that professional but in a way important in maintaining relationships as I can't expect others to keep giving [information] and me to never talk about my feelings.*

Questions of neutrality and whether researchers should talk about themselves have been the subject of much debate and there are different views on this matter (see Oakley 1981; Baum 1988; van Maanen 1991: 39, Hammersley and Atkinson 1993: 3–14). I struggled a lot with this issue, particularly towards the end of the project. Deciding when to reveal information about myself was always difficult. However, by the end of the project I was agreeing with the views of those such as Griffin, who writes:

> It is seldom possible for a researcher to make a neutral intervention: Respondents will usually read positive or negative connotations into your

words or actions. Even a stance of detachment serves as a form of intervention, because to remain silent and do nothing is likely to be read as agreement or a sign that particular attitudes or actions are condoned.

(Griffin 1991: 115–16)

If I had spent three years never giving my own opinion or talking about myself I think I would have appeared very stand-offish and would have had much more difficulty in gaining access and trust, particularly because of the culture of personal commitment which I mentioned earlier. As Gans (1968: 305), notes people often forget why the researcher is there and expect them to participate and express feelings of interest as other members would.[6] Asking questions of me probably seemed quite natural to participants, particularly as several people in MESMAC already knew me from my previous involvement in the HIV field. (Hugh Masters, Chapter 5, found himself in a similar situation as an ex-nurse already known to some of his respondents.)

Indeed, many project participants also knew each other before they started work with MESMAC. These existing networks and friendships obviously impacted greatly on relationships and played a large role in information sharing about the project. In turn this could make the development of new identifications and professional roles difficult. For me, then, deciding when to participate involved thinking about boundaries and the competing identifications of me as researcher, colleague and friend.

Identities are multiple and the particular identity asserted or accepted at any one time depends on context. (Rutherford 1990; Brah 1992; Gatter 1993). Because researchers have more than one identity, they often face dilemmas and tensions from their competing identifications. In the next section I discuss this in more detail with reference to some examples of identity juggling.

THE RESEARCHER AS ACTIVE PARTICIPANT

Given the nature of MESMAC work and the fact that most of the project members were men, some interesting issues arose concerning the relationship of my occupational role to my gender. For example, as the only female full-time member of the project, I sometimes felt that my fieldwork role and the nature of qualitative research reinforced stereotypes about women which in other areas of my life I would be keen to challenge. Listening, encouraging others to talk, being attentive and supportive involves a lot of invisible and emotional work (Hochschild 1983; Star 1989). Although other researchers would say that by doing this I was being a good fieldworker I sometimes felt I was being a good girl! For this reason I was concerned that I would be seen in ways that contradicted my identification with feminist ideas. This extract from my diary notes:

> . . . does being the only woman in a room full of men and being quiet and taking notes reinforce a notion of women as passive, voiceless and supportive?

Some have suggested that the fieldwork role is naturally female. Women are seen to be good researchers because of their skills of listening, communication and empathy; and because they are less threatening (for example, Warren and Rasmussen 1977). I do not think that any of these skills are naturally female. However, in a society where men and women are socialised and positioned differently, doing qualitative research may have different implications for male and female researchers. (See Jill Bourne, Chapter 6, who comments on possible differences between male and female researchers with regard to expressing their feelings.)

In MESMAC it was relatively rare for me to be undertaking research with women, and this no doubt exacerbated my concerns about reinforcing feminine stereotypes and not challenging sexism. Interestingly, similar tensions have been noted by women interviewing heterosexual men. For example, Green *et al.* (1993) discuss their experiences of sexual harassment and sexual innuendo when interviewing heterosexual men about sex. In order to preserve the research relationship they would rarely challenge their interviewees: this meant putting up with offensive comments or behaviour which in other areas of their life they would not tolerate:

> Forming an appropriate relationship with research subjects to get the data without compromising oneself . . . or undermining one's sense of self-esteem thus often involves an intricate juggling act, especially if, at the same time, one is trying to take on board feminist critiques of interviewers' power.
>
> (Green *et al.* 1993: 6)

Guro Huby (Chapter 10) and Brian Heaphy (Chapter 2) also discuss the implications of the researcher appearing to condone respondents' views and decisions.

Although I discussed issues of gender in supervision and occasionally with individual workers and co-ordinators, I was never sure whether or how I should address them within the project as a whole. Given that MESMAC was a community development project with a philosophy of challenging inequalities I felt a responsibility to raise such issues. However, as a researcher I was concerned not to damage research relationships or focus on my own personal issues. This again raised issues around boundaries and identifications. How much should I involve myself as a project constituent? Should I hide my personal dilemmas as a neutral researcher? In the end, I found a suitable compromise by writing a paper together with another female worker, detailing our experiences (Deverell and Bell 1993). This was presented at the final whole project meeting, which meant that we were able to discuss our experiences with other project members at a time when the fieldwork was complete. Interestingly, this paper led to a wider discussion of issues relating to gender within MESMAC, which in turn led to greater coverage of these issues in the final report. Thus, by becoming an active participant, rather than a neutral researcher, the data collection was enriched. (Interestingly, too, we have had repeated requests for this paper, and a discussion of the issues in it led to my inclusion within this collection.)

My acceptance within the project occurred in part through taking the role of an honorary gay man, and this raised further issues around identification. I would often receive comments such as: 'We don't mean you, we see you as one of us' when negative comments were made about heterosexuals. I also engaged in gay-related sexual banter and joking behaviour. Although this role had its pleasures and rewards (there is a certain honour attached), it could often create difficulties and frustrations, particularly as it led to a denial of my own sexuality and experiences as a woman (Gorna 1996). At times, such as national training weekends when I was playing a more participative role in the project, I found that I sometimes silenced myself in group exercises.

Interestingly, my own sexuality and relationships were hardly ever discussed, even though many of the workers would talk with me about their own sexual encounters and relationships. Of course, this situation was in part a result of my role as a researcher. I was there to listen and observe. However, I think the lack of interest in this area of my life was also related to my gender and heterosexuality.

Most of the discussions in the project regarding my own sexual experiences took place with other heterosexual women. It frustrated many of us that our sexuality and sexual experiences were seen to be uninteresting or irrelevant to the work of the project. This disinterest and reluctance to talk about opposite-sex relationships was also mentioned by men in the project who were having sex with women. It is also an issue for bisexual workers working with gay men.[7] Nevertheless, in order to develop rapport it often seemed necessary to avoid drawing attention to my gender identity.

An established role for straight women in gay male company is that of the 'fag hag' (Maitland 1996) and to some extent I feel I played, was seen to play, or asked to enact this role. For example, I received comments such as: 'You are the most glamorous evaluator in the world,' and I was frequently complimented on my clothes and jewellery. At times this was flattering, and it was encouraging to feel that I had been accepted into the project and was trusted. However, it could also feel sexist and demeaning. In addition, playing this role sometimes separated me from other women in the project who would be cast in other roles.

This identification of me may have been a way of attenuating my power as an evaluator, or of incorporating me as a woman into the project in a way which fitted current gay subcultural codes. After all, although it was my job, I was a straight woman hanging around with gay men; the stereotypical 'fag hag'. The identification of me in this way clearly drew on reference points outside the project and my role in it. Indeed, the external context of the project often impacted on the research process and the conflicts which I felt. For example, within the broader politics of HIV work, debates about the re-gaying of AIDS (King, 1993) led to criticism from others over the place of women in a project concerning men who have sex with men. This exacerbated my anxieties about my appropriateness in doing the work.

My dilemmas and anxieties parallel wider discussions and hot debates about 'who should research whom'. For example, can only gay men work with gay men, and can people classed as ethnic minorities be studied only by people who are similarly classed?[8] It is a difficult area, involving complex understandings of identity and identity politics, and is a subject requiring much more attention and research. Personally, I felt that my involvement in MESMAC enabled me to contribute to the development of HIV prevention and to highlight the needs of men who have sex with men. However, I sometimes wondered how appropriate it was for me to be evaluating the project. As MESMAC became more politicised around gay issues I began to feel less comfortable with my role. When the project was more widely focused around MWHSWM (some of whom were having sex with women) my involvement seemed easier to justify. Although it was sometimes argued that 'straight women' would not be credible, be able to understand 'gay' and HIV issues, or be told anything by respondents, I found that developing a good research relationship did not necessarily rely on sharing identities. I was able to establish rapport not just with project members but also with users. For example, I was asked back by one youth group I interviewed because they said they had enjoyed talking to me and had more to tell me. In addition, the following comment was made in an interview with a worker from whom I had a different gender, sexuality, ethnicity, age and educational background:

> There is a level of trust between us and I feel comfortable talking about anything . . . all the consultation has been very important, not only to build up trust but to make us feel more comfortable about telling the truth, so the evaluation is accurate, true.

At times being a woman may have prevented men from telling me certain things or initially made them unsure or uncomfortable. However, others have noted that questions of identity and relationships are complex and it is simplistic to think that there will be automatic alliances between people with the same sexuality, ethnicity or gender. These identities are not necessarily interpreted and understood the same way (Haraway 1990: 197; Brah 1992; Deverell and Prout 1995; Rhodes 1995). Individuals have more than one identity with which to relate to others:

> . . . so many dimensions of sameness and difference can be operating at any given moment. And where two people may claim commonality on one dimension, they may fall apart on another.
>
> (Song and Parker 1995: 246)

Reflecting on my own experiences in MESMAC has highlighted for me the importance of not taking a simplistic approach to issues of identification in research. I feel that important but subtle aspects of affinity between researchers and participants have been obscured by a concentration on more obvious identities such as sexuality, gender and ethnicity. For example, I sometimes felt that my taste in music, clothes, political beliefs and age were equally important signifiers of identification which helped in building trust. I am not sure that it is ever possible to parcel out what identifications or affinities will lead to good rapport.

It seems that good research relationships yielding good quality data do not depend solely on the researcher and respondent sharing certain identifications.[9] In fact, a lack of fit may be an advantage. However, who you are does affect what you get told. Warren, discussing her fieldwork with gay men, points out that she

> had access to areas of biographical experience less open to gay males because of the male sexuality focus of the world. Many of the gay men had had past sexual and marital experience with women which were rarely or never a topic of conversation in the gay world. However, they were legitimate topics of conversation on a one-to-one interview basis with a female researcher with whom sexual interaction was not an issue.
>
> (Warren and Rasmussen 1977: 356)

Rhodes (1995) has also discussed being told different things as a white researcher interviewing black respondents. I also found that I would get told different things, particularly by newly out young gay men who sometimes said they felt intimidated by older, out gay men and appreciated the chance to talk to a woman. In the next section I compare our own views about our role and the purpose of our research with the needs and understandings of other project constituents. Discrepancies between different views led to other tensions which we had to manage as part of the evaluation.

'JUST GIVE US THE FACTS': DIFFERENT VIEWS OF RESEARCH

Given my background (volunteering at THT; helping to run buddy training weekends; completing an HIV/AIDS counselling course; knowing a lot of people in the HIV field), I would often regard myself more as an HIV worker than an academic. This meant that in some ways I felt like a colleague as much as an external evaluator. On reflection, I am sure this is why I would talk about 'the people I work with' and feel very uncomfortable if people talked about my 'respondents', or 'those I was studying'. I like to think that this was not about a denial of my role but about the way I identified myself (as a fellow HIV prevention worker) and my desire to address relationships of power within research. I was not interested in exoticising, objectifying or studying the men I worked with. I was involved in a project, with a distinct role, but a definite sense of being part of a team. The urgency of the epidemic and the small and networked nature of the HIV field have led to close relationships between many researchers and practitioners. At times our shared aims take on more importance than distinct roles.

The main role of the research was to support and develop the work of MESMAC rather than add to academic theory from a position of neutrality (Prior 1989: 27; Aggleton *et al.* 1992: 18; Prout 1992: 83). For this reason, I felt more a part of MESMAC than the Sociology and Anthropology department at Keele University. No doubt this feeling was exacerbated by the fact that I spent most of my time in the field and was hardly ever in the academic department.

Therefore I was sometimes surprised to find myself being relied on by project members to present the 'objective, authorial voice' on the work of the project. This was not how I saw myself or my role at all. In fact, such recourse to the power, prestige and objectivity of academia was at odds with my own feelings about the nature and purpose of research.

On reflection, the way other project members clearly identified me with academia seems quite logical. This was where my office was and this perception was also linked to my role in the project. However, the identification of the evaluation team with academia shifted according to time and context. For example, jokes and references about our interest in theory, or being able to understand complex ideas were occasionally made, but this happened most often in contexts where our research role was emphasised, for example conferences.

This lack of control over how I was perceived seems quite common, as Shaffir notes:

> ... the researcher does not simply appropriate a particular status, but discovers that he or she is accorded a status by the hosts that reflects their understanding of his or her presence.
>
> (Shaffir 1991: 79)

Indeed, participants themselves may resist the researchers' collaborative attempts at being a 'fellow' and instead prefer them to take on the role of 'fact-finder'. An interesting tension emerged between the project's need for us to play a stereotypical 'ivory tower' academic role and our desire to break down and question notions of the objective expert. Indeed, our methodology drew on methods of self-evaluation and participatory action research which themselves question such roles.

In my academic role as a researcher at Keele I was involved in an interdisciplinary qualitative research group. This forum was set up as a space to discuss issues and to share experiences. Much of the discussion that took place here concerned issues of reflexivity, research relationships, writing and politics. Interested in many of these ideas, I was keen to explore critiques of objectivity and power within my own work. However, this seemed at odds with what was needed by the project. Because they were working in a bureaucratic and contract culture, project members relied on us to produce information with which they could gain future funding, as well as 'facts' to support and validate their work (see Edwin van Teijlingen and Guro Huby, Chapter 13). Therefore they had a vested interest in us taking a more traditional, authoritative role which saw research as scientific and objective, which meant we were often portrayed as the holders of 'facts' about the project. However, despite having regular access to all levels of the project, like other researchers our views were still only partial. At times our aim to identify, explore and represent different viewpoints contradicted the need for research which produced 'objective facts'.

This need for facts was related to the wider organisational context of the health services and the current dominance of an economic model of decision-making which seeks to compare services' performance according to narrow criteria of

inputs and outcomes (see Neil Small, Chapter 8). This situation affects expectations about what research is for, and what it is likely to produce, with research
increasingly being viewed as providing information on which to base funding
and managerial decisions. This means that it can be hard to develop a more
collaborative approach and to gain credibility for other types of research.
Furthermore, researchers can find themselves identified in ways which contradict
their own beliefs about the nature and purpose of their work.

Despite the importance placed upon evaluation from the start of MESMAC,
project participants seemed fairly uninterested in the methods we used or the
complexities of research relationships and design. This situation seems fairly
common. For example, Ann Oakley (1995) has reported being under pressure to:
'Forget all the methodological stuff, just tell me what works.' Her experience is
echoed by Secker et al.:

> . . . it appears to be common for methodological aspects of the research to be
> reported as a hurried preliminary before moving on to the 'real' business of
> reporting and discussing findings.
>
> (Secker et al.1995: 83–4)

The complexity of the project meant that it was sometimes difficult to meet the
demands for 'the facts' in a concise form whilst still doing good quality research.
How does one address important issues about reflexivity and representation
where one has a role in supporting practical work? It sometimes feels inevitable
that the managerial need for research to be presented as a 'bullet-pointed executive summary with recommendations' will win out against the depth and
sophistication many researchers would like.

The pressure to come up with 'the facts', the need to write up the work before
my contract finished, and the fast turnaround of information demanded by the
context of the HIV pandemic all contributed to a focus on reporting which
excluded much consideration of the research experience. In many ways this
balance was correct. It is hard to see how a chapter such as this will directly
improve and develop HIV prevention in the way writing about MESMAC has.
However, this is one of the reasons why a collection such as this book is so
important. The opportunity to reflect on material in a way that is less driven by
actionable agendas can yield important insights. That these insights are of
interest beyond the narrow confines of academia was brought home to me when
a practitioner, reading a draft of this chapter, commented that it was refreshing
to read something about research that was about the researcher.[10]

In the final section I continue the themes of collaboration, fact-finding and
boundaries in a discussion of the writing and reporting of MESMAC work.

'IT WILL BE INTERESTING TO SEE WHAT YOU MAKE OF ALL THIS': WRITING UP

From the beginning of the project we agreed that information would not be disseminated outside the project without the prior consent of those involved. We felt that the opportunity to negotiate accounts was not abused or used to hide aspects of the work, but instead used productively to clarify detail and find the best way of anonymising sensitive information. Members of the project were open about the work because they knew they would be consulted about the use of information. Indeed, we were often encouraged by the workers to write detailed 'warts and all' accounts rather than 'bland corporate statements'.

This meant that people were often prepared to be very honest, or discuss quite personal issues. For example:

> When I read in the report that there are gender issues for me being involved in the project at first I felt a bit uneasy seeing it there, I thought: 'Everyone else will be reading that as well [and] it would be a lot safer for me if I could just get that scrubbed off.' Then I thought: 'That is not being honest enough, there are issues there so why shouldn't everyone else know about it?' You have to take responsibility. Overall I think it's [the report] great. I get sick of reading reports that are really glossy and cover up all the problems for the sake of publicity.

However, this tension between being 'truthful' and providing good PR was manifest throughout the project, and was a frequent source of frustration. As researchers we felt a duty to provide a fair and detailed account which addressed both the successes and failures in the work. However, for others it was important to have information with which to promote and demonstrate the success of MESMAC. I sometimes felt that we were put under pressure to compromise professional principles for the sake of producing needed publicity for the work. This tension between competing needs is a common concern and related to different stakeholder's roles (see Cottam 1995; and Edwin van Teijlingen and Guro Huby, Chapter 13):

> . . . district health authorities, for example, need evaluations to help manage programmes effectively, and to support bids for extended funding. The regional health authorities, on the other hand, need evaluation to develop and guide policy. Both of these agencies, however, have a vested interest in demonstrating the success of programmes. Academics, on the other hand, need to produce scientifically acceptable evaluations, to publish papers, and to appear politically neutral in interpreting results.
>
> (McEwan and Bhopal 1992: 24)

As evaluators we clearly felt our role involved showing the variety of views and experiences within the project. However, as noted earlier, others felt that evaluation should present 'the facts' of what had happened. These different ideas about the purpose of research could create conflicts. For example, when asking for feedback on reports we would occasionally receive comments from participants about quotes from others, such as: 'This is not true, I don't agree with this.' This lack of understanding of our approach could prove quite exasperating.

On the other hand, our desire to represent different points of view could prove frustrating to participants who wanted an agreed line on what had happened, proof that the project had worked, or a particular view put forward. Our socio-logical interest in the social processes involved in producing a 'fact' (see Deverell and Prout 1995) often seemed irrelevant to a busy practitioner needing to make quick decisions. However, in other contexts, such as the bar, more theoretical discussions were often welcomed. Rosaline Barbour and Guro Huby, Chapters 1 and 15, interestingly make the same point about informal exchanges between academic researchers.

The differing expectations of the evaluation help explain the mixed reactions to our first report. This document described the processes involved in setting up the project and documented the thoughts and the experiences of different project participants. Although liked by the workers for providing a clear context to the work, the co-ordinators and HEA felt that it was too negative in tone and concentrated too little on the actual detail of the local work. Of course the wider context of the project was also important. At that time the work was regarded as very new and innovative and there was a lot of anxiety about unwelcome press attention. Furthermore, there was a desire for the project to show that commu-nity development can be a successful way of working and for the evaluation to give MESMAC support and credibility. This put great store on the outcomes of the research and no doubt added to anxieties that the evaluation was not producing what was expected. The intensity of feeling which the first report generated suggests a greater need for initial dialogue with all constituents about the role and nature of evaluation. As McEwan and Bhopal write:

> An influential factor in evaluation is the view of both the evaluators and eval-uation users about what evaluation is and how it should be conducted.
>
> (McEwan and Bhopal 1992: 24)

On the other hand, strong reactions to first reports seem fairly common (for example, Finne *et al.* 1995: 18). There will always be tensions which arise from constituents' different understandings and expectations of research and, hence, from their differing responses to it. This will create dilemmas for the researcher who is trying to develop Baum's (1995) 'sense of balance'.

I was writing about other people's work and I was constantly aware that my writing might affect the people about whom I was writing. By writing about things that did not work so well or addressing difficulties, a few members were concerned that they would appear to be incompetent, or that the project would be seen to have failed, which could have implications for future project work, funding or careers. As the HIV prevention field is well networked it was felt that it would be relatively easy for others to read a report and guess who was likely to have said what. Therefore, some workers were anxious that quotations appearing in reports would count against them in the future, either within MESMAC or in other HIV prevention jobs.

In this respect it was interesting for me writing this chapter. I decided to write about tensions which I had not really discussed elsewhere and I use quotes from my own project diary. As a result, I found myself feeling personally vulnerable.

Like other project members I was anxious that people may read this partial account, which concentrates on difficulties, and decide that the research had not been done well. This experience gave me a better insight into project members' vulnerability and a deeper appreciation of why there had sometimes been a desire not to include some issues/findings in reports. Hugh Masters, Chapter 5, and Jill Bourne, Chapter 6, both stress the importance of harnessing our own emotional reactions and using them as an analytic tool.

My anxieties regarding my rights as a straight woman to represent the views and perspectives of men who have sex with men were not echoed by the workers. They said they felt proud hearing the work being talked about; that it gave them a better understanding of the overall context of their work; that it was important for others to hear about their work and learn from it; or that they needed the evaluation team to provide support for the project with facts, numbers and reports. The reservations that did surface concerned competition between sites and the fear that other sites were going to look better in the final evaluation.

One of the key issues for me in relation to writing was that it shifted me from the role of listener to talker; from fellow to fact-finder. I was very aware that this was the time when participants would find out in detail what I thought. I had some anxiety about what they would think and how it might change my relationships with them. In addition to communicating our own viewpoints, writing also meant disclosing the views of others. Through reporting information which we had not previously revealed because of confidentiality, different project constituents discovered what the others had said. Although at times this helped bring participants together, on occasion it exacerbated mistrust or anger between them. Of course the research was just bringing into focus existing difficulties and anxieties, but how responsible were we for the consequences caused by bringing these tensions to light?

A final issue related to writing concerned finding ways to incorporate project members into the writing process. In recent years there has been some discussion of new ways of writing, particularly in anthropology, but also in sociology (for example Clifford and Marcus 1986; Atkinson 1990). This has paid attention to the way in which texts are constructed, and in particular the role of the researcher in creating accounts. More collaborative approaches to writing have been discussed, although there seems to have been little practical guidance as to how this is best done. Having collaborated with project members in the design, collection and analysis stages of the evaluation, I was keen to continue this relationship into the writing. This however, did not prove easy. We did receive some feedback on what we had written, and I occasionally co-wrote and presented papers with project workers. However, most of the writing fell to us and I began to see this as a pragmatic solution, regarding my desire for more involvement as idealistic. Often others felt that they did not have the time, skills or interest to write; or felt daunted by the prospect. Furthermore, they saw this as my job. In the same way that the project members found it hard to encourage men who have sex with men to develop their own HIV prevention initiatives and become more involved in the organisation of MESMAC (see Prout and Deverell 1995), we found it hard to generate more detailed engagement with the research. Indeed, it is salutary to reflect on the fact that encouraging more direct involvement in writing may be experienced by participants as the exercise of power, even though some researchers have advocated this technique as a way of addressing power imbalances. Rosaline Barbour, Chapter 11, also suggests that researchers who seek to involve respondents at this stage in the research process may be motivated, in part, by the desire to 'duck' responsibility. On balance, I conclude that the quality of the relationship, the feeling of ownership and the opportunity for members to get involved are more important than the mechanics of who writes:

> . . . the primary goal of [community-based research] is not finding an inventive way of adding the Others' voice to the anthropological text, as it appears to be for post-modern anthropologists, but assisting in the process of having this voice actualized in locally controlled community development initiatives and responded to by the dominant society.
>
> (Singer 1993: 17)

CONCLUSION

Writing this chapter has provided a good opportunity to reflect on the experience of undertaking the MESMAC evaluation and to address issues which it has not seemed appropriate to write about elsewhere – even though they had a major impact on the research. Indeed, my memories of doing the work are as much tied up with the issues of boundaries and identification, and the tensions, delights and dilemmas which they produced, as with the detail of what was found. Reflexive 'navel gazing' has often been seen as a luxury, fit only for academics removed from the demands of the epidemic and the necessary focus on quick analysis and reporting. Therefore, issues which are important to the production of research 'findings' have often been discounted or ignored because they do not fit the utilitarian desire for 'facts'. Although writing of this kind may serve a less immediately useful purpose, it is important not only in giving a fuller picture of how the research findings were produced, but in providing an opportunity to share experiences to which others may relate or from which they may learn.

In this chapter I have described how issues of identity and boundaries are highly pertinent to the production of knowledge. Through a discussion of my actual experiences I have shown that the complexity of the research process (including the methodologies used and theoretical perspectives underpinning the research) interweaves with the negotiation of a constantly shifting set of identities. I have described how researchers cannot control how they are seen and may be identified in ways they do not necessarily recognise or like. Indeed, they may find that identifications important to them are ignored or seen as irrelevant by research participants. Finally, I have argued that in order to understand the dynamics within a research project researchers will often need to look beyond its boundaries to the wider world.

As researchers we tread wary paths between different perceptions of our work and we are constantly negotiating boundaries and juggling identities. Our success or otherwise at this profoundly affects the kind and quality of knowledge produced. In terms of Baum's acrobatic metaphor, I would argue that in addition to developing a good sense of balance, researchers need to take a good look at the balls which they are juggling and attend to the diverse ways in which identifications, contexts and relationships impact on their work.

ACKNOWLEDGEMENTS

I would like to thank Kevin Eisenstadt, Philip Gatter, Jef Jones and Robin Vincent for useful comments on earlier drafts of this chapter. In addition, I would like to thank The HIV Project for enabling me to write this chapter, and in particular my colleague Chris Bonell for interest, encouragement and useful suggestions throughout the writing process.

NOTES

1 Much has been written about MESMAC already and therefore I will not go into detail here. The interested reader may like to consult the following publications: Deverell *et al.* 1994; Miller 1994; Prout and Deverell 1995.
2 For further detail on the evaluation of MESMAC see Prout and Deverell 1995: ch. 2.
3 I am grateful to Chris Bonell for pointing out this relationship to me.
4 For example, see Patton 1990; Maclachlan 1992; Altman 1994. For a different example see Deverell 1997.
5 Several workers have said that the fact that I did spend social time with them was crucial to their trusting and accepting me. Accompanying the workers to gay clubs also gave me first-hand experience of the kind of venues they worked in, which was important for the understanding and interpretation of data.
6 The context of the research also affects the researcher's feelings about participating (see Gans 1968: 305).
7 For more discussion of such issues see Deverell 1995.
8 These identity issues had many parallels within the work of MESMAC. See Deverell and Prout 1995 for a more detailed discussion.
9 Loretta Sweet Jemmott (1995) reported that the gender, sexuality and ethnic identity of facilitators made no difference in respect of reported outcomes for participants in an HIV prevention programme. What did matter were the communication, personal skills and training of the peer educators.
10 Writing this chapter provided an opportunity for project participants to learn about my experiences. For example, two of the workers to whom I showed a draft said that they were shocked to read about the dilemmas I had faced and of which they had been unaware. They suggested that as well as practical training in research and evaluation methods it may have been useful to encourage debate and discussion within

the project about wider methodological issues. This would give project participants an insight into what doing research is like, and provide greater understanding of what we were doing. I am not sure that this would have worked, been practical or appropriate. However, it is an interesting thought to reflect on.

REFERENCES

Aggleton, P. and Moody, D. (1992) 'Monitoring and evaluating HIV/AIDS health education and health promotion', in P. Aggleton, A.Young, D. Moody, M. Kapila and M. Pye (eds) *Does it Work? Perspectives on the Evaluation of HIV/AIDS Health Promotion*, London: Health Education Authority.

Aggleton, P., Young, A., Moody, D., Kapila, M. and Pye, M. (eds) (1992) *Does it Work? Perspectives on the Evaluation of HIV/AIDS Health Promotion*, London: Health Education Authority.

Altman, D. (1994) *Power and Community Organisational and Cultural Responses to AIDS*, London: Taylor & Francis.

Atkinson, P. (1990) *The Ethnographic Imagination: Textual Constructions of Reality*, London: Routledge.

Baum, F. (1988) 'Community-based research for promoting the new public health', *Health Promotion*, 3(3): 259–268.

—— (1995) 'Researching public health: behind the qualitative–quantitative methodological debate', *Social Science and Medicine*, 40(4): 459–68.

Brah, A. (1992) 'Difference, diversity and differentiation', in J. Donald and A. Rattansi (eds) *'Race', Culture and Difference*, London: Sage.

Clifford, J. and Marcus, G.E. (1986) *Writing Culture: The Poetics and Politics of Ethnography*, London: University of California Press.

Cottam, C.M. (1995) 'The anthropologist as grit in the oyster', *Anthropology in Action*, 2(2): 18–20.

Deverell, K. (1997) Sex, Work and Professionalism: A Qualitative Study of Boundary Construction by HIV Prevention Outreach Workers, unpublished Ph.D. thesis, Keele University.

—— (1995) 'Sexuality and HIV prevention: Experiences from a men who have sex with men Project', *Anthropology in Action*, 2(1): 14–17.

Deverell, K. and Bell, J. (1993) 'Some thoughts on being straight women in a men who have sex with men project', Keele University: Department of Sociology and Social Anthropology (mimeo).

Deverell, K. and Prout, A. (1995) 'Sexuality, identity and community: reflections on the MESMAC project', in P. Aggleton, P. Davies and G. Hart (eds) *AIDS: Safety, Sexuality and Risk*, London: Taylor & Francis.

Deverell, K., Prout, A. and Doyle, T. (1994) 'Issues for HIV prevention with men who have sex with men: the experience of MESMAC', in P. Aggleton, P. Davies and G. Hart. (eds) *AIDS: Foundations For the Future*, London: Taylor & Francis.

Finne, H., Levin, M. and Nilssen, T. (1995) 'Trailing research: a model for useful program evaluation', *Evaluation*, 1(1): 11–33.

Gans, H.J. (1968) 'The participant-observer as human being: observations on the personal aspects of fieldwork', in H.S. Becker, B. Geer, D. Reisman and R.S. Weiss (eds) *Institutions and the Person: Papers Presented to Everett C. Hughes*, Chicago: Aldine Publishing Company.

Gatter, P. (1993) 'Anthropology and the culture of HIV/AIDS voluntary organisations', in P. Aggleton, P. Davies and G. Hart (eds) *AIDS: Facing the Second Decade*, London: Falmer.

Gorna, R. (1996) *Vamps, Virgins and Victims: How Can Women Fight AIDS?*, London: Cassell.

Green, G., Barbour, R.S., Barnard, M. and Kitzinger, J. (1993) 'Who wears the trousers? Sexual harassment in research settings', *Women's Studies International Forum*, 16(6): 627–37.

Griffin, C. (1991) 'The researcher talks back: dealing with power relations in studies of young people's entry into the job market', in W.B. Shaffir, and R.A. Stebbins (eds) *Experiencing Fieldwork: An Inside View of Qualitative Research*, London: Sage.

Hammersley, M. and Atkinson, P. (1993) *Ethnography: Principles in Practice*, London: Routledge.

Haraway, D. (1990) 'A manifesto for cyborgs: science, technology, and socialist feminism in the 1980s', in L.J. Nicholson (ed.) *Feminism/Postmodernism*, London: Routledge.

Hochschild, A. (1983) *The Managed Heart: The Commercialisation of Human Feeling*, Berkeley: University of California Press.

Jemmott, L.S. (1995) 'Interventions for heterosexual young people: translating research into practice', paper given to Royal Society of Medicine Conference on HIV Behavioural Interventions, 21 June.

King, E. (1993) *Safety in Numbers*, London: Cassell.

McEwan, R. and Bhopal, R.S. (1992) 'Context, theory and practice in evaluating preventive health education about HIV/AIDS', in P. Aggleton, A.Young, M. Moody, M. Kapila and M. Pye (eds) *Does it Work? Perspectives on the Evaluation of HIV/AIDS Health Promotion*, London: Health Education Authority.

Maclachlan, J. (1992) 'Managing AIDS: a phenomenology of experiment, empowerment and expediency', *Critique of Anthropology*, 12(4): 433–56.

Maitland, S. (1996) 'Fag hags: a field guide', in *Angel Maker*.

Miller, D. (ed.) (1994) *The MESMAC Guide: A Practical Resource for Community-Based HIV Prevention with Gay and Bisexual Men and Other Men Who Have Sex with Men*, London: Health Education Authority.

Narayan, K. (1993) 'How native is a "native" anthropologist?', *American Anthropologist*, 95: 671–86.

Oakley, A. (1981) 'Interviewing women: a contradiction in terms', in H. Roberts (ed.) *Doing Feminist Research*, London: Routledge & Kegan Paul.

—— (1995) 'Evidence of effective behavioural interventions', paper given to the Royal Society of Medicine Conference on HIV Behavioural Interventions, 21 June.

Patton, C. (1990) *Inventing AIDS*, London: Routledge.

Prior, L. (1989) 'Evaluation research and quality assurance', in J.F. Gubrium and D. Silverman (eds) *The Politics of Field Research: Sociology Beyond Enlightenment*, London: Sage.

Prout, A. (1992) 'Illumination, collaboration, facilitation, negotiation: evaluating the MESMAC Project', in P. Aggleton, A. Young, M. Moody, M. Kapila and M. Pye (eds) *Does it Work? Perspectives on the Evaluation of HIV/AIDS Health Promotion*, London: Health Education Authority.

Prout, A. and Deverell, K. (1995) *Working with Diversity: Building Communities – Evaluating the MESMAC Project*, London: Health Education Authority.

Rhodes, P.J. (1995) 'Race of interviewer effects in qualitative research: a brief comment', *Sociology*, 28(2): 547–59.

Rutherford, J. (ed.) (1990) *Identity, Community, Culture, Difference*, London: Lawrence & Wishart.

Secker, J., Wimbush, E., Watson, J. and Milburn, K. (1995) 'Qualitative methods in health promotion research: some criteria for quality', *Health Education Journal*, 54(1): 74–87.

Shaffir, W.B. (1991) 'Managing a convincing self-presentation: some personal reflections on entering the field', in W.B. Shaffir and R.A. Stebbins (eds) *Experiencing Fieldwork: An Inside View of Qualitative Research*, London: Sage.

Singer, M. (1993) 'Knowledge for use: anthropology and community-centred substance abuse research', *Social Science and Medicine*, 37(1): 15–25.

Song, M. and Parker, D. (1995) 'Commonality, difference and the dynamics of disclosure in in-depth interviewing', *Sociology*, 29(2): 241–56.

Star, S.L. (1989) 'The sociology of the invisible: the primacy of work in the writings of Anselm Strauss', prepared for D. Maines (ed.) *Social Organisation and Social Processes: Essays in Honor of Anselm Strauss*, Berlin: Aldine de Gruyer.

Stenhouse, L (1975) *An Introduction to Curriculum Research and Development*, London: Heinemann.

van Maanen (1991) 'Playing back the tape: early days in the field', in W.B. Shaffir and R.A. Stebbins (eds) *Experiencing Fieldwork: An Inside View of Qualitative Research*, London: Sage.

Warren, C.A.B. and Rasmussen, K. (1977) 'Sex and gender in field research', *Urban Life*, 6(3): 349–69.

Part III

Narrative exchange

Chapter 8

The story as gift
Researching AIDS in the welfare marketplace

Neil Small

INTRODUCTION: THE GIVING OF GIFTS

The arrival of AIDS has prompted much social research. In the early days of the epidemic the emphasis was, understandably, on gathering and publishing hasty findings to help inform policy-making and service delivery. By now more research that is both reflexive and theoretical has emerged. However, the development of the subject area has occurred over a time period in which the organisation of social research and the environment of the welfare marketplace into which it reports have also changed. Moreover, that change, to an increased emphasis on utilitarianism, has been in an opposite direction to the maturing trajectory of the AIDS social research agenda, which has recognised the strengths of alliance and reciprocity.

Research involving people with the diagnosis of an incurable condition offers a particularly charged scenario for the researcher. When that condition is being lived within a social context of stigma and marginalisation we have a responsibility to consider the politics of research as well as its morality. This involves asking why our respondents agree to participate in our research ventures. I will argue here that their acquiescence or active participation can be viewed as a gift to the researcher or to the community more generally. In the context of the gift exchange, it is also pertinent to ask whether we, as researchers, can reciprocate by ensuring that the gift is received and passed on in the spirit in which it was given.

Whilst carrying out a research project concentrating on the post-diagnosis experience of people living with AIDS I was invariably welcomed by those approached to take part in the study. Respondents optimistically spoke of how, through talking to me, they were 'giving something back' and 'making a contribution that others would benefit from'.

Occasionally, however, respondents alluded to a felt pressure to participate. One of them told me:

> Of course you have got fear on your side. The poor bastards who have got AIDS, I mean, will be frightened of crossing you because they won't want to cross the hospital so they, within certain limits, have got to be cooperative.

Others were unsure of the etiquette of a research relationship they were experiencing for the first time. After thanking one couple with whom I had tape-recorded an interview, one of them said:

> You're more than welcome. As I say it's only a small way we can help for what we've received. We've got a till out there ready for you to put your money in. [*Laughter*]

In general, though, the interchange of researcher and researched was without expressed ambiguity. The gift they were giving me of their time and their story involved a sense of my then being a conduit to pass on what this gift had taught me so that it would help others. It was a gift given in good faith in which the giver was in no real position to evaluate the potential gains, or to consider possible losses, to themselves or to others. It involved trust in the judgement of the researcher, there being an assumed community of interest between researcher and researched.

But can that community of interest ever be assumed? It is currently challenged by a welfare marketplace shaped, at best, by utilitarianism and at worst by a philosophy of the survival of the fittest. There are winners and losers. One cannot assume everyone is on the same side. Giving a gift, particularly in such a context, involves the possibility of disappointment or loss. Perhaps those few respondents who jokingly mentioned the possibility of charging for their time, or who chose to talk about power and possible retribution, had sensed the zeitgeist better than the unequivocally enthusiastic amongst my respondents.

What follows in this chapter owes much to my reflecting on Richard Titmuss's study of the gift relationship involved in blood donation (Titmuss 1970). However, blood, given in good faith, became the route by which some people contracted HIV. In the context of HIV, then, the gift relationship becomes both poignant and ironic. I will suggest that, in the context of research, the gift is a story. In offering this, people hope their stories can be used to make a difference; sometimes to their own circumstances, sometimes for others like them, sometimes for people in general (Mor 1988).

My concern will be with both sides of the gift relationship. How and why the gift is given will be considered alongside a concern with the good faith of the person who elicits and accepts the gift. In order to explore these issues it is necessary to look at the relationship between human motivation and different forms of gift exchange. The research relationship will be located in the context of social change in British welfare policy and practice: in particular, an erosion of the social contract by a resurgent individualism. The extent to which such an individualism exercises a new hegemonic ascendancy and how far it is contingent on the interests of the Conservative government is being tested since the Labour Party's election victory on 1 May 1997. The rhetoric of the new administration is certainly more about public spirit and community

In seeking to incorporate the research relationship within the metaphor of the gift I am entering a wide-ranging area of debate on the 'gift' that has long been extant within sociology and anthropology. I will use the contributions of Titmuss (including the writers on whose work he drew) (1970) and Derrida (1995) as borders to frame my discussion.

Titmuss's analysis of the 'gift relationship' is essentially about the connection between gifts, social institutions and the objectives of social policy. He refers to the accumulating knowledge about gifts developed by anthropologists and sociologists and the

> vivid sense of the immense pervasiveness of the social obligation – the group compulsions – to give and to repay, and the strength of the supporting sanctions: dishonour, shame and guilt.
>
> (Titmuss 1970: 72)

> If it is accepted that man has a sociological and biological need to help, then to deny him opportunities to express this need is to deny him the freedom to enter into gift relationships.
>
> (Titmuss 1970: 243)

Titmuss is concerned not just with human motivations but with the assumptions public policy makes about these motivations. Le Grand has summarised the nuances of the interface of motivation and structure:

> . . . a welfare state constructed on the assumption that people are motivated primarily by their own self-interest . . . would be quite different from one constructed on the assumption that people are predominantly public-spirited or altruistic.
>
> (Le Grand 1997: 154)

Policies designed on the basis of a pervasive public spirit would have disastrous consequences if people were simply self-interested, and vice versa. Indeed Titmuss was pointing out that natural altruistic impulses might very well be suppressed in a policy context in which a narrow pursuit of self-interest was presumed to be the norm.

Arguments as to whether altruism or self-interest is the driving force of human interaction and exchange have fuelled public and policy debates about a range of issues, including the advisability or desirability of making payments to surrogate mothers. Similar debates have taken place within the research community, with some interesting outcomes, whereby payment in money is more likely to be offered to middle-class professionals and payment in the form of vouchers – or equivalent – is more likely to be offered to respondents such as injecting drug users (Barbour and Kitzinger, forthcoming). The debate about altruism versus self-interest has also been a feature of economic theory from its earliest days.

ECONOMIC OR SOCIAL VALUES?

Although dated, Tönnies' distinction between *Gemeinschaft* and *Gesellschaft* is a useful starting point for discussion. These are terms usually translated as, respectively, 'community' and 'association'. *Gemeinschaft* relationships are seen as characterised by affectivity, mutuality and naturalness, but they are dissolved by phenomena like the division of labour, individualism and competitiveness, that is, by the growth of *Gesellschaft* relationships. Tönnies regarded *Gemeinschaft* as the expression of 'real' organised life, with *Gesellschaft* as an artificial social arrangement based on the conflict of egoistic wills.

Subsequent research, particularly within economic anthropology, presents an explanation of the gift and the context in which it is given which is more complex than the simple distinction between 'altruistic' and 'economic' man suggests. Polanyi (1968) is critical of what he sees as a Western tendency to separate out something which is identified as 'ideal' from something 'real', and he sees this tendency as a product of a market economy. Man in general, he argues, values possessions to the extent that they ensure social goodwill and status, but in a society where the economy is predominantly market-driven these social values are subordinated to the value of production and are attributed a pejorative meaning.

Economic anthropology has long encompassed debates between 'substantivists' and 'formalists' which concerned how much difference there really was between the way different societies organise economically. The formalists argued that it was possible to see some economic exchange as profit-driven and context-free, and fitting within a narrow paradigm of the economic. The substantivists argued that all exchange is embedded within a social context and is about status and power as well as maximising material gain (see Firth 1967; LeClair and Schneider 1968).

Giving a gift in a *Gemeinschaft* relationship or carrying out a transaction in a *Gesellschaft* relationship involves engaging in a complex of motivations, reciprocities and meanings that problematise simple formulations of 'the altruistic' or 'the economic'. It is clear that social giving and economic exchange exist in complex juxtapositions and a primacy of the market as mode of exchange does not eradicate the social – just as the social contract leaves scope for negotiations of cost and gain within complex bonds of obligation and reciprocity.

Sahlins' work on the nature and quality of economic activity in small-scale societies offers a spectrum of reciprocities which range from gratuitous gifts to exploitative relations (Sahlins 1974). There are concealed, balanced or explicit, and negative reciprocities. Concealed reciprocities exist where the material side of the transaction is repressed by the social. Giving your children gifts at Christmas, for example, generates counter-obligations, but these are not stipulated by time, quantity or quality. Balanced or explicit reciprocity most closely approximates the 'economic': we give and in so doing expect something equivalent in return. This is not the simple relationship of purchasing from a stranger, however; rather, it is the sort of interchange that exists over time and implies a sense of relationship between parties – for example, a relationship with a local grocer that incorporates more than the simply commercial. Negative reciprocity sees two partners each seeking to exploit the other but each needing the other to exploit:

> The participants confront each other as opposed interests, each looking to maximise utility at the other's expense. Approaching the transaction with an eye singular to the main chance, the aim of the opening party, or of both parties, is the unearned increment.
>
> (Sahlins, quoted in Pocock 1975: 118)

Sahlins' main interest was in stone age man, but he could have been talking of today's Stock Exchange

Particular modes of exchange are considered appropriate in particular circumstances. Thus the exchange of Christmas presents among family members uses a different currency and is conducted according to principles of gain and reciprocity which are different from those according to which the Stock Exchange is run – even when the same individuals are involved in the two types of exchange. Strong sanctions – both internalised and externally reinforced – exist to prevent the blurring of boundaries between different types of exchange. Social change often entails a shift of such boundaries. Often, this shift is spurred by entrepreneurs with an eye for opportunities to convert one form of exchange to another whilst avoiding the invoking of sanctions and maximising their own material advantage.

Two examples from the NHS will help illustrate how a 'social' and 'economic' contract exist side by side and how social obligation among 'the many' can be converted into economic gain by 'the few':

1 By 1995 the welfare marketplace was impacting on the National Blood Authority (NBA). While they were not paying donors – indeed the service still relied on an average of 10,000 men and women a day giving freely – for internal accounting purposes a price had been put on their blood. The figure, representing the cost of collecting, testing and processing each unit, varied across the country, from £28 in Wessex and £37 in Cambridgeshire for a unit of blood. The calculated cost was charged to hospitals getting the blood. Commercial firms were also seeking access to the NBA mailing list in exchange for supplying drinks and biscuits to donors (*Guardian*, 23 September 1995).

2 With an increase in the number of medical students and clinical contact from day one of medical training, there are now greater demands on both inpatients and outpatients in teaching hospitals. While a majority of patients do want to help, a growing number are saying they are unwilling to afford students direct training opportunities (*Times Higher Education Supplement*, 24 January 1997). Most persons with AIDS are cared for in teaching hospitals and have extensive and prolonged involvement both as inpatients and outpatients.

Given that clinical research into AIDS has attracted an especially high profile and large amounts of funding, AIDS patients are very likely to be invited to participate in research projects. Generally, access to the new drugs or treatment regimes offered in trials is limited to those who sign up for the clinical trial – and, hence, its associated research components. In the broader medical research community – and certainly within research ethics committees – there is also a growing concern as to why patients join clinical trials. Their co-operation is given for a variety of reasons that include hope (see Brian Heaphy, Chapter 2), altruism, social obligation and a sense of the inevitability of conforming to the hierarchical structure of contemporary health care. Procedures are in place for seeking informed consent and in some places for more active consultation with patients about ongoing research work (see, for example, Bailey 1996). But many clinical trials are effectively about drug companies seeking market share – and hence profit. They are not only – or even, perhaps, primarily – about the development of new treatments and associated patient benefit. Those who unequivocally benefit from medical training are those who complete it and go on to well-paid and prestigious jobs and many drug trials benefit shareholders of one company as opposed to another. Should patients' contributions, then, be seen as transactions that ought to be based on payment, a contracted service rather than a gift relationship? Certainly, there have been developments in the AIDS field – such as the publication in 1991 of a consumers' guide to taking part in AIDS clinical trials (Mihill, 1991) – which suggest that patients are critically examining their role in such exchanges.

Given the different forms of reciprocity which can co-exist in any one society, any one exchange may serve a range of functions for the various parties involved. Schwartz (1967) identified four features of the gift where giver and receiver were known to each other:

1 the gift as a generator of identity;
2 the gift as a personal tool in our search for status and control;
3 the gift as a gratitude imperative, as something that compels reciprocity;
4 the gift exchange as a technique for the regulation of shared guilt.

These motivations and outcomes are not necessarily mutually exclusive, and any one actor may derive or bestow more than one of these in the course of an exchange. Giving, receiving, altruism and reciprocity can be understood only in relation to the conditions of exchange in which they are practised. If the context of any exchange problematises a simple conceptualisation of the gift, so too does the prevailing nature of social obligation.

We need to disentangle the gift and the general contract of the altruistic. Auguste Comte defined altruism as 'action taken for another's good'. It might be that the implied other is in a similar situation to one's own. How far solicitude extends in society and the stance of both the individual and the collective to the stranger changes both circumstantially and over time. Titmuss asks, 'Who is my stranger in the relatively affluent, acquisitive and divisive societies of the twentieth century?' (Titmuss 1970: 11). It is likely that the reasons people give for gift giving will change also. Titmuss surveyed why people in the UK gave blood. He found that altruism was the strongest motivation (26.4 per cent), followed by responses to general public appeals (18 per cent) or personal appeals perhaps from a friend or a nurse visiting the workplace (13.2 per cent). The latter two categories perhaps reflect a sense of obligation, a wish for approval and some feeling of inclusion in society. Reciprocity was identified as manifest when people said they gave blood after having received it themselves at some point in the past (9.8 per cent).

Kayal (1993: 131) uses the expressions, 'kin altruism' and 'collective charity' where a community acts on its own behalf. This puts action like volunteerism at an opposite pole to doing charity, with its implied hierarchical relationship of giving something to the poor or unfortunate. Similarly, Fox (1993, 1995) argues that informal care can be offered in a way that is not calculated and which does not involve the idea of repayment at a later date. Kayal (1983) in his analysis of the US voluntary sector organisation Gay Men's Health Crisis develops a typology of motivations that bring together the personal and the social. Individuals contact and work for the organisation for the following reasons:

- pure – people need help;
- political – the world needs changing;
- personal – after an experience of one's own;
- self-serving – put your involvement in your C.V.;
- social – a way to meet people;
- organisational – a wish to be associated with a high status organisation;
- communal – an assertion of belonging to a gay community.

For some volunteers, their involvement confers a sense of having shored up credit, and acts as an unspoken 'insurance policy': they hope that, by helping others today, they will ensure that someone helps them, if and when they themselves contract a terminal illness/develop AIDS (Paradis *et al.* 1987). Thus, even volunteering – located at the extreme end of the altruism continuum – may also confer benefits to the individual who gives of his/her time and energy.

Altruism may involve making a gift to a 'known other'; to an 'unknown' and 'unknowable other' (as in donating blood); or to an 'unknown other' who becomes 'known' through the exchange (as in 'buddying'). In this last situation the gift's function in linking people together becomes apparent.

In all cases, however, the bestowing of gifts both acknowledges and creates a social relationship. There is a political dimension to the exchange of gifts in the exclusion of certain individuals or groups who are denied the opportunity to take part. The opportunity to give a gift resonates with one's sense of social inclusion. It is about being given permission to act altruistically. If one's offer of a gift is not wanted or the gift is not used, then one's sense of self and social worth are damaged:

> I don't know if you were aware but I was a blood donor and have been for years, and then Doctor A [HIV specialist] rang up the blood transfusion centre. I'd only given blood three weeks before that. I've been stopped, which has really hurt me. It's as if they are saying I have got it [HIV]. My understanding

is that they test [the blood]. Then its free, then why . . . ? You know what I would have liked? Someone to have said: 'Thanks for all you've done.' It sounds silly . . . that's what brought things home to me.

(Seronegative partner of a man with AIDS)

The ability to be altrustic is, thus, contingent upon the social and political context. The closely related concept of 'the stranger' is also a matter of social construction and political exclusion. 'The stranger' is an important icon in the context of the AIDS epidemic, which is invoked in complex and even contradictory formulations. The message of HIV prevention exhorts us all to 'know your partner' and asserts the imperative of responsible communication about past intimacies. However, the exclusion of the stranger from our sphere of concern is manifest in stigmatisation, neglect and hostility to people living with HIV and to those assumed to be at increased risk of contracting the virus. It is also manifest in immigration controls, retrenchment of foreign aid budgets and an identification of AIDS with the foreign and the different (Small 1988).

THE COMPLEXITIES OF THE RESEARCH ENCOUNTER AND POSTMODERNIST IDEALS OF GIFT EXCHANGES

The relationships and exchanges established by research are caught up in the same complexities as is any other gift relationship. Research is a social act and more than 'data' or information is exchanged during a research encounter. There is the possibility that respondents will view the interview which gives them the opportunity to air their concerns as a therapeutic session. The impact and outcome of research can, thus, be said to be 'in the eye of the beholder': respondents may view a research interaction very differently from the way in which the researcher sees it. Whilst sharing one's views or concerns may, in itself, be therapeutic, serendipitous positive outcomes are not assured. As Clark and Haldane (1990) point out, interviewing people about sensitive topics may expose emotional problems whose interpretation and handling may ideally require the interviewer to possess therapeutic skills. Thus the interview becomes, inadvertently, something that neither party felt they were contracted for and neither may be ready or able to satisfactorily pursue. There may also be a more complicit pursuit of the therapeutic possibilities, the 'it's good to talk about it' scenario. Sometimes the intervention of the study itself is seen as positive. Fallowfield *et al.* (1987), in carrying out a psychological study of people with breast cancer, reported that the subjects saw the psychological study as a helpful extension to their treatment.

In my study, as well as 'giving something back' and 'wanting to help others', a number of other motivations were identified, including the possibility that the research interview would provide a therapeutic opportunity:

[From the beginning of an interview with a man with AIDS and his wife] I think one thing that may be missing is where can me and [wife] talk about it really. You know, with an independent person, you know, because . . . once or twice I wanted to talk and I sort of hold back. Sort of marriage guidance. . . . I think this is going to be the real first time between us that we can really really talk in any depth on it.

[Towards the end of the interview]

Husband: Maybe once a fortnight or once a month, there should be somewhere where, I mean, you can go and have a chit-chat, like what is happening tonight. . . .
Wife: We wouldn't do this if it wasn't for you. We wouldn't sit down and talk like this.

Another person saw the arrival of the researcher as a welcome diversion, a bit of human contact in a quiet day:

It would do to motivate myself a bit more. . . . Like if you hadn't have come down this morning I'd have sat down or laid down upstairs watching television.

As a respondent in an interview carried out in early March put it:

Well I'm pleased to see you. After Easter the cricket season will be on and the TV will get better.

There are, thus, mixed motives and gradations of emphasis possible in the encounter between researcher and researched. The agenda of the researcher and of the research subject are unlikely to exactly coincide. Studies will have different, hopefully complementary, goals and some will have more resonance than others for the research subjects. For example a recent study (Young *et al.* 1994) of the meaning of friendship and its relationship with families for people at the end of their lives explored two areas: (1) How might changes in policy and practice overcome the experience many friends have, for example at the time someone with AIDS dies, of being disenfranchised? (2) How does the relationship between family and friends illuminate Anthony Giddens' explorations of the changing nature of intimacy in late modernity (Giddens 1992). One can hypothesise that the first area was more likely to be closer to the agenda of the research subjects while the second was of concern to the researchers as they sought to frame the research question and locate the significance of their findings in the context of contemporary social theory. Negotiating and agreeing an honest and clear contract of exchange with research respondents is a crucial and elusive task which, nevertheless, remains an ideal.

Derrida (cited in Fox 1993: 92) saw subtle calculations that are obscured in many donor/recipient relationships, for example, 'I give you this then I will be seen in this way and she will be grateful. . . . ' He deals with this complexity by removing volition: the true gift is one that someone does not realise s/he is giving.

Post-structuralist feminist Cixous (1986) takes the gift further and poses a gift relationship as a paradigm for a new realm of relationship. Relations based on control and dependency may be seen as a form of property relationship – the empowered party possesses the dependent. Such 'Proper' relationships (Moi 1985), characterised by male possessive desire, can be opposed with what Moi calls 'Gift' relationships – these are open-ended, trusting relations of generosity in which a person invests another with the gift of his/her desire – a positive desire, a feminine desire based on generosity.

The gift, here, stands in place of discourse – even a discourse of liberation or emancipation – which, like all other discourses, closes down options. The need is not to just define a new subjectivity but to allow subjectivity the freedom to wander before it settles back in a different configuration. This is achieved through disrupting the mentality that imbues a subjectivity. For Cixous, scholarship – ways of teaching, writing and reading – can contribute to this disruption. Perhaps the research encounter, in raising new questions and exploring potential meanings, can also do so. (For a contribution to this debate from outside the post-structuralist school see Williams [1961], who, in his writing and teaching, utilised the technique of 'unlearning the inherently dominative mode'.)

Writing from a postmodern perspective, Fox offers words that describe what is entailed in the gift relationship: generosity, trust, confidence, love, benevolence, commitment, involvement, delight, allegiance, esteem, accord, admiration. Relationships easily slide into possessive relations: trust becomes dependency, esteem becomes reverence, generosity becomes patronage, and curiosity becomes 'the gaze' (Fox 1993: 92).

As researchers, we operate in complex and shifting political contexts and we do not have full control over the interpretation and use of our research products. The possibility is always before us that our carefully negotiated research relationships mutate from intimacy and equality to exploitation – at least in the eye of the independent commentator or respondent, who may be affected by the revelations which we make. This is certainly the case for those of us who conduct research in areas associated with welfare (see Guro Huby, Chapter 10). Welfare provision entails especially subtle and morally sensitive forms of exchange. Current welfare policy, based on narrow concepts of 'the market', overlooks those less visible forms of exchange on which the informal system rests and depends. Similarly, a narrow research focus on 'cost-effectiveness' and 'value for money' of welfare provision misses valuable opportunities for understanding the shifting social context within which criteria of success or failure are negotiated and determined.

THE WELFARE AND POLICY CONTEXT OF AIDS RESEARCH

I have suggested, in discussing Titmuss, that the gift's construction as a manifestation of a sociological and biological need is mediated by the policy context that frames it. Indeed, Titmuss was seeking to contrast an arrangement for providing blood according to market principles with one based on altruistic giving. In the

USA the poor sold their blood which was then used by relatively richer people. In the UK altruistic exchanges – with no direct reciprocity – meant blood transfusion could be based on medical need. As such the gift of blood offered a vignette for the wider altruistic exchanges and collective risk-sharing of the welfare state.

Mauss (1954) saw a system of social security as a way of expressing solicitude or co-operation and as a renaissance of the theme of the gift. Titmuss (1970: 209) comments that had Mauss been writing some years later he might have included the socialised medicine of the NHS as another example. If he had been writing much later, by the early to mid-1980s, he might have been less inclined to assume solicitude or co-operation.

The changes in the welfare state in the UK – most notably from the mid-1980s – both draw on and contribute to perceptions of the relationship between individual motivation and social provision which differ from Mauss's version of social security. Welfare state reforms sought to infuse the provision of welfare with the philosophy of the economic marketplace. As such the individual was cast as the agent of his or her own success or failure. The able should be encouraged to make provision for themselves, so that private education, pension plans and health care would supplement public provision. The market, it was argued, would maximise wealth creation, which, whilst benefiting the most entrepreneurial, would also generate a trickle-down effect such as to make all better off when compared to the standards of the past. We would have greater inequality but with the mean level of wealth at a higher level than would be possible without the market. At best such a system can be termed utilitarian; at worst it manifests the 'greed is good' credo of the film *Wall Street*.

The idea that the welfare state is a site for the gift relationship becomes problematic in this emergent scenario. If solicitude, co-operation or reciprocity have value it is surely as ends in themselves. But the idea of the marketplace subsumes such 'process' considerations – it is the cash value of welfare, and not its social role that becomes most important.

Le Grand invokes eighteenth-century philosopher David Hume's advice that in contriving any system of government, every man ought to be supposed a 'knave' and to have no other end than private interest:

> By this interest, we must govern him and, by means of it, notwithstanding his insatiable avarice and ambition, co-operate to the public good.
>
> (Hume, quoted in Le Grand 1997: 149)

The generation of welfare based on markets assumes a different view of human interest and seeks to unleash individual ambition for the public good. In the UK the election of the Labour government on 1 May 1997 invoked the possibilities of a new social paradigm in which social inclusion and the centrality of community replaced the business metaphor of UK PLC or UK Limited. If this change begins to take place then we might look to the 'knights' offered by David Hume as an alternative to his 'knaves'. He describes 'knights' as public-spirited and altruistic individuals who need very different public policy frameworks.

As social and policy rhetorics change, there is a time lag as auxiliary systems adjust to, and reconcile themselves with, new orthodoxies. The layered effect produces anomie; the norms that govern social interactions break down (Merton 1957). In the research environment the relationship between funder, researcher and research subject offers an example. The goals that these different parties have in mind might differ and the means to achieve these goals might not be in place. The situation is somewhat akin to a dance with elaborate steps in which one is never sure everyone is dancing to the same tune.

Research into aspects of health and of social care provide examples. An examination of strategy or principle – or even the scrutiny of something that has not been ordained from on high as relevant – is increasingly difficult. For example it is possible to fund research into effectiveness but more difficult to look at equity (Small 1996; to guard against a nostalgic 'golden ageism', see Carr-Hill 1984). What is the basis of our ethical encounter with the subject of our research in an ethically impoverished environment that emphasises neither solicitude nor co-operation but the narrow pursuit of cost-effectiveness? If research concentrates on the extent to which predetermined outcomes are being met, do we not diminish the possibility of critiquing causality and locating here and now concerns within a more wide-ranging scrutiny of meaning? Do we not also accept the demise of the redistributive ethic of welfare? How do we engage in that encounter with the disadvantaged in the context of this demise? What happens to concepts of need or justice in a utilitarian environment where the greatest good of the greatest number may well require further marginalisation of, say, the sick or the 'deviant' (see Rawls 1972; Doyal and Gough 1991).

Responses to the HIV epidemic have provided both challenges and opportunities for social research. By 1990 research into HIV and AIDS was the area attracting by far the highest level of funding within British medical sociology with approximately £2,763,436 allocated to thirty-two different projects. The next largest category was mental health with £1,620,002 on eight projects (Field and Woodman 1990). By 1994, although the cash value had gone up slightly to £2,809,500, HIV and AIDS research now occupied third place behind chronic illness, and at the top general practice/primary care (Barbour and Van Teijlingen 1994).

There have been many critical observations that the level of HIV funding is too high either in relation to the apparent size of the epidemic or to the levels of funding available for other medical needs (Craven et al. 1994). But to what does 'too high' relate – is it the identified size of the epidemic, the size of the epidemic in comparable countries, or the potential size and impact of the epidemic? If the relative low levels of the epidemic in the UK are used as justification for cuts in expenditure on support services, it is also possible to use low levels of actual incidence as justification for high levels of expenditure on prevention.

We could seek to develop policy via cost-effectiveness analysis: how much would it cost to treat people compared with the costs of prevention programmes? Or we could accept that, in relation to an infectious disease, we have to include risk as well as incidence in carrying out a needs assessment and deciding expenditure policy. Again, we could accept that to understand and effectively intervene in the prevention of HIV infection we need a research approach that allows us to theorise risk, to examine critically the way the public world impacts on the intimate, to look at disparities of power in society, and so on. Indeed it is in some of these areas of critical research that progress has been made by those working on aspects of the HIV epidemic (see the contributors to Boulton 1994 and, on risk, Hart and Boulton 1995 and Rhodes 1995).

REFLEXIVITY, COLLABORATION AND POWER IN THE RESEARCH ENCOUNTER

Nevertheless, the imperatives of the policy context have meant that many such insights have been over-looked. Thus both policy and debates are based on tried and tired assumptions, resulting, for example, in surveys that end up showing a supposed link between unsafe sex and the use of alcohol or drugs. Do we really need to do such surveys in every part of the world? As Simon Watney has pointed out:

> . . . most of the social science research ostensibly concerned with gay men and HIV amounts to little more than a kind of academic scenic tour through the worst hit areas of the epidemic.
>
> (Watney 1994: 235)

Likewise, an unproblematised use of terms like 'the gay community', 'denial' or 'relapse' means that one not only misunderstands but also cannot engage with the challenge of AIDS in a praxis sense.

There is a long-standing debate within social research about the extent to which the researcher can and should be an advocate for the researched. In the 1960s Becker (1967) and Gouldner (1968) took opposing positions via articles titled, in turn, 'Whose side are we on?' and 'The sociologist as partisan'. Gouldner was concerned with the limits put upon the academic discipline of research if the researcher was manifestly seeking to promote the interests of, or write in sympathy with, the researched. Further, such an approach risked romanticising a group of people or privileging the voices of some in the way recently criticised by Atkinson (1996), who urged researchers to subject their own analyses to the rigorous critical scrutiny which they reserve for examining respondents' accounts.

The influence of critical theory and of feminism on research methods, combined with the accumulated experience of anthropologists and the developing critical stance of ethnographers, has led to an emphasis on reflexivity.

Lee (1993) has looked at the extent to which research encroaches on people's lives, and on the life of the researcher, when s/he is concerned with what he calls 'sensitive topics'. He defines a sensitive topic as one that inspires dread or awe, poses a threat, or has broad social implications. One trend within such research has been an increased awareness of the potential collaborative relationships between researched and researcher (Merton 1990).

Cannon (1989), in a study of women being treated for breast cancer, considers issues of involvement, detachment and personal responsibility. She draws on feminist research, including Graham (1984; surveying through stories as a device for overcoming traditional power imbalances), Oakley (1981), Finch (1984) and Cornwell (1984; the recognition that there are public stories told to researchers and private feelings attached to both the story, the telling and the researcher doing the interview). Cannon also examines 'collaborative interviewing and interactive research' (Laslett and Rapoport 1975) and the counter-transference this generates.

Cannon speaks of women expressing what they had got from the opportunity to talk – an opportunity that was not always available elsewhere. She discussed what Oakley (1981: 44) has called the 'transition of friendship' – cups of tea, small gifts, the interchange of personal information, the decision to keep in touch after the research finished.

After all that, researchers might, nevertheless, still be seen as 'half-hearted, and therefore unreliable partisans' who are 'necessarily a disappointment to the person(s) they are studying' (Barnes 1984: 103). Stanley and Wise (1983) have argued that collaborative research does not go far enough because the results are presented by the researcher and not the researched. Once given, we lose control of our story, as blood donors lose control of their blood.

In the narrative generated in the research experience there is that selection, editing and interpretation that reconstructs the told story in the context of the narrative of the researcher (see Rosaline Barbour, Chapter 11). Marshall and O'Keefe (1995) had a person living with AIDS tell his story to medical students and then had the students recount it. The story was changed in ways consistent with the affective world of the students. We have encapsulated here the problem of relying on reflexivity or collaboration as a route to reconciling either the objectification or romanticisation of the research subject. In the natural sciences there is an axiom that looking at a phenomenon changes the phenomenon that you are looking at. The same is happening here. Indeed, returning to Marshall and O'Keefe, we can assume that when they tell us of the changes from the original story in the medical students' accounts these changes are interpreted in a way consistent with the narrative world of Marshall and O'Keefe. I then read the findings and interpretations, change them myself, offer them to my reader and that person changes them . . . and so on.

Researchers studying AIDS also face specific problems in developing collaborative research with the dying. As Ricoeur says about research in the areas of birth and death:

> Now there is nothing in life that serves as a narrative beginning; memory is
> lost in the hazes of childhood. As for my death, it will finally be recounted

only in the stories of those who survive me. I am always moving toward my death, and this prevents me from ever grasping it as a narrative end.

(Ricoeur 1992: 160)

Current theories, as a part of narrative exchange, offer a way out of these dilemmas. Kleinmann's work (1988, 1992), sees one of the central tasks of the doctor as helping the patient develop a narrative out of illness (see also the 'Narrative Study of Lives' book series, for example Josselson and Lieblich 1993). Sometimes that narrative helps locate the subject in what Kleinmann calls the 'local world of suffering'. The same perspective has been applied to the research encounter (Good 1994). Telling one's story to a researcher may also help elucidate the relationship between the individual and the context within which s/he lives and dies (Costain Schou 1993). Such approaches can, however, be problematic. Atkinson has recently argued, in the context of discussing Kleinmann's work, that this risks abandoning the critical stance of not taking anyone's account at face value. They privilege particular accounts and in so doing risk romanticising them (Atkinson 1996).

It might be that if we shift from the individual to the social we can see narratives as contributing to a process of bearing witness. This is the imperative Primo Levi identified in relation to the Holocaust. It was only through bearing witness that the events could be kept real. It was only in continuing affirmation of its reality that it could remain meaningful, and thus bearable (Levi 1989; also Clive Foster, Chapter 9). As researchers, part of our task consists of documenting our contribution to this bearing witness.

While reflexivity can help make explicit the conditions in which we mediate between the private world of our subjects and the public world in which we place our research, our encounters, as researchers, are shaped by constraints of understanding and interpretation as well as by systems of power and influence as we look, Janus-like, in both directions. Just as I have argued that the social context in which blood is given and the prevailing understanding of altruism and reciprocity frame that gift, so too do such concerns frame the research subject's gift to the researcher. This means that our reflexive gaze needs to extend beyond the research interaction to encompass the wider context in which this encounter takes place. A much neglected area is the conditions of exchange which structure academic work at any one time.

CONCLUSION

Methodologically a way forward, and one consistent with the argument developed above, would be to look to the contribution of postmodernism:

> To be effectively and consequentially present in a postmodern habitat sociology must conceive of itself as a participant (perhaps better informed, more systematic, more rule-conscious, yet nevertheless a participant) of this never ending, self reflexive process of reinterpretation and devise its strategy accordingly. In

practice this will mean in all probability, replacing the ambition of the judge of 'common beliefs', healer of prejudices and umpire of truth with those of a clarifier of interpretative rules and facilitators of communication; this will amount to the replacement of the dream of the legislator with the practice of the interpreter.

(Bauman 1992: 204)

The problem here is not the methodological challenge this poses – although that is difficult enough, especially in areas such as the ones we are concerned with here – but the social context of research. Titmuss (1970: 217) was writing within a welfare tradition he identified as incorporating the 'Paretian optimum' – any change is for the better as long as nobody is worse off and at least one person is better off, each in his or her own estimation. Paradoxically, in our age of relative plenty that sounds like a luxurious approach we choose not to afford. It is luxurious because funders want a return for their money; the instrumental is in the ascendant.

It is also luxurious because social research has few certainties. You don't know what research will have an impact before you do it: it's like adding to a pile, a heap of debris. Occasionally something is picked off this mound by wandering prospectors and at times something just seems to find its way onto the pinnacle. If only there was a way of knowing which would emerge from the heap before you do it – but there isn't so you just keep going. It is the 'Aztec' theory of academic production: akin to sacrificing someone every night to ensure the sun comes up the next day. Although they were not sure that this really worked, the stakes were too high to try an experiment one night and not do it. It also kept the priests in work.

If social research is of debatable benefit to those researched it is of immediate benefit to those employed to do it, although those so employed might bemoan the conditions in which they work. The Red Queen tells an out of breath, running Alice in the world 'through the looking glass' that she must go this fast to stay put: 'If you want to get anywhere else you have to go a lot faster.' With an increasing number of researchers, a prevalence of short-term contracts and a paramount concern within higher education for the sorts of output that will lead to further funding via the Research Selectivity Exercise, there is an agenda for researchers that is not concerned solely with the needs of their research subjects. This may have always been the case – Gouldner in the 1960s did suggest that Becker's interest in the underdog and the disadvantaged worked such that he, Becker, received professional advancement. One might surmise that Gouldner's high profile in entering the lists against Becker and colleagues did him no harm either. My intention is not to suggest that all was once good and has now been corrupted by invidious 'knavery', but to underline the importance of considering both motivation and structural features in seeking to scrutinise the context in which the researcher encounters the researched.

In considering the gift of a person's story, offered freely to a researcher, we have complex interpersonal nuances, an institutional context that shapes what are considered appropriate research questions and useful answers, and a social structural domain characterised by a market ideology to consider. Bauman wants what we might call a modest research enterprise. If we pursue this I think we are right to still ask for and receive the gifts of stories like those told me. If, however, we are instrumentally pursuing the interests of utilitarian welfare, we ask for and receive such gifts in bad faith.

REFERENCES

Atkinson, P. (1996) 'Narrative turn or blind alley? Reflections on Narrative and qualitative health research', plenary paper presented at the Third International Interdisciplinary Conference on Qualitative Health Research, University of Bournemouth, 30 October–1 November.

Bailey, C. (1996) 'Ethical issues in multicentre collaborative research on breathlessness in lung cancer', *International Journal of Palliative Nursing*, 2(2): 95–101.

Barbour, R.S. and Kitzinger, J. (eds) (forthcoming) *Developing Focus Group Research*, London: Sage.

Barbour, R.S. and Teijlingen, E. van (1994) *Medical Sociology in Britain*, Durham: British Sociological Association.

Barnes, J.A. (1984) 'Ethical and political compromises in social research', *The Wisconsin Sociologist*, 21: 100–10.

Bauman, Z. (1992) *Intimations of Postmodernism*, London: Routledge.

Becker, H.S. (1967) 'Whose side are we on?' *Social Problems*, 14: 239–47.

Boulton, M. (ed.) (1994) *Challenge and Innovation: Methodological Advances in Social Research on HIV/AIDS*, London: Taylor & Francis.

Cannon, S. (1989) 'Social research in stressful settings: difficulties for the sociologist studying the treatment of breast cancer', *Sociology of Health and Illness*, 11(1): 62–77.

Carr-Hill, R. (1984) 'The political choice of social indicators', *Quantity and Quality*, 18: 173–91.

Cixous H. (1986) 'Sorties', in H. Cixous and C. Clement (eds) *The Newly Born Woman*, Manchester: Manchester University Press.

Clark, D. and Haldane, D. (1990) *Wedlocked?* Oxford: Polity.

Cornwell, J. (1984) *Hard Earned Lives*, London: Tavistock.

Costain Schou, K. (1993) 'Awareness contexts and the construction of dying in the cancer treatment setting: "micro" and "macro" levels in narrative analysis', in D. Clark (ed.) *The Sociology of Death*, Oxford: Blackwell.

Craven, B.M., Stewart, G.T. and Taghavi, M. (1994) 'Amateurs confronting specialists: expenditure on AIDS in England', *Journal of Public Policy*, 13: 305–25.

Derrida, J. (1995) *The Gift of Death*, Chicago: University of Chicago Press.

Doyal, L. and Gough, I. (1991) *A Theory of Human Need*, London: Macmillan.

Fallowfield, L.J., Baum, M. and Maguire, G.P. (1987) 'Do psychological studies upset patients?', *Journal of the Royal Society of Medicine*, 80: 59.

Field, D. and Woodman, D. (1990) *Medical Sociology in Britain*, London: British Sociological Association.

Finch, J. (1984) '"It's great to have someone to talk to": ethics and politics of interviewing women', in C. Bell and H. Roberts (eds) *Social Researching: Politics, Problems, Practice*, London: Routledge & Kegan Paul.

Firth, R. (1967) *Themes in Economic Anthropology*, Association of Social Anthropologists Monographs, No. 6, London.

Fox, N. (1993) *Postmodernism, Sociology and Health*, Buckingham: Open University Press.

—— (1995) 'Postmodern perspectives on care: the vigil and the gift', *Critical Social Policy*, 44(5): 107–25.

Giddens, A. (1992) *The Transformation of Intimacy*, Oxford: Polity.

Good, B. (1994) *Medicine, Rationality and Experience*, Cambridge: Cambridge University Press.

Gouldner, A.W. (1968) 'The sociologist as partisan', *American Sociologist*, 3: 103–16

Graham, H. (1984) 'Surveying through stories', in C. Bell and H. Roberts (eds) *Social Researching: Politics, Problems, Practice*, London: Routledge & Kegan Paul.

Hart, G. and Boulton, M. (1995) 'Sexual behaviour in gay men: towards a sociology of risk', in P. Aggleton, P. Davies and G. Hart (eds) *AIDS: Safety, Sexuality and Risk*, London: Taylor & Francis.

Josselson, R. and Lieblich, A. (1993) *The Narrative Study of Lives*, London: Sage.

Kayal, P.M. (1993) *Bearing Witness*, Boulder, CO: Westview Press.

Kleinmann, A. (1988) *The Illness Narratives: Suffering, Healing and the Human Condition*, New York: Basic Books.

—— (1992) 'Local world of suffering: an interpersonal focus for ethnographies of illness experience', *Qualitative Health Research*, 2(2): 127–34.

Laslett, B. and Rapoport, R. (1975) 'Collaborative interviewing and interactive research', *Journal of Marriage and the Family*, Nov.: 968–77.

LeClair, E.E. and Schneider, H.K. (1968) *Economic Anthropology*, London: Holt, Rinehart & Winston.

Lee, R. (1993) *Doing Research on Sensitive Topics*, London: Sage.

Le Grand, J. (1997) 'Knights, knaves or pawns? Human behaviour and social policy', *Journal of Social Policy*, 26(2): 149–69.

Levi, P. (1989) *The Drowned and the Saved*, New York: Vintage Books.

Marshall, P. and O'Keefe, J. (1995) 'Medical students' first-person narratives of a patient's story of AIDS', *Social Science and Medicine*, 40(1): 67–76.

Mauss, M. (1954) *The Gift*, London: Cohen & West.

Merton, R.K. (1957) *Social Theory and Social Structure*, New York: Free Press.

Merton, V. (1990) 'Community based AIDS research', *Evaluation Review*, 14: 502–13.

Mihill, C. (1991) 'AIDS "guinea pigs" guide may open up medicine', *Guardian*, 10 December.

Moi, T. (1985) *Sexual Textual Politics*, London: Methuen.

Mor, V. (1988) 'The research design of the National Hospice Study', In V. Mor, D.S. Greer and R. Kastenbaum (eds) *The Hospice Experiment*, Baltimore: John Hopkins University Press.

Oakley, A. (1981) 'Interviewing women: a contradiction in terms', in H. Roberts (ed.) *Doing Feminist Research*, London: Routledge & Kegan Paul.

Paradis, L.F., Miller, B., and Runnion, V.M. (1987) 'Volunteer stress and burnout: issues for administrators', *The Hospice Journal*, 3(2/3): 165–83.

Pocock, D. (1975) *Understanding Social Anthropology*, London: Hodder & Stoughton.

Polanyi, K (1968) *Primitive, Archaic and Modern Economics*, New York: Academic Press.

Rawls, J. (1972) *A Theory of Justice*, Oxford: Oxford University Press.

Rhodes, T. (1995) 'Theorising and researching "risk": notes on the social relations of risk in heroin users' lifestyles', in P. Aggleton, P. Davies and G. Hart (eds) *AIDS: Safety, Sexuality and Risk*, London: Taylor & Francis.

Ricoeur, P. (1992) *Oneself as Another*, Chicago: University of Chicago Press.

Sahlins, M. (1974) *Stone Age Economics*, London: Tavistock Publications.

Schwartz, B. (1967) 'The social psychology of the gift', *American Journal of Sociology*, 73(1):1–11.

Small, N. (1988) 'AIDS and social policy', *Critical Social Policy*, 21: 9–29.

—— (1996) 'Critical social research', in N. Lunt and D. Coyle (eds) *Welfare and Policy*, London: Taylor & Francis.

Stanley, L. and Wise, S. (1983) *Breaking Out: Feminist Consciousness and Feminist Research*, London: Routledge & Kegan Paul.

Titmuss, R.M. (1970) *The Gift Relationship*, Oxford: George & Unwin.

Tonnies, F. (1887) *Community and Association* (1957 edn), Michigan: Michigan State University Press.

Watney, S. (1994) 'AIDS and social science', in S. Watney (ed.) *Practices of Freedom*, London: Rivers Oram Press.

Williams, R. (1961) *Culture and Society*, Harmondsworth: Penguin.

Young, L., Bury, M. and Elston, M.A. (1994) 'Prospective work with dying people and their friends: at the boundaries of social exploration?', paper presented at Palliative Care Research Forum, Dublin, 9–10 November.

Chapter 9

Of tales, myth, metaphor and metonym

Clive Foster

INTRODUCTION

In my study into families' reaction to HIV/AIDS and drug use on an Edinburgh estate I have used narrative as both a methodological and an analytical tool. From this perspective narrative appears as an essentially diachronic device, valorising the past and providing idioms against which the helplessness of the present may be reflected and managed. It becomes a vocabulary devised to cope with suffering and deprivation and a stratagem by which individuals reflect the beliefs and hopes of their world. It is, in one form, a Barthesian discourse.

Anthropology differentiates several approaches to the notion of myth, from Malinowski's interpretation as a kind of social charter to be understood within its present-day context, to the complex Lévi-Straussian analysis of myth as an elaborate discourse on social relations. Drawing from both these paradigms I situate myth within a time span delineated by the lives of those who took heroin and who were eventually to die of AIDS; the mythic past for those I studied is short. In order to explain how narratives were constructed, it is necessary to define the terms 'metonym' and 'metaphor'. The first I define as the substitution of the name of an attribute or adjunct for that of the entity itself. Thus, the word 'turf' recalls the sport of horse racing, or 'the ring' that of boxing, 'Westminster' the processes of government and 'the crown' those of royalty. 'Metaphor' I take to mean the application of a name or descriptive expression to that which it is not literally applicable. Typical of this practice would be the way in which medical processes may be comprehended in terms of a battle: *invasive* therapy, *attacking* the virus, or how tales of its past glories represent Scottish nationhood. However, within this definition it is the elements which metaphor discards that form the basis of my argument.

It is my intention to show how the processes of narrative, by placing the inchoate within existing frameworks of meaning, help those whose lives have become disorientated by drug use and HIV/AIDS. I examine the creation of contemporary myth from selective metaphor, and demonstrate the place of narrative in the strengthening of cultural norms and individual identity. Exploring this process further, I show how the significance of one particular myth enabled it to gain metonymic status. Finally, by situating ethnography within these paradigms, I examine the figurative and selective construction of metaphor, and show how these elements are told and retold in narrative form until they become the myths by which the individual may reconstruct reality within indigenous strategies.

A REASON FOR TELLING TALES

I have just spent half the morning looking for Nita to take her down to the hospital for her regular HIV check. I finally run her to ground in the car park at the back of the shopping centre. She and Len, her partner, and another couple are sitting with their backs against a wall sunning themselves. I sit down with them and we are joined by several others. The conversation eventually gets round to an overdose (OD) that had happened the previous week and this seemed to start off reminiscences of other similar incidents.

Of such situations is the telling of tales begun.

One of the ways in which drug users attempted to make sense of their lives was in the tales that they told of themselves and others. Tales which related to their values, their history, their heroes and villains, and their way of doing things. The analysis of these tales goes beyond an idiographic perspective and attempts to contextualise the narratives within their structural and historical settings.

Denzin suggests that tales tend to focus on key issues of people's lives and that, to interpret them, the researcher needs to become an informed reader of the tales themselves and of the biographies of the people to whom they refer. As well as the biographical details, it is necessary to have knowledge of the historical and cultural setting, not only of the tale itself, but also of the person telling the tale (Denzin 1989: 35–47). I would go further, and suggest that what we may have here is a 'chicken and egg' situation. While Denzin is right and that it is essential to be aware of the biographical, historical and cultural details of the tale and its teller, it is often from the very tales themselves that many of these details can be gathered.

Events had overtaken people in this community to the extent that they were often unable to express coherently their feelings and their awareness of reality. This resulted in a Durkheimian sense of anomie brought about by the realisation that many would soon die of AIDS. In an effort to deal with this they appeared to be creating an alternative vehicle, a new vocabulary with which they endeavour to cope with the crises of illegal drug use and AIDS. As Geertz suggests, they attempt to cope with suffering 'by placing it in a meaningful context, providing a mode of action through which it can be expressed, and, being expressed, understood, and being understood, endured' (Geertz 1973: 105).

This aspect of making meaningful the incoherent is also taken up by Myerhoff, where, quoting Lévi-Strauss as well as Geertz, she puts forward the notion that it is in the creation of meaningful categories that the individual can come to comprehend otherwise confused and subjective experiences. She suggests that a known, shared and intelligible set of events described in terms of a set of collective representations may relocate the person into a familiar, coherent and orderly world (Myerhoff 1982: 234). True, the drug user may not have recourse to the skills of a Lévi-Straussian shaman; nevertheless, the creation of narrative can – and does – inform a process of establishing a coherent world out of chaos.

Hannerz attempts to explain the male street-corner gatherings of a downtown Washington ghetto and suggests that this street-corner sociability has, at its base, moral and intellectual concerns. To compensate for the absence of fathers, and hence role models for young boys, a ghetto-specific male reality had to be worked out. He points out that the never-ending series of narratives were attempts at resolving these conflicts and ways of providing an awareness of self. They also provided the individual with a social anchor from which he could go on to build his identity within the accepted cultural norm. The tales delineated what experiences they had in common and enabled them to arrive at a consensus of normality. Each single recollection represented an individual's claim to a part of the collective identity and the telling of it replenished that identity as each new tale passed through a screen of cultural verification by which the events were assessed and interpreted (Hannerz 1969: 105–17).

Hannerz considers these tales as a form of myth making. The myths are not sacred neither do they deal with primeval time nor with men who are Gods. The time is yesterday and the protagonists are unemployed and in trouble with the law. The myths do, however, represent a reality, and through them the individuals are able to reflect on the conditions in which are grounded the beliefs and hopes of their world (Hannerz 1969: 115).

If myths are the ways by which we try to make sense of our world, then the tales I heard were indeed myths, for like Hannerz's ghetto, they seemed to be ways of resolving the moral and intellectual issues of this particular community. As Hannerz (1969: 116) suggested, myth is seen as the charter for social action, strengthening the individual's belief in cultural norms and identity within them.

In particular, the harm reduction policies brought about in response to the spread of AIDS by needle sharing resulted in a massive social change within the community. Heroin, and the concomitant structural elements on which its culture was based, had virtually passed into history, and with it the narratives of its devotees into mythic past beyond verification – a process not dissimilar from Barthes's notion of myth as a discourse that, at one level can transform historical events into nature, thus placing them into the eternal and sacred where they are no longer available to be challenged (Barthes 1972: 129).

In order to understand this process of storytelling or myth making, and the complex ways it was used by the community, I want first to examine a particular narrative of a mutilated body and explore the processes whereby it came to gain currency and significance to the extent that the place where it occurred was to attain the status of metonym. Within this story there is a convergence of text, boundary and violence which reflects the hegemony of the drug dealer, a cognitive awareness of social control, and the means of establishing the male identity. It is a tale of the appropriation of a conceptual boundary whereby, for those who transgressed the dealer's authority, there was always the possibility that this didactic, somatic text may also come to be writ large on their own bodies. It is a tale *pour encourager les autres*.

However, it is first necessary to examine the processes whereby the appropriation of a 'topologised space', in Thornton's (1980) terms, may lend authority to myth and empowerment to its narrator. Bruner and Gorfain suggest that the process of attaching a mutable story to an immutable place is a device to fix meaning and lend stability to authority and interpretation. Furthermore, they put forward the notion that as well as these prominent stories helping to constitute and reshape society, they also define and empower the storyteller (Bruner and Gorfain 1984: 57–84). For Bruner and Gorfain, no story is 'a story' nor 'the story', but a dialogic process of historically situated particular tellings. Narration is a *process*, not an entity; it includes voice, point of view and the positioning of a narrative within a discourse. A story becomes a processual text as each person engages in the 'dialogic narration, adding, interpreting and subtracting according to their own societal perspective, using the tale for their own ends' (Bruner and Gorfain 1984: 57). These are stories which exist in, and help to create, their social worlds; furthermore they are situated in named places whose permanence becomes the anchor for the elusiveness of their tales.

TALES AT THE BOUNDARY

Along the northern edge of this Scottish housing estate where I conducted most of my research is the coastal road. Although a bus route, it is not one of the major access points for those living there and it is fairly uncommon to see people using it on foot. On the other side of this road is a large expanse of green leading to a promenade and then down to the beach. When the estate was built in the late 1960s, it was considered a 'utopian dream' when compared to the inner city slums from which most of the new residents were to come. This stretch of green field, the golf course adjacent and the beach itself were seen by the town planners as an idealised amenity, and one that would greatly enhance the lives of those living on this 'dream' estate. Their calculations were wrong, for within some ten years much of the estate had become a ghetto.

The stretch of green is a strange piece of land for, despite its close proximity to the estate, I have rarely seen people on it. This is even more curious when one considers the high proportion of families with young children who live nearby. The beach itself is rather stony even at low tide and it is little used. Occasionally some older couples drive down for a walk along the prom and, at lunchtime, there might be a few company reps who have come down for some peace and quiet while they make up the morning's sales list. At times, there was also an anthropologist writing up some field-notes.

Thornton suggests that

Boundaries are literally imaginary; they consist of images of continuity and closure applied to a continuous reality. Boundaries are communicated in 'practical' acts (e.g. scientific survey, of the Australian aboriginal 'walkabout', or the Masay ceremony). Once constituted they may be related to human individuals or groups in many ways.

(Thornton 1980: 11)

Seen from this perspective, the 'constituted imagery' of the beach as boundary, communicated in the political acts not only of a local authority concept of a utopia, but also of a community's own notions of the limits of acceptable behaviour, becomes a vehicle in the construction of identity. Thornton (1980: 16) points out that Van Gennep's achievement was to show that territory was a cultural phenomenon, in that he recognised that boundaries were not 'natural', but collectively conceived and ritually established. Thus

Territory is the symbolic differentiation of space (topologisation) and the appropriation of this topologised space into a structure of meaning by attributing shared and public values to places, directions, and boundaries such that it may be graphically, cognitively, or ritually represented as a coherent and enduring image.

(Thornton 1980: 19)

Given the common usage of 'the beach' in my ethnography – in narrative if not always in fact – it would appear that, for them, it had indeed become a 'ritualised space' which was cognitively represented in the narrative surrounding it. Despite its apparent lack of use, the 'beach' had become a significant landmark to some of those I studied and it played an important role in 'constituting and reshaping' their society, as well as lending authority to its tales and empowering the storyteller. It was a place whose tales, like Bruner's processual texts, were used by the narrators for their own ends and to enhance their own authority, while at the same time reshaping and constituting the society in which they lived.

Yet these texts are not conscious processes, for there is a reluctance of cultures to treat their indigenous events as signifying anything beyond themselves. However, if they are just events, why then are they told, retold and embroidered, until in some cases they attain a metonymic value whereby a word or phrase becomes sufficient to recall the symbolic inferences of their telling?

THE MUTILATED BODY

There had been a particularly horrendous murder some years previously when a young woman's body had been found badly mutilated on 'the beach' and this formed the subject of a narrative that was told and retold complete with gory detail. According to the tale, the girl had been 'carrying the cutty' (it was quite common for a dealer to use young women to carry and look after a supply of heroin as, if stopped by the police, they were less likely to be searched) for one of the big dealers and had been dipping her fingers into the stash (the supply of heroin) to the tune of several thousand pounds worth of smack. Quite early into fieldwork, I had heard several references to the 'beach' as being the place where those who transgressed the boundaries of acceptable behaviour would be taken to be shown the error of their ways.

There was obviously a reason why this particular narrative had become a 'processual text' to be recalled and interpreted as though part of some hermeneutic circle, taken down from the shelf once again, dusted a little, and retold. I have already suggested the significance of the beach as a place of retribution. I now put forward the notion that the mutilated body has become a means of reinforcing and sustaining that idea.

Feldman, referring to stories of the atrocities of a loyalist murder gang operating in Belfast in the mid-seventies, suggests that the 'violent location of political codes in a somatic space . . . is in effect a statement about social space', and that violent incidents and the particular persons involved 'function as condensed symbols of historical possibility'. Thus, the acts and figures mark an outer limit to the performative logic of paramilitary violence (Feldman 1991: 59).

The body on the beach narrative reflects a similar discourse in the violation of somatic space. In Bruner and Gorfain's terms, the immutability of the place of its mutilation – the beach – now attains metonymic status representing the violence of the drug culture and the limits of its performance, for to be threatened with 'the beach' does indeed recall the consequences of transgressing these limits. The veracity of the narrative is immaterial, for the more harrowing the detail, the more the somatic image is abstracted from the self to become a political token: a token to be read and acknowledged by others who they may learn and obey.

This aspect of the legitimating of violence is also taken up by Foucault, when, in explaining a public execution with all its attendant horrors, he suggests:

> Its aim is not so much to re-establish a balance as to bring into play, as its extreme point, the dissymmetry between the subject who has dared to violate the law and the all powerful sovereign who displays his strength.
>
> (Foucault 1979: 49)

For the sovereign, we may read 'dealer'. The horrors attributed to the killing on the beach and their subsequent embellishment in narrative serve to re-establish the power of the dealers and the 'dissymmetry' between them and the user. Foucault goes on to point out that

> the atrocity of a crime was also the violence flung at the sovereign; it was that which would move him to make a reply whose function was to go further than this atrocity, to master it, to overcome it by an *excess that annulled it*.
>
> (Foucault 1979:56; my emphasis)

There are two levels of explanation here: the notion of 'annulling' the crime by violence and atrocity – the mutilation of the body – and the concept of justifying that violence. The dealer was the 'anti-hero', his power was acknowledged and legitimated, and, as such, it must be seen to be upheld. Within a violent community where disputes could be, and were, resolved with the knife or a beating, the notion of excess by those with 'sovereign' power would be maintained as a process of defining community in their terms. While the actual crime may be deprecated, by using it at the level of narrative it performed its didactic purpose. Thus, the narrative of a past violent excess, fed by the tales of other acts of retribution attributed to the anti-hero, is passed into myth, and, now beyond verification, serves to legitimate this sovereign violence.

> *Olive, the mother of one of the drug users, and I were combing the estate trying to locate her son who she knew was ill but who, for various reasons, had 'gone to ground'. At one point we were witness to an altercation directly across the street from us where Bill, a 'small-time' dealer was punching and kicking another man quite violently. Eventually the man hobbled away with Bill yelling at him that he would be round the following day for his money.*
>
> *This done, Bill then crossed the street towards us. His manner to both Olive and myself was very friendly and respectful, and, on being asked by Olive what the fight was about, he was off-hand and dismissive, as though the incident was of little consequence and merely an adjunct to his business. There seemed to be an assumption on his part that as a dealer he had the right to 'uphold his sovereign power', in Foucault's terms, and that this right should be, if not actually condoned, then at least recognised. Olive went on to ask Bill if he knew anything of her son's whereabouts. He did, and was most helpful and considerate in then escorting us to the block of flats where her son was now living.*

I detail this incident because it seems to show quite clearly the attitudes and assumptions of the dealer hegemony and the presumptuous manner in which violence is meted out. It is, as Fernandez suggests, 'a "revelatory incident" . . . those especially charged moments in human relationships which are pregnant with meaning' (Fernandez 1986: xi). Fernandez points out that these incidents often contain colloquialisms, expressed in a Bernsteinian restricted code, which consist of evocative figurative expressions of images and tropes. They are not so frequent in the flow of everyday life as to be easily noted by a tourist, and in any event the awareness of them and their significance is the fruit of participation over the long term (Fernandez 1986: xii).

The significance, however, of the 'revelatory text' inhering in this violent incident is in the manner in which it is quickly discarded by the perpetrator. Fernandez points out that this long-term participation enables us to give these moments of a 'sudden constellation of significances' an adequate reading. My reading here is that the off-hand manner in which the violence took place, amplified and exaggerated by the sharp contrast of Bill's subsequent respectful behaviour towards Olive and myself, reflect only too clearly the dealer's sense of 'sovereign power'.

I have suggested that the retelling of the stories of the mutilated body is a significant element in the narratives surrounding the notion of the beach as a didactic text. There is, however, another element in this hermeneutic circle, for, while each gory version upholds dealer authority, it is also an attempt to justify violence within the community *per se*, and to valorise the narrator's position as one who is able to operate successfully in this environment. There is an iconicity surrounding this somatic discourse that becomes an essential element in community identity. Reference to it, even in metonym, is a means of acknowledging the dangers of participating in the drug culture. It is a way of saying, 'you gotta be tough to make it round here', for it is an element in the processes of sustaining the macho image.

> *It is about eleven thirty in the morning and the centre for drug users, most of whom are HIV+, has been open for an hour or so. The usual routine is for the users to drift in as soon as the place opens. They are given a cup of coffee and sit around waiting to score. At this stage some of them are quite tense and strung out, the atmosphere is subdued and there is little talking, apart from the occasional greeting as they huddle round the small table in the centre of the room sipping their drink and cadging the odd cigarette. Eventually, somebody will arrive who has a supply of 'rugby balls', 'Up-Johns', 'DF's', 'meth', or whatever happens to be available that morning, and they will go outside to do some trading. More coffee is made and the pills are swigged down. The tension relaxes and the gossip of the day begins.*

Schwartzman suggests that storytelling is much more than a pastime. Stories shape and sustain the image of the organisation and the roles within it and furthermore it is a form that individuals use to interpret each other and their experiences (Schwartzman 1984: 81–91). Although her studies were of the staff in a community mental health centre, it would seem that her observations are pertinent to the situation here. This too is an organisation which meets daily and has, for the most part, a regular clientele, to the extent that one of its major criticisms was that it operated virtually a closed shop and was little more than a 'gang hut' for the exclusive use of a few junkies.

Gossip and storytelling are an integral part of the centre's role and, as Schwartzman (1984: 87) goes on to suggest, provide the individual with a means of interpreting, constructing and reconstructing events, discovering meaning in what they are doing and, most importantly, creating a way for individuals to legitimise their actions to each other. This getting together to engage in a sort of collective storytelling is a way for the users to cope with the chaotic lifestyle brought about by their drugs, and the underlying fears of their HIV/AIDS status.

The previous week some of the people from the centre had been taken to a local sports complex for the afternoon and later that morning there was to be a group meeting to discuss some trouble that had occurred and which resulted in the centre being banned from further visits. The conversation became quite heated at one point over the issue of what would constitute suitable retribution for those whose actions led to others being denied access to these various facilities. Two of the men were very much for them being, 'taken down to the beach and given a "doing"', while one of the women put forward a very strong argument that much of the unacceptable behaviour is the result of drugs and the individuals concerned could hardly be held responsible for their actions. She recalled an incident concerning one of the people she was arguing with and where, in this instance:

> You were so full of bloody speed that you wrecked the soddin' place. The way you're going on it's you we should be taking down to the fucking beach, you're bloody mad, that's your trouble.

The talk changed from collective storytelling and got rather too personal. It wouldn't have been the first time that this sort of situation developed into a fight and, since it was not beyond the bounds of possibility for the odd knife to be tucked away somewhere, it was time for the staff to step in before things got too far. Another round of coffee was served, and with a considerable degree of skilful manipulation on the part of one of the staff, plus calls of encouragement from some of the users, calm was restored.

Tales about the 'beach' were obviously important to those sitting around the table for, despite a risk of further aggression, they held on to the subject even after calm had been restored. A story was told of a small-time dealer who had set up his customers to be mugged as they left the empty house that was being used for dealing and so get back the heroin he had just sold them. The tale goes on to tell how he was eventually taken down to the 'beach' to effect retribution. Descriptions of the process of his being 'dealt with' varied from having his legs broken with an iron bar to just a general beating up. Like Bruner and Gorfain's dialogic narration of historically situated particular tellings (Bruner and Gorfain 1984: 57), each person was engaged in the process of adding, interpreting or subtracting from the original version according to his or her own perspective.

Some of the men, for instance, used the tale as a base from which to launch into narratives or their own experiences of the days of heroin dealing. Stories were told of flights to Amsterdam and of the techniques of passing heroin through customs. Others recounted their experiences of the 'big dealers' and how they obtained their 'stash' direct rather than lower down the hierarchy of drug supply. Not all the stories retained the drug theme and at one point the experiences were related of the athletic prowess of two of the men at an outward-bound course the centre had visited the previous summer. Yet the themes were the same, each version becoming a manifestation of the macho image that was no longer viable now that the skills of dealing were replaced by the whining and sometimes aggressive negotiations with medics in an effort to obtain an increase in prescribed drugs.

The women's place in these narratives appeared at first to be that of cheer leader, for in this setting they seemed to have no tales of their own. Their stories reinforced those of 'their man', helping him to retain his image and reflecting their own identity in his macho past. They too claimed their place among the anti-heroes of the days of heroin. Yet outside this narrative domain they seemed

to perform a more positive function. It was the women who became the controlling element in this dialogic process for it was they who called for constraint
when accusing the narrator of 'being full of bloody speed', and it is they who
took the lead in calming down the potentially violent situation. This perspective
was also reflected in the other tales they told in the more domestic setting, tales
which reflected the realities of their lives as mothers and home-makers.

Repeated references were made to the 'beach' and to examples not only of its
past use and the murder of the young woman, but of where the transgression of
the social code deemed it to have been an appropriate response. Interestingly,
there appeared to be more of these tales than of actual incidents, and I was left
with an impression that it is the beach itself that is the significant entity for these
people. It is indeed a metonym being used as an immutable place, fixing
meaning and adding authority to the tellers of other narratives that now
surround it.

What also appears to be happening in this process of communal storytelling is
a reshaping and reinforcing of the role of the 'beach' in the collective identity.
The extent to which it is actually used is probably of little importance, and
indeed I have very few reports in my field-notes of specific violent incidents
taking place on the beach, for most of them have occurred in somebody's flat or
stairway. What I do have are quite a few recordings of the 'beach' being used as
a threat in the context of unacceptable behaviour or as a mark of what others
deem as an appropriate response. It is an indicator of what is, or is not, acceptable to the community and its tales constitute and reshape the role that it serves.
It would seem that in the telling and retelling of 'beach' narratives, its specific
place as a construct of the margins of societal behaviour is being reinforced.
This construct is important; it must be maintained in order that the disruptive
behaviour brought about by a culture of illegal drug use is kept within some
acceptable bounds. The beach is a marginal zone, defining both physical and
symbolic boundaries.

Later that year there were several particularly violent incidents that were
eventually laid at the door of one of the more chaotic and aggressive individuals
in the community. I heard several references to the fact that he was going 'over
the top' and that eventually somebody would have him taken down to the
'beach'. In fact he was dealt with in an empty flat and was to spend some time in
intensive care at the local hospital. The beach, however, had served its purpose:
it had defined the margins of behaviour and its physical situation had lent
authority and justification to an act of retribution.

MANAGING AND HARNESSING POWERLESSNESS

My examination of these tales so far has been about the ways they are used to
voice the social and ideological positions of the narrators, and their role in maintaining and reaffirming the society from which they came. As well as situating
narrative as myth, at least in Hannerz's and Barthes's terms, and showing how

Bruner and Gorfain's notion of the immutability of space enabled one specific story to attain metonymic status, I now contend that as a construct of meaning and action these narratives may equally well be construed as metaphor; indeed, a metaphoric form which ultimately informs contemporary myth.

Fernandez (1968: 8) defines metaphor as a strategy for dealing with an inchoate situation. By expressing the lived reality of drugs, AIDS, and deprivation in terms of a metaphoric narrative, the individual can distance him/herself from this reality. Hence, a tale of the incompetence of the drug squad becomes a metaphor within which the powerlessness of the individual may be dealt with. As Fernandez (1968: 7) states, these metaphoric assertions make manageable objects of the self or of others, and facilitate performance. It becomes easier to accept the power of others through metaphor since, in so doing, the person is not denying the lived reality of the self.

These assertions make the self and others manageable at an individual level, and there is also a sense in which this metaphoric form of non-figurative description comes to attain its own ontological status. It is as though the tales themselves, be they related to values, history, heroes, villains, or merely the way-of-doing-things, become their own truth and, in so doing, serve some overarching purpose.

Parsinnen, in examining Malinowski's ethnography, suggests that his use of metaphor

> is not surprising, for it effectively frees him to concentrate on the distinctive aesthetic properties of his formulation, rather than the uncapturable qualities of his private experience. The result is a creation accessible to the reader because it is complete, concrete and immediately susceptible to comparison and judgement. One might in fact argue that metaphor lies closer to the 'truth' of individual experience than non-figurative description, since it bears the individuating mark of the experiencing self.
>
> (Parsinnen 1982: 215)

In using metaphor we may not translate it back into this 'non-figurative' reality, and interpretation then takes place only at this metaphoric level. If this is so, then the 'overarching purpose' may well be that the unwanted elements of reality can be ignored. As Lakoff and Johnson argue:

> . . . the very systemacity that allows us to comprehend one aspect of a concept in terms of another (e.g. comprehending an aspect of arguing in terms of battle) *will necessarily hide other aspects of the concept.*
>
> (Lakoff and Johnson 1980: 10; emphasis mine)

Thus, by not retranslating the metaphorical discourse back into its non-figurative description, the indigenous processes of denial, common to communities under considerable trauma and distress, are maintained. Given the positive aspects of this process in terms of restructuring identity in the face of AIDS, these elements of narrative play an important role.

I have promised to take Nita some clothes for her youngster that I have been given by a local church charity and am hoping that her partner, Len, is not too stoned this time as I want to get him to tell me about the days of heroin dealing and how he, and others, were able to bring the heroin in from the continent. There is no answer to my knock at the door, a not unusual situation which could mean anything from their being too 'gouched' to be bothered to open it, to the fact that they've forgotten I was coming.

Eventually I find them at another flat and when I arrive I am introduced to the others as the bloke that's writing the book about AIDS. There's a polite enquiry as to how the book is going and I mumble something about my still talking to people and how they are giving me information. A tall emaciated looking man asks if anybody's told me the one about the steel door.

This tale takes place in the older dock-lands part of the city. It seems that in an effort to prevent the police raiding a flat that was used as a distribution point and storage facility for one of the bigger dealers, the front door had been lined with steel and a reinforced architrave fitted (a common enough procedure in those days). When the police did eventually raid the property, and after spending some considerable time and effort trying to break the door down with their sledge-hammers, they found that the door opened outwards instead. The telling of this particular narrative raises a fair amount of humour for it is obviously well known by those present. It is also the prompt for other tales of the same genre like the time they raided a house to find the owner busy papering the living-room. The 'stash' of heroin had been emptied into the bucket of paste and, despite a thorough search – for the police were convinced there were drugs in the house – they didn't think to look in the paste bucket. This tale sets everybody wondering if the room has been redecorated by now or if it would be worth having a lick at the old wallpaper.

These particular tales of reinforced doors and walls laced with heroin may be seen as boundary markers. They are symbols of the drug using community's defence against outsiders, in this case the police. The following narratives, also about the police, concern responses to the invasion of the self with the injecting needle becoming a symbol of this defence. There is also the story of the community's ultimate victory over authority.

In the first instance there are other tales about 'junkies' and how they would leave their used works in their pockets in the hope that the police officers searching them would get a needle-stick injury and become infected with HIV. This particular tale was quite common and I heard different versions of the story repeated several times. Towards the end of fieldwork I had arranged an interview with the then head of the drug squad, and was told that there had been no incidents of this kind reported by his officers. There had been situations in the cells where infected prisoners had attempted to contaminate the police. On one occasion a man had scratched an officer's face and then spat on him and there was also an incident where excreta had been thrown in an officer's eyes. There were, however, no cases of infection.

Finally, of course, there has to be a tale about the police that caps all the rest and of which everybody makes sure the anthropologist is aware. This one concerns a female dealer who sets up a kinky sex session for some of the drugs squad and, unbeknown to them, has the whole thing videoed. I was never told exactly who this person was, although there did seem to be a pattern of accusations being made against individuals who, despite being known to be successful dealers, never seem to be raided. I am certainly in no position to sanction the truth of this tale, neither do I think its veracity or otherwise is all that important. Its significance lies in the role that it plays as yet another metaphor enabling the narrator to create a distance between self and threatening other and thus deny the implications of a non-figurative reality.

What is being brought into play here is the way that metaphor can hide certain aspects of reality; aspects which, were they not removed, would deny the individual this ability to reconstruct identity. These stories of one-upmanship conveniently forget the fear and panic as the fourteen-pound sledge-hammer crashes into the front door and the drug squad rush through the flat, bursting into each room and tearing it apart in their efforts to find the stash of heroin before it is disposed of. They also forget the aggression and violence, the prison sentences, the awful invasion of self and the final humiliation and reduction of that self into a prison number. It is the good times the metaphor remembers, the heroic times, the times when 'we won and they lost'. These metaphors serve a very positive function, for it is this selectivity of their construction that serves to inform the idioms from which the present is reflected and managed, and suffering and deprivation endured.

It would seem that in the creation and telling these stories myth and metaphor are conflated. Indeed, I would argue that this selective construction of the figurative form is one of the building blocks of the contemporary myth, now beyond verification and thus relieving all necessity for the non-figurative reality to be confronted.

A similar construction of narrative takes place in relation to other agencies whose activities impinge on the lives of people in this community. Here, instead of the often physical and aggressive relationships with the police, it is the capacity of agency authority to create feelings of powerlessness that must be dealt with.

Thornton suggests that claims to agency provision, if validated and legitimated, give power to those who make them since the client/patient has, without access to prerequisite knowledge, difficulty in constructing viable counter discourses which permit effective challenge (1989: 150). Under these circumstances other less convincing dialogues are brought into play and the recipient resorts to a condemning narrative which berates those whose offers of support are considered, at least for that moment, inappropriate. The relative powerlessness of the individual leads to feelings of passivity in the face of authority. This passivity is also reflected in Foucault's notion of the 'normalisation' of power, where he points out that:

> The judges of normality are present everywhere. We are in the society of the teacher judge, the doctor judge, the social worker judge: it is on them that the

universal reign of the normative is based; and each individual, wherever he may find himself, subjects his body, his gestures, his behaviour, his attitudes, his achievements. This carceral network, in its compact or disseminated forms, with its systems of insertion, distribution, surveillance, observation. has been the greatest support, in modern society, in the normalising of power.

(Foucault 1979: 304)

Given a community where, as I suggest, there is a limited access to discourses of effective challenge, then the panoptic functioning of agencies such as police, social work and the medical profession, in adopting this 'normalising' stance, leaves those they serve an essentially passive role. Yet this role is not wholly accepted, for despite the lack of a counter-discourse on the agency's terms, other alternative discourses are created in the form of narrative.

For instance, there is an undertow of guilt within the community which requires a response. There is the guilt of parents who watched their teenage sons and daughters descend into a world of heroin, some to die of an overdose, and, now that the allotted span of infection has been reached, others to die of AIDS. There is the guilt too of the drug users, now somewhat more 'rational' in their thinking because of harm reduction, as they watch the deaths of their contemporaries yet are unable to give up their drug habit. To make sense of these feelings other past experiences are translated into selectively constructed metaphors, their figurative form invoked as these tales too are told and retold until they pass into the mythic world beyond.

In this instance the stories concern the deeds of the 'Mr Bigs' of the drug world: the major heroin dealers. Stories are recalled of the ready availability of heroin, names are named or implied and specific incidents are defined and situated as these anti-heroes of the past are valorised. Forgotten now are the violence and the beatings, the mornings 'strung out' because there isn't a hit to kick-start the day, the shakes and the fevers as yet another attempt is made to dry out. Forgotten too, for the moment, is the anguish of parents combing the estate for their 'wains' yet again, lest they be the next to OD.

One such tale tells of the house across the street where BMWs, Range-Rovers and powerful motorbikes arrive and depart in the small hours, and how the drug squad also arrive and catch no one despite a whole fleet of police cars in attendance. The theme running through these stories implies a negation of guilt, for if the heroin was that close to us (just across the street) and the dealers that powerful (symbolised by the power of the vehicles used) how could we possibly have prevailed against this onslaught of heroin, when even the police have failed?

Yet the guilt still remains, for today the plethora of pills available through harm reduction policies has, if anything, exacerbated the problem. True, there is a reduction in the stealing and the violence, but individuals are still dependent on drugs and many still die of overdoses. The difficulty is that today there is no illegal drug dealer, at least not in the accepted sense of the big heroin dealers of the past, and certainly not one whose actions are horrendous enough to be able to shoulder all this blame. It would seem that a curious transference has taken place and that these harm reduction policies have now cast the GPs in the role of dealer, albeit a legal one, and along with their role of providing the pills has come that of assuaging the community's guilt.

So too must this new dealer assume this burden, as tales are told of the GP who deliberately arrived too late to prevent the fatal OD, or the doctor who over-prescribed and took a cut, or the one who will increase your prescription if you grass on who is 'selling on' their pills. I was discussing these and other varia-tions on stories about the 'horrendous' behaviour of the GPs with a group of drug users and expressed my scepticism. At one point one of the women present suggested that perhaps she should make up a story of her own and see if it 'did the rounds'. It did, and three days later I was retold this same tale by the mother of one of the users who was somewhat at odds with her GP over the treatment received by her daughter.

CONCLUSION

My intention has been to show how narrative enables the community to meet specific needs and thus inform a process of establishing a coherent world out of the chaos of multi-deprivation, illegal drug use and HIV/AIDS. As Hannerz reveals of his 'ghetto-man', 'he gets together with his peers in a cultural process where their shared problems are made the basis of shared understandings' (Hannerz 1969: 117). So, too, the drug users get together and engage in this cultural process as they examine and attempt to make sense of the shared prob-lems of their lives, creating and re-creating their myths and in so doing attempt to survive.

I began this chapter by examining the work of Hannerz, Bruner and Gorfain, Denzin, Thornton and others in order to establish the notion that storytelling and gossip are meaningful activities which enable people to constitute, reshape and strengthen cultural norms, establish and reaffirm identity, and 'make sense' of each other. I examined a specific story in some detail to show how, through the linking of myth with immutability of place, it attained metonymic status representing the boundaries of societal tolerance and the hegemony of dealer authority. I then contextualised this narrative by situating it against others in the same genre that were told one particular morning in the local drugs 'drop in' centre.

However, these contemporary myths must have a basis upon which they are constructed. I contend that the realities of the past are translated into figurative descriptions which, in eliminating unwanted elements, become part of the indigenous system of reconstructing of self and community. They become narratives told and retold in a dialogic process until their metaphoric form passes into myth and frames the new reality upon which this reconstructed life is predicated.

REFERENCES

Barthes, R. (1972) *Mythologies*, New York: Hill & Wang.

Bruner, E.M. and Gorfain, P. (1984) 'Dialogic narration and the paradoxes of Masada', in E.M. Bruner (ed.) *Text, Play, and Story: The Construction and Reconstruction of Self and Society*, Washington, DC: American Ethnological Society.

Denzin, K. (1989) *Interpretive Interactionism*, London: Sage.

Feldman, A. (1991) *Formations of Violence*, Chicago: University of Chicago Press.

Fernandez, J. (1986) *Persuasions and Performances: The Play of Tropes in Culture*. Bloomington: Indiana University Press.

Foucault, M. (1979) *Discipline and Punish: The Birth of the Prison*, Harmondsworth: Penguin.

Geertz, C. (1973) 'Religion as a cultural system', in C. Geertz *The Interpretation of Cultures*, New York: Basic Books.

Hannerz, U. (1969) *Soulside: Inquiries into Ghetto Culture and Community*, New York and London: Columbia University Press.

Lakoff, G. and Johnson, M. (1980) *Metaphors We Live By*, Chicago: University of Chicago Press.

Myerhoff, B. (1982) 'Life history among the elderly: performance, visibility, and re-membering', in B. Myerhoff and J. Ruby (eds) *A Crack in the Mirror: Reflexive Perspectives in Anthropology*, Philadelphia: University of Philadelphia Press.

Parsinnen, C. (1982) 'Social explorers and social scientists: the dark continent of Victorian ethnography', in B. Myerhoff and J. Ruby (eds) *A Crack in the Mirror: Reflexive Perspectives in Anthropology*, Philadelphia: University of Philadelphia Press.

Schwartzman, H. (1984) 'Stories at work: play in an organisational context', in E.M. Bruner (ed.) *Text, Play, and Story: The Construction and Reconstruction of Self and Society*, Washington, DC: American Ethnological Society.

Thornton, R. (1980) *Space, Time and Culture among the Iraqw of Tanzania*, New York: Academic Press.

Chapter 10

On networks and narratives
Research and the construction of chaotic drug user lifestyles

Guro Huby

INTRODUCTION

This chapter concerns social scientists' part in the construction of the social settings and phenomena which we then proceed to make into objects for our studies. I draw on material from an action-research project concerned with co-ordination of service provision for people with HIV/AIDS in Lothian. HIV infection in Lothian has come to be associated with drug use and deviant drug user culture and lifestyles. I examine in detail encounters between researchers and respondents in various situations and contexts where identities are traded and boundaries between 'us' and 'them' are negotiated. My aim is to explore ways in which research in this particular setting often contributed to constructing drug user lifestyles as 'chaotic'. With Tsing (1994), I suggest 'marginality' as an analytic position from which to explore boundaries between 'researcher' and 'researched' and the social consequence of our interactions. With Herzfeldt (1997), I suggest 'social poetics' and 'cultural intimacy' as a way of engaging practically, experientially and intellectually/analytically with research settings.

MARGINALITY AS A STRUCTURAL POSITION

I begin with theories of the social construction of 'the other', 'deviance' and 'marginality' in anthropology and sociology. Social anthropology as a discipline was born as the study of 'the other' and has fed on ethnographies and fieldwork carried out in places far away and very different from the ethnographers' own home ground. The political and conceptual status of anthropologists' research subjects has changed with theoretical and political shifts in the discipline as a whole. The founding fathers (and mothers) often saw the appearance, behaviour and thoughts of their exotic research subjects as objects of scrutiny, classification and comparison and thereby fixed the latter into categories of 'different', 'exotic' and 'primitive'. By implication, these characteristics came to be associated with 'inferiority' by the anthropologists' audiences, if not by the anthropologists themselves. Moreover, the subjects of research appear passive and 'to be known' rather than active and 'knowing' (for discussions of an ethnographic classic, see Denzin 1992). Anthropologists now see 'researcher' and 'subject' and associations of superiority/inferiority as symbolic and social constructs emerging from the very act of doing research. New forms of research and writing are developing which seek to address these imbalances and represent subjects of research as active and knowing participants in research encounters. As several contributions to this volume testify, a 'maturing trajectory' (in Neil Small's words) in AIDS research draws heavily on these traditions.

The construction of 'the other' in anthropological fieldwork and writing is particularly interesting, and raises particular issues, in studies carried out in the social setting which the anthropologist calls his or her own and involving relationships where the anthropologist's non-professional selves are more subtly entangled with the role as an ethnographer than is the case with fieldwork in the ethnographer's 'abroad'. Unlike studies of Third World peoples, anthropology 'at home' has no easy recourse to a conceptual space or time where the 'other' existed outside of contact with colonial/research discourse (Taussig 1987, referenced in Tsing 1994). The 'other' is often created, or creates him/herself, as 'marginal' in daily contact with the 'dominant society' and its agents: police, social and medical services, the media and, importantly, research.

The 1960s and 1970s saw a whole discipline emerging within sociology which adopted the loose label 'sociology of deviance' and explicitly analysed 'deviance' as forms of behaviour and lifestyles labelled as such by custodians of dominant mainstream society and processed into a social reality through (symbolic) interaction between labelled groups and representatives of 'social order' (Becker 1963; Cohen 1971; Young 1971, for a description of the production of a 'drug user' culture).

HIV/AIDS has become a powerful marker for the construction of 'deviant others' (defined by class, sexual behaviour, race) against whom society defines its normality (Frankenberg 1992) and social science research into HIV affords a particular example of the production of 'marginality'. This research has been driven by the urgency of acquiring an understanding of the epidemic and its likely spread. Social scientists in the HIV/AIDS field have been given the explicit brief to define and describe 'the marginalised other' in the guise of, for example 'sex worker', 'gay man', 'drug user', rather than reflecting on these labels as social constructions. It is difficult to avoid confirming their 'otherness' through work and writing which at times must, in order to satisfy job descriptions and aims of research proposals, exaggerate their stigmatising characteristics as linked to risk of infection and transmission.

If we thus see 'the other' as constituted politically and historically, the kind of situations and relationships through which our knowledge of 'the other' is being produced become a topic of scrutiny in its own right (Okely and Callaway 1992). I will suggest that such a scrutiny is best attempted from what Anna Tsing terms marginality as an analytic position:

> . . . an analytic placement that makes evident both the constraining, oppressive quality of cultural exclusion and the creative potential of rearticulating,

enlivening and rearranging the very social categories that peripheralise a group's existence.

(Tsing 1994: 279)

Inherent in this problematic is the issue of structure versus agency and the relationship between macro and micro social process. This is an ongoing concern in social sciences which appears in slightly different guises according to the theoretical and conceptual trends of the times and particular field with which we engage. It certainly is a concern in much social research into AIDS and, as contributions to this volume suggests, there is a powerful personal dimension to this concern. HIV and AIDS engage emotions and imaginations in a way other topics may not. We struggle to reconcile, on the one hand, the inevitability of economic and structural development which arrange social relationships into 'powerful majority' versus 'powerless minority' groups and, on the other, agency – individuals' creative response to structural contingency and determination. The issue here is the solidity or otherwise of social categories and the extent to which research confirms or destabilises these. Tsing addresses this problematic from 'zones of unpredictability at the edges of discursive stability' (Tsing 1994: 279) and imagines such a zone in a debate between Gramsci, 'who assumes too much' about the potential for reflective and political self-interest in producing social transformation, and Foucault, who assumes too little and thus 'obscures the suspense that infects the possibility of change' (Tsing 1994: 279).

The problematic of agency concerns the researcher no less than it does our respondents, of course. Research encounters are politically and historically contingent and structured by the very forces which we set out to understand and analyse (Marcus 1992). If we see research subjects' selves as historically and socially contingent, then the selves through which we as researchers engage with subjects of research are similarly constituted (see Philip Gatter, Chapter 4). To harness the tension of debates about agency and let subjects of research stand out as active agents, researchers need to look to the ambiguities of their own private and professional selves as precariously balancing the 'structure/agency' dichotomy. Warning against the dangers of essentialising the social categories with which we engage during our research, Herzfeldt (1997) suggests that agency is found in the subtle interplay between, on the one hand, confirmation of and, on the other, challenge to the stereotypes and categorisations around which social life revolves. He develops perspectives on 'social poetics' to catch hold of the irony and self-recognition which social actors 'play around with' the roles and stereotypes which structure their interactions with others. As a form of practical engagement with our own positions as researcher, 'social poetics' implies a similar intimate and (seriously) playful recognition of the forces that shape this engagement.

Much has been said, both in this volume and more generally, about the way private biographies shape our research histories. Warnings have been issued that we have gone too far in this direction and that we are losing sight of the research encounter as a social, rather than private, event (Rosaldo 1989; Spencer 1989; Tierney 1995). The selves with which we meet respondents in the field are also a product of academic socialisation (see, for example, Downes and Rock, 1982: Introduction), together with demands and expectations placed upon us as researchers. The challenge and the value of reflexivity lie in coming to grips with our own contingency and our reactions to it.

I proceed to explore these issues in a description of the setting in which I worked during the study of co-ordination of services for people with HIV/AIDS. I describe the *networks* which structured the field socially, and the *narratives* which circulated through these networks. I then go on to demonstrate a particular consequence of the exchange of tales in the constant scrutiny, commentary and interpretation of drug users' lives. Images of 'chaos' emerged as an inevitable consequence of this commentary. Finally, I discuss the social positioning of myself as researcher and the drug users who became my informants and ways in which 'drug user' identities were part of researcher–respondent encounters.

NETWORKS: SERVICES FOR AND RESEARCH ON PEOPLE WITH HIV IN LOTHIAN

HIV arrived in Lothian in the 1970s and manifested as a trickle of infections among gay men. In the mid-1980s, an HIV epidemic among intravenous drug users was discovered virtually overnight with data suggesting a 50 per cent rate of infection in certain younger age groups (Robertson *et al.* 1986). This was a dramatic discovery, particularly as little was known about clinical management of HIV infection, transmission and infection risks at the time. The discovery had potentially serious practical implications. A large number – more than a thousand people – might become seriously ill around the early to mid-1990s and need care and support which were beyond the capacity of services at the time.

There was a swift response, in terms of both management and prevention of HIV among drug users. This response revolved around the Infectious Diseases Unit at one Edinburgh hospital, which became the main centre of management of HIV in drug users. A range of new and dedicated HIV services were drawn in or established (Brettle 1990). Management of drug use was developed in order to prevent spread of HIV through needle sharing. Edinburgh pioneered the prescribing by general practitioners of methadone as an oral substitute to injectable heroin (Greenwood 1992). The voluntary sector services for people affected by HIV and drug use expanded through extra funding. Local authority social services responded with both specialist services and an increased awareness of the implication of HIV for general provision.

The AIDS field in Edinburgh, as in other places in Britain, attracted people with skills, ambition and commitment. There was money going into AIDS work when other sectors experienced cut-backs. There was also room for innovation, and people saw a chance to create services which were exceptional in that they were non-discriminatory and user-centred. People tended to stay on within the field. They might change jobs or leave and come back, but when our research project started in early 1992, many workers had been around for a long time. The Edinburgh HIV/AIDS field developed slightly apart from mainstream provision, with separate and stable networks of people operating with specific norms and ideals of service provision. One of these ideals concerned service user participation in the development and planning of services.

Boundaries between roles and categories were often blurred. The same people met in various capacities, in different fora of service provision and planning. Some service providers met and visited clients outside working hours. And often, the boundaries between the personal and the professional became vague as service providers, researchers and clients of services met in the same geographical space: in the school playgrounds, on the streets, in the shops and public places of the city and its neighbourhoods.

The feared uncontrolled HIV epidemic spreading from drug user networks did not happen. Infection rates have slowed and the pattern of transmission has changed. Men infected through sex with men, together with women infected heterosexually, now account for the largest numbers of new infections. The expected sudden and overwhelming influx of ill people did not materialise. Improved clinical management of HIV has resulted in increased control of disease progression, and terminal illness and death are staggered in the group of people infected around the same time. The comprehensive system of care thus came to cater for fewer people with HIV infection than expected.

When our research project started, a complex service system was in operation, with several service providers involved in one person's care. Co-ordination of services was seen as an issue. It was difficult to meet expectations of the present community care philosophy: to streamline co-ordination so that everybody works together, equipped with the right and appropriate information about what goes on and working with the service user's wishes at the centre of action. As in any setting, service providers worked to different obligations, interests and perspectives. Service users were not always seen to use the system 'appropriately'. They did not turn up for appointments, did not tell their service providers who was involved in their care and why and they 'dipped' in and out of services as crises occurred. Our research project became part of the scene and added to the complexity.

The project started in early 1992 and lasted for three years. It was an action-research project concerned with co-ordination of services for people with HIV in the region. Our aim was to provide continuous feed-back to providers and managers of services in order to inform both provision and development.

The project was divided into four studies, each building on the findings from a previous study and allowing for feed-back of results and refinement of aims between each stage. Two of these studies are of relevance here. One was a study of discharge from hospital into care in the community of forty-nine people with HIV. This study ran from late 1992 until the spring of 1993 and aimed to look at co-ordination of care between specialised hospital care and community-based care, importantly primary care. We used a combination of quantitative and qualitative methods to record and describe contacts between people with HIV and their service providers and also among providers (Huby *et al.* 1997). The other was a long-term prospective follow-up of a smaller group of people with HIV and their service providers. It overlapped with the study of discharges and ran until late 1994. This involved studying relationships and interactions between people with HIV infection and their service providers over time and studying specific events where these relationships were activated. The service users were recruited from a variety of settings and represent diverse personal and social characteristics, lifestyles, patterns of service use and stage of illness (Huby *et al.* 1995).

The findings from the studies suggested marked discrepancies in the providers' and users' perspectives on co-ordination. The providers of services, who had instigated the project, perceived the difficulties to lie in lack of co-ordination of everyday medical and social support systems, especially between hospital and community-based care. They perceived the system as stressful and 'chaotic' and they often blamed the lifestyles and personalities of patients, particularly drug users: 'These people are so chaotic – they make us chaotic too,' one service provider said.

Service users, on their part, did not experience the day-to-day co-ordination of care as an issue, mainly because of the commitment and dedication of their care workers, who went out of their way to deal with problems of co-ordination before they filtered down to service users. The majority of service user respondents were unemployed and living off state benefits. For them, the slow, arbitrary and inefficient nature of the state benefit system, together with a lack of co-ordination of welfare benefits and welfare rights services with medically focused systems of care, was the main problem (Huby 1997; Huby *et al.* 1997).

From the complexity of the setting and its interactions, there was ample scope for perceptions of 'chaos' to impinge on the experience of both service provision and use, and, as I will go on to describe, also the research thereof. The question I will go on to address is to what extent the 'chaos' experienced by researchers and service providers was a product of individual characteristics of service users, and to what extent the experience of disorder was a product of the system of service provision and research on which many people with HIV are forced to rely.

NARRATIVES

In the close-knit networks stories circulated constantly in the guise of information, gossip and rumours. Service providers told each other stories about colleagues and clients, who, in their turn, told each other and their service providers stories both about other service users and providers. Everybody was invited and coaxed to tell stories to researchers (of whom there were many) and no doubt everybody told 'researcher stories' behind our backs. Often stories simply passed our way by virtue of our position in the networks. Researchers used and are still using some of the stories to produce papers, reports and presentations to various audiences. The stories have been changed and re-created at every stage in the process. Plummer's (1995: 5) description of 'society as a textured but seamless web of stories emerging everywhere through interaction' seems peculiarly apt for Edinburgh HIV/AIDS settings.

To a large extent, this exchange of information was a necessary part of service co-ordination. At its most 'proper' and formal this exchange happened by letter, by phone, in meetings and encounters of varying degrees of formality set up explicitly for the purpose of service co-ordination. In many settings, however, the informal and casual exchange of information was an intrinsic part of service provision and co-ordination:

GP: This 'junkie' comes in and says: 'Have you heard about NN?' [another of his drug-user patients]. And I try and keep my head down and piece it all together.

(Field-notes, March 1994)

The informality of the exchange often closed gaps in communication and made for easier access to good service provision. Thus, early on in the longitudinal study a welfare rights worker told me he was going to see a client of his in hospital in order to help him sort out funeral grants, a will, and so on. His client was very ill and did not expect to get home again. The welfare rights worker had been told about him by another client of his and had phoned him up to ask if he could be of help.

Similarly, people with HIV acquired information about benefit entitlements and sources of help and support in applying for benefits by comparing notes with other people they met in hospital wards and in the hospice or with friends and relatives. Such information is not routinely available to clients, although many workers have benefits training. Also, the actual practice of benefits allocation does not fit the official information which *is* available: the system is experienced as arbitrary, unfair and inefficient. Clients must, therefore, piece together their own knowledge base. Thus snippets of information relating to benefits are eagerly seized upon and discussed in order to develop a coherent body of information.

Although the express purpose of passing on of stories may be to convey information, a lot else is being conveyed with it. The stories passed around in the name of information exchange contain all sorts of information extraneous to the main purpose at hand, but revealing much more about the identities and experiences of the individuals involved. Thus, the exchange of notes about benefits entitlements and experiences included comparisons of various people's 'rights' to benefits and moral evaluations about 'fraud' and 'scrounging'. This information was not anonymised as it would have been in a handbook, the absence of which thus contributed to 'benefit fraud' as an intrinsic element of the 'drug user chaos'.

Similarly, in the name of service co-ordination a lot more was exchanged than necessary 'facts' about individuals. The information was evaluated and assessed from different professional perspectives, each with particular views on the kind of 'fact' which was important and significant in shaping treatment and care decisions. These different views often became the object of intense inter-professional rivalries about whose version of 'fact' was to be the basis for decision and action. Thus, there were regular disputes between 'medical doctors' and 'community staff' (social workers, voluntary organisations, community psychiatric nurses) concerning service users' motivations for help seeking. Doctors often interpreted behaviour as manipulation to wrestle more drugs and benefits out of the system, whereas 'community staff' interpreted the same behaviour as a combination of lack of resources and lack of ability to manage available resources efficiently.

Service users' evaluations of their own motives and interests were often lost or, at best, distorted, in this constant exchange and evaluation of information about them. One of my respondents said:

> . . . I don't want all different stories getting bounced back off walls, fae a tennis ball to a football. Cause it snowballs . . . 'Watch her for this'. . . . Because I hate all this feed-back from this one, that one, 'You said this' I says 'No!' That's why I would have loved to have one of them [points to the tape recorder] you know, 'cause I forget what I've said.
>
> (Interview, February 1994)

Even allowing for professionally grounded discrepancies in views regarding relevant information, it was clear that more information than was strictly speaking necessary would often be exchanged. The danger of breaking confidentiality is a particular issue with HIV because of the stigma. This danger increases with the density of the networks, and Edinburgh networks are nothing if not close-knit, even outside the HIV field. It is all too easy for researchers to become involved in potential or actual breaches of confidentiality.

Thus, during data collection and writing up, I discussed my material regularly with my two co-grantholders as a way of enhancing the rigour of both data collection and analysis and also in order to make sure that we were meeting the aims of the study. One of them was herself a worker in the Edinburgh HIV/AIDS field, and she knew many of the participants in the study. However, we took great care to protect the anonymity of the people whom she did not know. Thus, we discussed one particular person for one year without my colleague knowing either her name or her circumstances. My colleague then attended a co-ordinating meeting at the hospital where the respondent received her care. Even with an outsider present at the meeting, the staff did nothing to restrict the amount of information exchanged and within five minutes my colleague knew the person's name, profession and life history. This was at a time when the woman was particularly concerned to control information regarding her seropositivity for both professional and personal reasons. My colleague was connected to the woman's professional networks and an unguarded word or comment on her part could have had grave consequences indeed.

Stories exchanged had different purpose and function. Some were told for mutual support, some were gossip, some were tales of woe, warning and heroism. The purpose varied with the circumstances of the telling and the motivation of the teller and the audience. A tale of woe told in one situation could become a tale of bravery and endurance in another context. Breaches of confidentiality could be idle gossip in one context and a vital source of support in another.

In the spring of 1993, I was talking to the adoptive mother of a child who has HIV infection. Suddenly, I realised that I knew the child's biological mother. I asked, and the woman confirmed. 'Ha!' I said, 'It's a small world!' (A bit sheepish, realising that I had played hard and fast with confidentiality rules.) 'Yes,' she replied, 'it's a small world!' She went on to tell me that she and her husband went on holiday with a colleague of the husband and his wife, who works as a home help. The two women had never met. They talked about their work and its stresses and difficulties and after a while they realised that the child's biological mother was a client of the home help. 'So much for confidentiality!' the adoptive mother told me. 'So we were able to share this and talk about it' (field-notes, April 1993).

The density of the Edinburgh networks is reflected in my own position and my many-stranded relationships to informants. I carried several roles, each of which was a potential avenue of information and carried implications for confidentiality. For example, as a member of a university Department of General Practice, I had been involved in evaluating a policy of drug use management in an Edinburgh practice. I interviewed drug users about their views and experiences of this policy. One of the drug users I interviewed, 'John', told me he was HIV positive, but that he did not use any services and that he did not use the hospital. Later, as I was writing up the AIDS study and reading through field-notes and interview transcripts, John was mentioned as somebody who had been a heavy user of services. Then one evening, my GP husband came home and asked me what was going on in the practice where I had done the evaluation. One patient had come from there to him and asked to join his practice. My husband did not know how to tackle the situation. The patient was giving mysterious reasons for wanting to change and told stories about his drug prescriptions which were difficult to make out. It was obvious that it was John he was talking about.

My own and my colleagues' position in this constant exchange of information and evaluation of information affected the way we saw our role as researchers. There was an expectation among many of the funders, users and respondents of the study that we were there to provide an objective and 'factual' description of the service system and its outcomes. However, it soon became apparent that it was impossible to separate 'the truth' from people's interpretation of what actually happened. It was obvious that people told me their own versions of events. Sometimes informants deliberately manipulated me by telling me a politically strategic interpretation of events or relationships. Usually, however, this 'manipulation' was more subtle and less obvious and it was difficult to determine who was being 'manipulated' – me or the story's author. The stories were part of interpretive work to make sense and order out of complexity. Halliday (1973, cited in Riessman 1993) suggests that the meaning of stories is conveyed by three 'distinct but interdependent functions of language'. She terms the first 'ideational', that is, the content in terms of the speaker's or community's experience. The second she calls 'interrelational', that is, the context of the telling which allows the nature of relationships to be expressed and interpreted. The third, which she terms 'structural/textual', refers to the syntax which structures the story. It is the circumstances of the narration, in the specific constellations of personal/ideational/textual factors, which structures the telling of a story and determines its meaning.

Although he writes specifically about illness narratives, Good's (1994) perspective applies to storytelling in other contexts. Good suggests that the story, as a product of the intersection between the personal and the social, sets up dialogues between characters narrated and the audiences of the telling, one of whom is the narrator him/herself. Stories thus have 'openness' and 'indeterminacy' (Good 1994: 164). We live, rather than simply narrate, our (illness) stories. We try out different plots and endings and the story changes course and potential according to new experiences, new knowledge and new situations of telling. Stories are always 'open to reinterpretation as life goes on – revealing hidden aspects unavailable to the blindness of the present' (Good 1994: 164).

We were obviously a part of this collective storytelling. Small wonder, then, that we had to give up our role as 'objective' researchers producing 'facts' about the system and its outcome and began to see ourselves as participants in the setting. The notion of 'fact' or 'truth' is a cultural and social product (Tonkin 1990), and the way people change, select and distort events is itself a social fact and has explanatory value in terms of the dynamics of interaction between service providers and users staging episodes or histories of care. It was obvious that we were a part of these dynamics, rather than outside observers, and we also had a part to play in their outcome. A social consequence of the narrative exchange was the processing of drug user clients as 'chaotic'.

THE 'GAZE'

The exchange of tales constituted a running commentary of people's lives where their every action and utterance were subjected to scrutiny, interpretation and evaluation. The stories or narratives which circulated, long since disembodied from actual events and persons, subtly selective in focus and changing their meaning with each telling, thus took on a 'life of their own'.

One day in the autumn of 1993 I was waiting for 'Scott' in the outpatient clinic of the hospital unit which he attends for his HIV infection. He was late for his appointment. The outpatient staff told me he turned up unexpectedly last week. He was stoned, and smelt of booze. They said he was 'always around – always wanting things', particularly when things were going badly for him. I remarked that I thought this was a shame, his being drunk. He had done so well, lately. 'Oh, yes, but that's the way he is,' a nurse replied. 'He begins drinking and becomes suicidal. He is probably down in Accident and Emergency, now!' After an hour of this I decided that Scott probably was seriously off the rails and unable to talk to me about his service use in any coherent manner. I decided to leave. I met him outside the clinic. He was shaven, smiling, cheerful and well dressed. He smelt of nothing stronger than soap. He had been for lunch and a therapy massage, he said, and he was running a bit late. He had lost his diary and obviously forgotten the time of his appointment (field-notes, October 1993).

There were few possibilities of escape from this scrutiny because absences and silences were noted and interpreted as 'inability to cope' or 'abnormality and deviance' (Huby 1997).

From the safety of these pages it is easy to judge such interpretations as 'misguided' and 'controlling'. However, in the thick of specific situations which could be both confusing and threatening, such interpretations came quite naturally, even to an anthropologist well versed in theories of labelling and control.

At one time during the study of discharges, my colleague (a man) asked me to visit a potential respondent in a certain high-rise block outside the city centre. This man had seemed very happy to take part in our study when my colleague spoke to him in hospital, but he had moved from the address he gave us and he was difficult to locate. My colleague found his new address through the hospital and wrote to him saying that I – a female researcher – would come to see him. Under the circumstances we thought that a woman might be less intimidating than a man and that I was more likely to elicit his co-operation. What follows are extracts from my field-notes:

I found the address without difficulty and located the right high-rise entrance. However, the door was locked. A woman returning home from the shops told me the block had been equipped with security intercom doorbells to the flats because vandalism had been a problem. She let me in and showed me the lifts. I was reassured by the friendliness and domestic activity which surrounded the woman who let me in. The flat I wanted was on the ninth floor.

As soon as I entered, all signs of routine everyday life evaporated. The entrance hall and lift were empty and the building filled with an eerie silence. Although it was clean, freshly decorated and free of the smell of human waste and Jeyes fluid (which greets the visitor to many council blocks of flats), this absence of life was threatening and sinister, rather than reassuring. I clutched my alarm canister as I went into the lift, which took me to the right floor. The corridor was empty, the only sound was from the wind whistling around the outside corner and through the emergency stair entrance. I located the door and knocked. A dog started barking, there was a sound of a chair scraping and a muffled voice told the dog to be quiet. I shouted my name and errand through the letter box, but there was no response apart from the sound of the dog moving and the whispering voice urging it to be still. I waited ten minutes or so, then I wrote a message on a piece of paper and shoved it through the letter box. I wrote that I would be returning the next day at a certain time, but when I did, there was obviously nobody in the flat.

(Field-notes, February 1993)

We did not try to make contact again. Had I been to the wrong door? If not, what had happened to this man to make him hide like this? Was our study so imposing that he could not tell us to our face that he had changed his mind about taking part? Or was he on the run from things more dangerous and decided not to take any chances? The police? Drug deals gone wrong? Social security frauds? Fear of his disease? I was filled with an urge to see him and to make contact, to submerge this threat or suggestion of fear, secrecy and rejection in the humdrum activity of our research project.

The information I collected as a researcher also touched on non-professional areas of my life, something which made a dispassionate interpretation difficult.

Resp.:   You know that time Cameron was assaulted? He always said they were drug dealers. But I have heard another story – that it was a vigilante attack. He had been selling to kids in the area and some people decided to do something about it. Who told me? It was NN [another service user; I knew this person, who had been passing information on to us about other people participating in our research]. These stories are told to me, and it is impossible to know what is the truth.

(Interview, August 1994)

To me this information was of more than academic interest. I had met 'Cameron' in places where my own children go. I had once left my youngest at a party in a public place where he was also present. I trusted him fully on his own, but theoretically, vigilantes or dealers might have turned up and violence might have developed.

The question arises, whether the drug users in this setting were 'chaotic' or whether we – that is, the researchers and providers of care – created them as 'chaotic' by looking at them 'too closely'. The exchange of narratives constituted a constant 'gaze' (Foucault 1979) in the glare of which a person's everyday life with its inconsistencies and unreflected or unarticulated responses was magnified into 'chaos' and 'disorder' and our research project was a part of this. There were several dimensions to our part in 'processing' of people as 'chaotic'. I have tried to describe how some were rooted in my personal background and social position which, in turn, conditioned my responses to situations I encountered in the field. Others lay with the organisation of research generally and this particular project in particular.

There was scepticism about the planned method of data collection for the study of discharges, namely diaries given to respondents when they left hospital. They were then sent stamped and addressed envelopes in which to return the completed diaries. This scepticism was entirely justified – there was an appallingly low return rate in spite of apparent commitment to the survey when we recruited people in hospital. The lack of response was by some service providers – and occasionally ourselves – put down to people's 'chaotic lifestyles' and their inability to structure time and follow through plans and commitments. However, as we followed people home and collected information through personal interviews, we were forced to question this notion of 'chaos'. For example, we found that inadequate material base of existence was an important factor in service users' response to offers of treatment and care and also to requests for research participation. The slow, inefficient and apparently arbitrary DSS system of processing benefit applications structured people's existence to an extraordinary degree and influenced decisions about how to spend and prioritise time. Thus, chasing up a giro or concluding a drug deal might have taken precedence over sessions with a counsellor, attending a medical appointment for a routine check-up, or spending time with a researcher. The discrepancy between, on the one hand, routines and concepts of time on which clinics and management of caseloads often rest, and, on the other, the time management of people who live a hand-to-mouth existence dependent on welfare also played a part. Finally, evasion of services and research was clearly often a form of resistance to the intrusion of a system too overwhelming for refusals to be negotiated face-to-face (Huby 1997).

Sometimes, what we concluded was a lack of co-operation had nothing to do with respondents' behaviour at all, but resulted from the inefficiency of the postal system. For example, two respondents whose diaries we had not received claimed to have posted them, and we had no reason not to believe them. Post office disorganisation seems a perfectly plausible explanation.

As pointed out by Neil Small elsewhere in this volume, both the meaning and manifestation of 'altruism' shifts with economic and social conditions of exchange. In view of the amount of research to which our respondents were exposed we wanted to give them something in return for their participation in the discharge study. However, we did not have the budgets to offer a substantial recompense to all. We were also wary of raising expectations among research participants in ways which put future publicly funded research at a disadvantage. In the end, we approached an Edinburgh cinema and asked if they would donate weekly free tickets which we then raffled among those who returned their diaries. Although the tickets were appreciated by those who got them, there was clearly no incentive for people to take part. I note with interest that we had replicated the tendency to offer non-monetary rewards to working-class respondents (see Neil Small, Chapter 8).

In describing 'the chaotic drug user' as a social construction I am, of course, not implying that none of the drug users we met during our study conformed, in one way or another, to this stereotype. The point I wish to make is that so do many people not classed as 'drug users'. Ideas about 'time' and 'time keeping' are themselves specific cultural values. Lack of ability or motivation to structure time and organise life in certain ways is equally distributed throughout the population. The power to interpret one's lifestyle according to own values and preferences, however, is not. A certain 'chaos' in an academic or an artist is a virtue and a sign of creativity, even when this chaos is drug-induced (cf. Burroughs' [1977] *Junkie*). The 'chaos' associated with the drug users in our study was considered a character deficit. It was also class-specific. Drug use, in the form of cocaine and cannabis, is prevalent in certain middle-class milieux, for example the City professions, but it is not deemed 'chaotic' and abnormal in the way the drug users in our study were stereotyped.

'US' AND 'YOU'

'Chaos' was thus constructed as an attribute in specific populations. As another research project in the setting we contributed to this attribution, no matter how much we might deconstruct it academically and theoretically. For example, the (initially – we increased the response rate through personal follow-up of respondents at home) low response rate to our survey was automatically put down to the behaviour of our respondents and became another proof of their 'chaotic lifestyles'. Moreover, I have tried to describe how my reactions to events flowed from subtle interweavings of personal and professional engagements with the many situations I encountered in the field. The attribution of 'chaos' was thus a complex process, the deconstruction of which required more than academic and theoretical detachment. The process of attribution involved the negotiation of social boundaries *in practice*, and the research encounters were one forum where boundaries between 'us' and 'them' were drawn, redrawn and negotiated.

In my dealings with informants, it was obvious that although we might live in the same locality, we did not share social space. We talked about and compared children, schools, family and so on, but it soon became obvious that the similarities we might identify did not go very deep. For example, at one time it looked as if the eldest child of a woman with whom I was almost a 'neighbour' would start at the same secondary school as my eldest daughter. We discussed the school and its reputation with the same fears and hopes that any parents would do whose eldest children were about to embark on secondary education. I sometimes wondered how I would handle confidentiality in the (unlikely – the school is very big) event that they ended up in the same class. However, our two children ended up in different schools divided by the same differences in ethnic, political and religious affiliation which separated us and our families despite the rapport which might have developed between us.

These differences were a constant backdrop to the dynamics of individual research encounters. One of my 'drug user' informants once said in surprise: 'You come here to the likes of us, Guro, and you fit in! How come?' I was, of course flattered, and I really liked this woman and her partner and valued my time with them. However, I did not 'fit in'. I might have bantered a bit about cheating the DSS and asked her and her partner how much they would give me not to 'grass on' them, but that was how far it went. For example, I did not, like them, smoke hash, neither was any seriously offered me. 'Don't be silly, you *know*

Guro doesnae smoke,' she would say when her partner offered to pass me a joint. (I was also careful not to put myself in a position where I would be obliged to accept. Given the visibility of the field and the speed with which information travelled, there was a good chance that the Scottish Office as funders of the project would find out that the researcher smoked hash with informants. The funders were unlikely to take kindly to this.) The couple also talked to me about their financial matters and the 'mess' they were sometimes in and they told me stories about their creativity and resourcefulness in getting money – occasionally by less than regular means. However, it was never suggested or even implied that I would be in even worse difficulties without an income, which, in turn, gave me access to credit and an overdraft. How they talked about me when I was gone I do not know. However, in my presence, neither they nor any other of my informants discussed or questioned other researchers' or service providers' survival skills if they, like my two informants, were forced to rely long-term on a hand-to-mouth existence which reliance on welfare engenders.

Clive Foster in the previous chapter discusses ways in which the people on the housing estate where he did his fieldwork purposefully used inverted and exaggerated drug user identities to their own advantage. I did my research among the same people and networks as Clive. Often, subtle play with 'drug user' identities was an intrinsic part of my research encounters. The woman described above was particularly skilled at, and took great pleasure in, this game. In fact, this was one of the reasons why I and several of her service providers found her such good company. Thus, when she marvelled at my ability 'to fit in', I was never entirely sure whether she was mocking or complimenting my social skills.

Less subtle were the macho boasting in heroic tales about 'the heroin days'. Early on in the study of hospital discharges I had introduced myself to a respondent, 'Paul', on one of the hospital wards. He had been admitted to hospital because of a drug overdose and an incident in the outpatient clinic where he fell out with his doctor over the amount of substitute drugs he was being prescribed. Paul looked at me suspiciously and asked: 'Are you the psychiatrist? They say the psychiatrist is coming – I don't want to see her' (his behaviour in outpatient was being put down to his mental instability, and he resented this). I assured him I was not the psychiatrist, and he relaxed and invited me to sit down in his room. We talked at length, but not about what mattered to me. Paul was stoned and very talkative.

I had come to ask him to take part in our study of hospital discharges. I needed him to understand the study, to sign a consent form and to commit himself to completing the diaries and send them to us by post. His agenda was altogether different. He wanted to boast to me about his exploits in 'the heroin days'. He described in great detail his job as a minder to one of the big dealers to finance his £120 per day habit. He told me of narrow escapes down dark alleyways with police or with rival gangs armed with knives in hot pursuit. He painted grisly pictures of 'shooting galleries' in derelict flats with syringes being passed around. Occasionally, a youngster who was too green and inexperienced to take heroin responsibly slumped down dead and was carried out in the night to a lift or a flight of stairs for their parents to find him. He talked of death:

> You know, death is not new to us. We have always lived with death. Before AIDS it was Hep[atitis] B. We have always taken risks. You walk along, so desperate [for a fix] that you draw water up from puddles on the ground. See – we're used to it.

(Field-notes, November 1992)

It seemed he was a man of considerable talent and promise in many areas, both sport and music. I grew increasingly irritated by his boasting, and I asked myself why he did not use these talents to help young people get their lives together, rather than selling them heroin? I also wondered if I should challenge him, but I did not get a word in edgeways. This was a monologue and no occasion for discussion and debate. More importantly, however, I desperately needed him in our study of discharges because our response rate was so low. If I responded to him like a fellow human being with whom I reserved the right to disagree, I would sidetrack him even more from the pressing matter of our survey and I was not prepared to – neither did I have the time or energy – to do this. After one hour, I left, exhausted and angry over the waste of his and other young lives, but, I must admit, equally exasperated over the waste of my own precious time.

The boundaries between 'researcher' and 'researched', between 'us' and 'the chaotic and irresponsible drug user', were firmly drawn. Paul and I, divided by gender, class and experience and each with different agendas, were pitted against each other in interaction which both constructed and confirmed him as 'deviant' and 'chaotic'.

However, there was a moment – albeit brief and fleeting – during our encounter when Paul appeared with a depth and understanding which went far beyond his cardboard replica enactment of a 'typical drug user'. Just before I was to leave, one of the ward nurses popped her head around the door and said: 'Paul, you can go home this afternoon. This is just to tell you that a community psychiatric nurse is coming around to see you at home on Thursday morning.' Paul turned to me and nodded knowingly, as if to say: '*See what I mean?*'

There was a wealth of possibility and ambiguity in this little gesture. At one level, he was perhaps passing comment on the fact that the ward staff were forcing unwelcome services on him. He resented the fact that his altercation with the consultant in outpatient was put down to his mental instability, rather than to a disagreement between him and the doctor where at least part of the responsibility fell to the latter. However, there was also an implication that his charade was nothing more than a disguise for his strategy of keeping me and my research project at bay.

I would have minded a straight 'No' less than his 'heroin days' performance. However, I can see that a person dressed in pyjamas and dependent on the ward staff both for his supply of substitute drugs and medical care for a life-threatening disease might see it in his interest to formulate his refusals in roundabout ways lest he offend somebody useful. However, I am also convinced that he took delight in his performance. He enjoyed the game of pulling the wool over my eyes. With his brief nod and telling glance he invited me to share in his complicity and his delight in it. It was an 'intimate' (Herzfeldt 1997) moment, in which he made clear to both of us the power and pervasiveness of the stereotypes around which our interaction revolved, and also the elasticity of the boundaries which separated us.

Such moments of 'intimacy' often occur between researchers also, and the story of Paul provides an example. Paul promised to take part in the study, to complete the diaries and return them to us. I somehow knew his promises to be false, and I was right. In the end, my colleague arranged to go to his home and conduct an interview. A few days before the planned visit, Paul died. I heard the news from one of his support workers and when I met my colleague the next morning I told him. The low response rate to our diary survey went through both our minds as we exchanged embarrassed grins and burst out simultaneously with a brief comment that might have seemed both uncaring and callous to the uninitiated (so I will not repeat it here). However, our embarrassed complicity contained poignantly, and with both sadness, compassion and resignation, our understanding of the relationship between us as researchers and Paul as a respondent, the forces that structured this relationship and the possibility that it might have been different.

CONCLUSION: MARGINALITY AS AN ANALYTIC POSITION

This chapter has explored issues around 'deviance' and 'marginality' as a social/structural position and I have described and discussed how 'marginality' in Edinburgh HIV/AIDS settings was constructed through exchange of narratives about 'chaos' and 'chaotic lifestyles'. I have also discussed my own position in this exchange and I have described how my personal biography and experience impinged on my work as researcher. The task remains to distance myself from the experience in order to engage analytically with my material. What I am aiming for is a research account which situates the narratives in the historically specific relationships and contexts wherein they were constructed, so that our voices – my own and the service users and providers who took part in my research – may be placed and heard (Marcus 1993).

With Tsing (1994), I suggest marginality as an analytic position from which to engage theoretically with the contexts of our research in ways which recognise the limits of any one theoretical framework in catching the complexities of social behaviours and human motivations. With Herzfeldt (1997), I suggest that we look to the 'intimate' moments of research interactions to capture the subtleties of our own and respondents' practical engagement with structural contingency and the forces that determine who we are, or are allowed to be, in specific situations.

ACKNOWLEDGEMENTS

The project on which this chapter draws was funded by the Scottish Office Home and Health Department and was based in the Department of General Practice, University of Edinburgh. My thanks to colleagues in the project: Edwin van Tejlingen (now Department of Public Health, University of Aberdeen), Mike Porter (Department of General Practice, University of Edinburgh), Judy Bury (Lothian Health HIV/AIDS and Drugs Primary Care Facilitator Team) and the research participants.

Ideas for the chapter started developing during my time as a Ph.D. student in the Department of Anthropology, University of Edinburgh. Thanks to supervisors Judith Okely (now Department of Sociology and Social Anthropology, University of Hull) and Sarah Cunningham-Burley (Department of Public Health, University of Edinburgh) and fellow students for help and suggestions.

REFERENCES

Becker, H. (1963) *Outsiders*, New York: Collier-Macmillan.

Brettle, R.P. (1990) 'Hospital health care for HIV infection with particular reference to injecting drug users', *AIDS Care*, 2: 171–81.

Burroughs, W. (1977) *Junkie*, Harmondsworth: Penguin.

Cohen, S. (ed.) (1971) *Images of Deviance*, Harmondsworth: Pelican.

Denzin, N. (1992) 'Whose Cornerville is it, anyway?', *Journal of Contemporary Ethnography*, 21: 120–32.

Downes, D. and Rock, P. (1982) *Understanding Deviance*, Oxford: Clarendon Press.

Foucault, M. (1979) *Discipline and Punish: The Birth of the Prison*, Harmondsworth: Penguin.

Frankenberg, R. (1992) 'What identity's at risk? Anthropologists and AIDS', *Anthropology in Action*, 12: 6–9.

Good, B.J. (1994) *Medicine, Rationality and Experience: An Anthropological Perspective*, Cambridge: Cambridge University Press.

Greenwood, J. (1992) 'Persuading general practitioners to prescribe: good husbandry or a recipe for chaos?', *British Journal of Addiction*, 87: 567–75.

Halliday, M.A.K. (1973) *Explorations in the Functions of Language*, London: Edward Arnold.

Herzfeldt, M. (1997) *Cultural Intimacy: Social Poetics in the Nation-State*, New York and London: Routledge.

Huby, G. (1997) 'Interpreting silence, documenting experience: an anthropological approach to the study of health service users' experience with HIV/AIDS care in Lothian, Scotland', *Social Science and Medicine*, 44(8): 1149–60.

Huby, G., Porter, A.M.D. and Bury, J. (1995) *Issues in Co-ordination of Services for People with HIV and AIDS in Lothian: An Ethnographic Study*, Edinburgh: Department of General Practice, University of Edinburgh.

Huby, G.O., Teijlingen, E.R. van, Porter, A.M.D. and Bury, J. (1997) 'The Chief Scientist Reports . . . : Co-ordination of Care on Discharge from Hospital into the Community for Patients with HIV/AIDS in Lothian', *Health Bulletin*, 55(5): 338–50.

Marcus, J. (1992) 'Racism, terror and the production of Australian auto/biographies', in J. Okely and H. Callaway (eds) *Anthropology and Autobiography*, ASA Monograph No. 29, London: Routledge.

Okely, J. and Callaway, H. (eds) (1992) *Anthropology and Autobiography*, ASA Monograph No. 29, London: Routledge.

Plummer, K. (1995) *Telling Sexual Stories: Power, Change and Social Worlds*, London: Routledge.

Riessman, C.K. (1993) 'Narrative analysis', *Sage Qualitative Methodology Research Series*, No. 30.

Robertson, J.R., Bucknall, A., Welsby, P., Roberts, J.J.K., Inglis, J.L., Peutheier, J.F. and Brettle, R.A. (1986) 'Epidemic of AIDS related virus (HTLV–ivILAV) among intravenous drug abusers', *British Medical Journal*, 292: 527–9.

Rosaldo, R. (1989) *Culture and Truth: The Remaking of Social Analysis*, London: Routledge.

Spencer, J. (1989) 'Anthropology as a kind of writing', *Man*, 24: 145–64.

Taussig, M. (1987) *Shamanism, Colonialism and the Wild Man: A Study in Terror and Healing*, London: Routledge.

Tierney, W.G. (1995) '(Re)presentation and voice', *Qualitative Inquiry*, 1(4): 379–90.

Tonkin, E. (1990) 'History and the myth of realism', in R. Samuel and P. Thompson (eds) *The Myths We Live By*, London: Routledge.

Tsing , A.L. (1994) 'From the margins', *Cultural Anthropology*, 9: 279–97.

Young, J. (1971) 'The role of the police as amplifiers of deviancy, negotiators of reality and translators of fantasy: some consequences of our present system of drug control as seen in Notting Hill', in S. Cohen (ed.) *Images of Deviance*, Harmondsworth: Pelican.

Part IV

Representation and agency

Chapter 11

Engagement, representation and presentation in research practice

Rosaline S. Barbour

INTRODUCTION

Janice Morse (1994) has dedicated her edited collection *Critical Issues in Qualitative Research Methods* to 'those who participate in our projects', adding, 'We are trying to find ways to communicate what you know so that others may understand.' At first glance, this seems a relatively straightforward and suitably humble explanation of the research enterprise. The simplicity and sincerity of the language, however, belie the enormity and complexity of the task involved. The 'knowledge' which we derive from our research is – as so many of the contributors to this volume have shown – the result of a process of social construction in which we, as researchers, play an active role. The sharing of such knowledge is also a social act. This aspect of the research endeavour, however, has not been subjected to the same amount of reflexive examination as has the process of fieldwork. Brettell observes that 'these issues relating to the politics of audience reception, whether real or imagined, [are] rarely treated in print with the kind of brutal honesty and exposure of self that is necessary', adding that the question is 'complex and multifaceted' (Brettell, 1993: 5).

In this chapter I examine some of the issues surrounding representation and sharing the products of our research with those whom we study and with others, drawing mainly on an interview study of 152 health and social care staff (in both specialist and generic posts) providing services for people with HIV/AIDS in four Scottish cities in the early 1990s. Guro Huby (Chapter 10) has described how, within Edinburgh, boundaries between researchers, service providers and clients were often blurred. With a relatively small number of specialist workers and even fewer researchers, the same could be said of the situation in Scotland as a whole at this time. The workers whom I interviewed were sometimes friends of friends and attended the same seminars as I did in order to orient myself to a new field of study.

In addition to the more standard expectations that I would publish the results of my research in peer-reviewed journals and present conference papers, the project had a commitment to providing dissemination sessions for staff members, eight of which were scheduled near the end of my funded period. In the discussion which follows I reflect on both the potential and limitations of attempting to share our research-generated insights with respondents, seeking to present their views, argue their cases, and engage with them in collaborative research, analysis and writing. Of course, writing for diverse audiences has long been a part of the academic enterprise. However, in this chapter I argue that it is only when circumstances force us to examine critically the assumptions and conventions which structure our writing and oral presentations and their interpretation that we begin to apply the tools of reflexivity to engage analytically with our own role in the social construction of knowledge. As Aldridge argues:

> Sociological method texts . . . deal . . . with what sociologists contend happens when research is carried out, and not with how sociologists go about the process of translating 'the research' – a multi-faceted experience in time – into writing. This latter experience is rarely written about in a standard research account, but is instead systematically stripped from it.
>
> (Aldridge 1993: 54–5)

It is crucial that the incorporation of such reflexivity into our writing amounts to more than consideration of techniques for conveying our thoughts and arguments: it requires a recognition that the assumptions and conventions which structure our research accounts are an integral part and product of the research process:

> Writing is also a way of 'knowing' – a method of discovery and analysis. By writing in different ways, we discover new aspects of our topic and our relationship to it. Form and content are inseparable.
>
> (Richardson 1994: 516)

RECIPROCITY AND REPRESENTATION

In a similar vein to Morse, Hughes (1992) talks of ethnography as involving 'process, product and promise'. He views the task of producing an ethnographic account – the 'promise' – as going beyond the 'etic' (that is, outsider's) description of the object of interest to provide an 'emic' frame of analysis, where 'internal' and 'subjective' data supplement the outsider's observations and measurements. Thus our research may serve the purpose of 'bearing witness' (Neil Small, Chapter 8).

In explaining why they had agreed to participate in my study, many of my respondents echoed the sentiments expressed by some of those interviewed by Neil Small (Chapter 8), saying that the study afforded an opportunity to 'set the record straight' and focus on the needs of staff members, which, they felt, were all too often overlooked. Although practitioners, in common with researchers, are nowadays often encouraged to be 'reflexive', their involvement in this activity has not generally led to the sort of over-indulgence of which Tierney (1995) accuses anthropologists. It was relatively unusual for staff members to be able to set aside forty-five minutes to talk exclusively about their own experiences and concerns. I was jokingly referred to as 'my therapist' by a number of my interviewees, who told me that they valued the chance of talking about their work to an interested outsider and stressed to colleagues that they did not want to be interrupted during their 'counselling session'.

As both Jill Bourne (Chapter 6) and Neil Small (Chapter 8) observe, taking part in a research interview may be a therapeutic or cathartic experience. McBeth says that 'the opportunity to tell one's story to an interested listener both validates one's life and helps one to discover its significance' (McBeth 1993: 150–1). Johnson (1996) argues that focus groups – in particular – can function an emancipatory tool, by affording participants the opportunity to voice their concerns and thus come to a fuller understanding of their situations. Such an argument echoes current folk wisdom which states that feelings are 'better out than in', or that, in Johnson's words, 'It's good to talk.' It is debatable, however, how lasting such research-generated insights are, or how easily they can be translated into strategies for effecting change. As Horowitz points out, respondents' consent to our analyses 'in no way guarantees their empowerment' (Horowitz 1993: 138).

There is, however, some limited evidence that, at least for some individuals, such insights *can* lead to action and enable them to change their situation. A worker whom I interviewed about her experience of providing services for people with HIV and AIDS told me immediately afterwards, 'I wish I could tell my line-manager all of this,' and then continued, 'Well, there's no reason why I shouldn't, now that I've got things sorted out in my own mind.' This individual later reported to me that she had managed to hold a similar discussion with her line-manager, who had turned out to be very sympathetic and willing to address the issues which she had raised.

As Brettell (1993: 4) has observed, ethnographic texts take on a life of their own that is beyond the ethnographer's control. Whilst this often culminates in criticism or vilification on the part of disgruntled readers and gives rise to much soul-searching on the part of the authors, texts may also be perceived in a sympathetic light – and may even be employed as a tool for effecting change:

> *After I had presented a paper at the Social Aspects of AIDS Conference in London I was approached by an individual who introduced himself as a specialist AIDS worker. He shook my hand warmly, saying that he was very pleased to meet me at last. He then recounted how he had distributed copies of a paper I had published (Barbour, 1993) to his co-workers and had used this as the basis for a discussion about organisational problems and tensions within his work setting. He had, he told me, been very relieved to read my article, partly because it confirmed that his concerns were not confined to him as an individual, and partly because he saw an opportunity to put these items on the agenda in the relatively un-threatening context of a staff seminar.*

(Researcher's diary, July 1993)

Whilst it was very gratifying, the experience cited above is, at least in my experience, very rare. We do not hear of those – probably more numerous – situations where respondents or other interested parties are less successful in their attempts to use our analyses to initiate discussion with managers or co-workers about difficult topics. For every reader who is reassured or enthused by our writing, there are probably several who find our 'insights' irrelevant, boring, inaccurate or even offensive.

My reaction to this colleague having found a practical use for my paper was one of unqualified pleasure. As an academic researcher I am not familiar with the experience of having produced something considered 'useful'. I wonder, however, what my reaction would have been had he chosen to use my paper in another way – perhaps in a way which encroached on what I saw as my own professional territory. Sheehan (1993) reports being both flattered and dismayed to see some of her ideas published under the name of an Irish intellectual who was one of her respondents.

Such rare triumphs as the one outlined above notwithstanding, we run a much greater risk of respondents being 'underwhelmed' by our insights. Davis, writing in 1971, commented on the widespread expectation that research findings will 'amaze and shock'. At the very least, respondents are likely to expect to be surprised or informed, as did the social work students with whom, as a Ph.D. student, I shared some of my preliminary findings relating to their experience of professional socialisation. As one told me and several others confirmed, 'Well, it didn't really tell us anything we didn't know already.' There is, then, a danger that, to 'insiders', our analyses are seen as 'common-sensical', reproducing – although usually also commenting upon – their 'taken-for granted' (Schutz, 1972) views. Thus we appear to be offering insights similar to those provided by John Cleese, in the guise of paleobiologist Ann Elk, in an often re-televised sketch, where, with considerable gravitas, 'she' expounds 'her' 'theory' that 'all dinosaurs are thin at one end, much, much fatter in the middle, and thin again at the other end'.

> The interactionists generally have adhered more closely to lay reasoning than have their competitors. They have not arrogated vastly superior understanding to themselves, and the contrasts between their assertions and those of everyday life are relatively slight in consequence.
>
> (Rock 1979: 232)

Whether we take an explicitly interactionist approach or not, this applies to most types of qualitative research, where we are concerned with presenting the world-views of our respondents.

In the dissemination sessions which I presented in each of the cities where I had carried out my fieldwork my decisions about content were informed by what I perceived as the need to provide information which had implications for policy and the organisation of work. I gave a breakdown of my sample; discussed the extent to which interviewees considered that AIDS work made unique demands of them; detailed the most important stressors/demands; described the support currently provided; highlighted shortcomings in terms of support provision and the neglect of organisational issues; and ended with consideration of the perceived rewards of working in this field (see Barbour 1995 for an indication of the material presented).

For some respondents these sessions confirmed that their personal concerns were shared by others. Often respondents would come up to me at the end of such sessions and thank me, firstly, for taking the time to share findings with them and, secondly, for showing that other people's experiences were similar, making comments such as, 'Thank goodness it's not just me!' Although they had no way of knowing whether those 'others' who shared their concerns were, in fact, members of their own work group, they seemed happy to air their views in front of colleagues, having perhaps been granted 'ceremonial permission' (Jill Bourne, Chapter 6) to admit their concerns in public.

Some respondents may be reassured both by evidence of widespread agreement with their views and the demonstration that the researcher is going about quantifying results in the manner associated with competent research. Others, however, may not react positively to the aggregation of what they view as their unique and intensely personal responses. There is a dilemma here and a balance to be struck between ensuring that anonymity is preserved and risking misrepresenting respondents by confusing a one-to-one interview with group settings. Being identified by a number – or as one of a larger number – may ensure anonymity but, in providing a collective voice for respondents, we may be privileging frequently mentioned concerns which, although raised by those we have interviewed, are not the issues which are most important to them as a *group*. In seeking to aggregate data from one-to-one interviews are we not just imposing the notion of a collective perspective whilst conveniently ignoring the context in which our data were collected: a one-off research encounter rather than a group process? However, perhaps where we feed back these findings to respondents and alert them to the extent of individual expressions of a particular perspective, this can act as a basis for them to further explore and construct a collective voice. Unless our work is embedded in a dialogical approach, we cannot, of course, guarantee that this will happen.

At these dissemination sessions I also made available to respondents all of the papers which I had published. It was with some trepidation that, at one particular session, I laid out a few copies of an article entitled 'I don't sleep with my patients – Do you sleep with yours?' This paper explored the tensions involved in AIDS-related work and looked at workers' accounts of the reactions of members of their own professional peer groups. These individuals were sometimes portrayed as being just as prejudiced and fearful as members of the general public, although interviewees considered that these individuals 'ought to know better'. The quote used, thus, summed up in a very concise way the resentments felt by staff in the face of a lack of understanding from their fellow professionals. The respondent who had made this memorable comment, which I found impossible to resist when searching for a title, was in the room and taking a keen interest in the material displayed. It occurred to me – admittedly rather belatedly

– that perhaps I should have sought permission to use this quote. I had not asked for permission at the time, my rationale being that I had used many quotes from respondents and had not considered it necessary to obtain clearance from any of the others, all of whom I had taken pains to anonymise.

ATTRIBUTION AND INTERPRETATION

In my own research methods teaching, I frequently remind students that part of the skill of interviewing lies in getting our respondents to do some of our analysis for us, by encouraging them to clarify their views, contextualise their statements, and make comparisons between themselves and others. Although the 'key informant' is a staple ingredient in traditional anthropological texts, we do not routinely attribute our analytical insights to respondents in other forms of writing about research. Sheehan asks:

> How do you correctly ascribe ideas that are offered within the context of an interview but which may also be the basis of new works, new publications? How do you separate the public thinker from the private, honour his confidentiality and intellectual property, and still offer a meaningful analysis?
>
> (Sheehan 1993: 81)

Perhaps our reluctance to attribute theoretical insights to respondents is justified, given that their explanations take a different form and serve a purpose somewhat removed from our own as researchers. Here, discussing the limitations of 'member validation', Bloor argues:

> . . . while laymen produce their own distinctive sociological accounts of their social worlds, these accounts will inevitably differ form the accounts provided by sociological researchers, since each is formulated in light of different purposes at hand. A member's sociological account will only have that degree of clarity, consistency, and elaborateness required by the member's purpose at hand, and hence cannot be directly compared with a sociologist's description compiled for different purposes.
>
> (Bloor 1983: 157)

Although, in the event, she seemed pleased that her comment had been considered insightful enough to warrant its use in the title of my paper (and went round telling the other people attending the dissemination session, 'That's my quote – I said that!'), my respondent would have had every right to have been surprised – and, perhaps, even displeased – by the resurfacing of this comment in such a prominent position. Indeed, although I had laughed with her when she recounted this incident during her interview, I had not considered using this quote for my title until I had actually written the piece and was searching for a title a couple of days before I was due to present the paper at a conference. (It was subsequently published as a contribution to an edited volume of conference papers.) Although I had asked for permission to tape interviews, I had not explicitly warned respondents that I might wish to quote them, but none seemed surprised that I used anonymised quotes in my papers and at the dissemination sessions. Munhall (1988) suggests that, since the focus of qualitative research unfolds throughout projects, the concept of 'process consent' may be more appropriate than 'informed consent', which tends to be viewed as occurring as a discrete event when access is negotiated at the outset. Since respondents – and, indeed, the researcher – cannot know at the start of a project exactly where interests and theorising may lead, it is, obviously, not possible to give guarantees as to how data are to be used in the analysis and writing up of research.

Hugh Masters (Chapter 5) recounts how he negotiated a move from nurse to researcher. He does not mention his other parallel role in the AIDS research endeavour – that of one of my respondents in his capacity as charge nurse at Milestone House. For me to feel that was ethically permissible to disclose this here necessitated a telephone conversation with Hugh, testifying to the somewhat vague and open-ended bargain we make with our respondents at the time – and to the somewhat unusual nature of this collection. We do not usually provide the names of our respondents or identify quotes, although, at times, it is not too difficult for others who have been involved to recognise – or think they recognise – individuals. In a subsequent letter to me Hugh commented, 'I was a "nurse" when you first saw me and asked for consent to interview; now you are asking me for consent to publish as a "fellow researcher" who (hopefully) has knowledge of the research process and can now give "informed consent".'

In many of the research situations which we encounter, however, to return to respondents to request further permission may constitute an imposition in their eyes and may undermine their faith in the research process – is it our respondents or ourselves that we are trying to reassure? Individuals will differ with regard to which situations they consider to merit renegotiation of the research bargain and it can be difficult, as a researcher, to get this balance right. Further, it may be hard to discuss such matters in the abstract and respondents may only become aware that a shift has taken place once material appears in print.

William Foote Whyte (1958, cited by Brettell 1993: 13) commented, 'There is a difference between public knowledge which circulates from mouth to mouth in the village and the same stories which appear in print.' Brettell (1993) reflects on the role of the press in drawing attention to published work and amplifying concerns about the accuracy or 'reasonableness' of research accounts on the part of participants or representatives of groups which have been the subject of study.

As researchers, we devote considerable energy to anticipating the reactions of our potential readership, whether it is the press, society at large, among colleagues or, indeed, our respondents. It is, of course, possible to test audience reaction, and 'member validation techniques' constitute an attempt to harness the critical power of our respondents to strengthen the rigour of our analyses. As Bloor (1997) points out, enthusiasm for member validation has been subject to wild swings in popularity as qualitative research fashions come and go. There are several approaches to respondent validation (described by Bloor 1997) and there is a continuum with regard to the extent of respondents' proposed involvement: we may ask them to comment on the accuracy of transcripts but continue to privilege the researcher's interpretation over respondents' (Brettell 1993); we may elicit their input in terms of commenting on our emergent analyses in broad terms or in detail; or we may seek to involve them in collaborative writing projects.

Emerson and Pollner suggest that, rather than using member validation to arrive at a 'final, determinate version of . . . members' perspectives', it is of value in that it allows us to study the ways in which members 'interpret, use or abuse a researcher's version', thus revealing a setting 'in new depth and dimension' (Emerson and Pollner 1988: 190). The approach which they advocate is, thus, a variant of 'returning to the field', incorporating respondents' reactions as new data which give the researcher further opportunity to explore and amend his/her emergent theories or explanations. This is, in some ways, similar to the injunction not to worry about upsetting events as 'It's all data', or 'There's a paper in there!' (Rosaline Barbour and Guro Huby, Chapter 15). Valuable though such further fieldwork may potentially be, it is important not to underestimate the impact for the researcher of exposing emergent and often hard-won embryonic insights to others who are unlikely to share his/her disciplinary or theoretical concerns. As Bloor observes,

> . . . aspects of the research which the researcher feels to be of relatively minor importance may be dragged centre-stage by the member, while the researcher's supposed central topic is disregarded.
>
> (Bloor 1997: 45)

Talking here of audience reaction to a body of published papers, Emerson and Pollner comment:

> . . . some of the most vitriolic criticism we received in the County presentation seemed to be in response to a paper we had *not* written.
>
> (Emerson and Pollner 1988: 191; my emphasis)

This suggests that, when recruited to comment on our transcripts or emergent analyses, respondents may be equally selective and may react to inferences which exist only in the eye of the beholder – and an individual beholder at that. Although we may be subject to injunctions to explore the possibilities of 'member validation' – at least when it is in fashion – there is relatively little guidance about how to make sense of and act upon respondents' reactions, even assuming that they assent to our overtures. Respondent may simply not be interested in collaborating with us to produce an account of the research process. Writing is a skilled activity and research participants may not have the necessary skills. Although we may aspire to the ideal of an equal partnership, this may be unrealistic. Indeed, respondents may mistrust our motives. Katie Deverell (Chapter 7) reports that her respondents' reservations in declining her invitation to join her in a collaborative writing project centred on the suspicion that she was seeking to 'control' them. Certainly, one of our aims in pursuing 'member validation', on which most attempts at collaborative writing are implicitly based, is to render participants' objections 'manageable' by incorporating them into our analyses and resulting text.

Interestingly, Emerson and Pollner (1988: 191) refer to the requirements made of respondents in reading draft papers as 'homework'. This is an apt description for what is involved of participants in all attempts at 'member valida-tion' and suggests that such requests may be something of an imposition. Asking those who have taken part in our interviews to read whole transcripts not only makes considerable demands on their time; it also raises ethical issues. It is one thing to provide an account in a one-to-one setting, but another thing altogether to see one's own experience graphically presented in black and white.

CONSTRUCTING THE 'OTHER'

The task of the ethnographer operating in his/her own society is frequently seen as making the familiar strange. S/he 'finds weighty significance in the apparently most trivial of scenes and activities' (Atkinson 1990: 165).

> No doubt some of the opprobrium heaped on sociological discourse reflects actual readers' sense of exclusion: they are constructed as naïve or mistaken outsiders by the text's contrastive rhetoric.
>
> (Atkinson 1990: 166)

In thus problematising the mundane under our sociological 'gaze', we also risk 'exoticising' or even 'ghettoising' our respondents. Rosaldo (cited by Brettell 1993: 16) comments that anthropological writing may seem 'parodic' rather than 'perceptive'. Concern about this potential danger was at the root of my difficul-ties in deciding how to incorporate into my analysis a particular story which I had uncovered in my research:

> *I was told several versions of a story about a client who was not too bright and who supple-mented her meagre income 'on the game'. She told a worker that she had also been removing coins from the gas meter installed in her flat. She had told a worker that she had evaded detection by providing sexual favours to the 'gas man', who came to read the meter. The punchline, however, is that her flat was all-electric.*

Like Clive Foster (Chapter 9), I do not intend to question the veracity of this tale. It may well, like many good stories, have a large grain of truth in it. The incident may actually have occurred and been considered too good a story not to pass on to other workers in the field. I hesitated to use this example, though, because I had been told this story as if each of my respondents had direct contact with the client concerned and thus, in its mode of telling, it bore one of the main characteristics of an 'urban myth'. I felt that to use this story as an example of an 'urban myth' would constitute a violation of the trust placed in me by the respondents who presented this information to me 'in good faith'. There was, of course, the option – which I did not take – of challenging respondents in the course of the interview or conversation in the field (see Guro Huby, Chapter 10).

I had, several years previously, made the mistake of pointing out to a friend of mine that the story he had just recounted to me was an 'urban myth'. He had told me of a friend of a friend whose grandmother died during a family outing, whose body was then wrapped in a carpet and tied to the roof rack of the family car to be returned home and thereby save considerable time and expense with regard to funeral arrangements. When the family stopped at a service station on their return journey, however, they returned to the car park to find that their vehicle – complete with deceased grandmother – had been stolen. My friend's reaction to my revelation was very far removed from the rueful gratitude which I had anticipated and I had to wait for some considerable time before he again trusted me with such intimate information.

Mindful of the unexpected hostility which my earlier attempt to share my sociological insights had occasioned – and reasoning that the uncovering of 'urban myths' was not a central concern of my research – I chose not to use this example in any of my dissemination sessions, conference presentations or published papers. Instead I used other examples to illustrate the 'picaresque' stories recounted by AIDS workers who found themselves in close contact with individuals from sectors of society very different from those in which they themselves socialised. Amongst these were comments which also contained analysis:

> We have a laugh sometimes . . . we don't mean it – it's a way of coping. It's the stories some of the drug users come in with. I mean, you just think, it's such a waste, really, they're incredible some of the things they tell you. They're so sharp – in other circumstances some would have made great lawyers.
>
> (Social worker – AIDS unit)

Like the drug users studied by Clive Foster (Chapter 9), 'my' AIDS workers also engaged in storytelling and these stories served similar functions for them in terms of making sense of their work and the place of this in their lives. Workers' stories took a number of accessible and popular forms including 'cautionary' tales, 'picaresque' tales, 'mysterious' tales, 'inspirational' tales, horror stories, humorous stories and 'urban myths'.

Both workers and clients engage in the telling of 'mysterious' tales. Workers in a number of settings spoke – tentatively at first, but with increasing enthusiasm – of individuals they had come across who remained seronegative 'against all the odds': for example, someone who was a long-term injecting drug user, had habitually shared needles, had unsafe sex, and had at least one previous sexual partner who had since died of AIDS.

I also collected a number of 'cynical' stories which questioned the motivation of workers in the HIV/AIDS field:

I feel that a lot of study days and counselling courses that people go on, they mention so much these days about burnout and stress and how people should cope with this . . . nurses . . . often take it on board too seriously, I think. . . . So many people these days say to you, 'Don't be frightened to show emotion', and, to me, it's not everybody that likes to show emotion when a patient dies or if they're in a stressful situation. But now I get this impression that they feel they've got to show emotion and be as open as that. . . . Sadly, some of the emotion I have seen [here] I have not always been convinced that it's genuine emotion.

(Charge nurse – specialist AIDS unit)

In examples such as the one above, workers are taking advantage of the relatively safe arena of the research interview to say things which they might not say to colleagues, who might well take a dim view of their 'de-bunking' of professional orthodoxies. Of course, sociology is the 'de-bunking' profession *par excellence* and interviewees may simply have been playing to a willing audience and telling the researcher what they knew she would love to hear. Perhaps our respondents have been quicker to understand and seize the opportunities offered by the essentially collaborative nature of the construction of knowledge than we ourselves have been, despite our theorising and posturing.

SELECTION AND PRESENTATION OF MATERIAL

Our research task may be to recount and examine the mundane, but when selecting quotes for presentation we tend to opt for those which, although typical in some respects, make the point more vividly, succinctly or humorously than do others in our store.
As Edmondson explains:

If . . . we regard such citations as rhetorical devices for enabling and encouraging readers to preceive the force of general remarks, we can expect examples to exhibit particularly concentrated cases of what happens generally but, perhaps, less remarkably.

(Edmondson 1984: 50)

We thus use the atypical to highlight the typical. Fine judgement is required and we do not always get it right. In selecting quotes for presentation to one's own professional peer group, however, one is usually on firmer ground. The reading of a common literature, ongoing engagement in theroetical debates and past informal sessions with colleagues in the bar have enabled us to 'tune in' to the same wavelength and give us a ready feel for what is likely to be appreciated. It is much harder to select appropriate examples, excerpts or quotes for other audiences, who may be unsympathetic with regard to both the form (viewing our enterprise as 'anecdotal' or 'journalistic') and content (seeing our examples as sensationalist, unkind or indicative of an 'unhealthy' or prurient interest). Despite a plethora of methods texts which advise us on the mechanics of assigning coding categories and building up theoretical constructs through our data analysis, there is little practical guidance available on choosing examples for our oral and written presentations. In many respects the selection of such materials for presentation is a matter of 'taste', with all the gradations and subtleties which this implies.

The craft of writing, however, can obscure as well as reveal:

> [In these traditional texts] the researcher proves his or her credentials in the introductory or methods section and writes the body of the text as though the quotations and document snippets are naturally there, genuine evidence for the case being made, rather than selected, pruned and spruced up for their textual appearance.
>
> (Richardson 1994: 520)

By contrast, we are unlikely to devote as much time or energy to 'sprucing up' quotes from our respondents as we do to perfecting our own prose. In our published texts we strive for cogent arguments and elegant structure; however, by contrast, we generally take pride in leaving the utterances of our respondents untouched, quoting them verbatim, frozen for ever in the inarticulacy brought about by our imperfect questions and need for on-the spot answers.

> In our postmodernist efforts to use the voice of 'the other' by quoting directly, we may in fact open ourselves to more criticism than when we embed what particular respondents tell us in generalities.
>
> (Brettell 1993: 7)

There is, however, no easy answer. Horowitz describes how he sought to edit a respondent's account, feeling that the verbal style employed might lead readers to doubt this individual's integrity. Having presented his respondent with the amended draft for approval, this was returned with the quotes rather uncannily – given that only the researcher was in possession of the recorded interview – restored to those preserved on the tape. Horowitz was still not certain that he had gone far enough in his efforts to rectify the situation, wondering 'if I should have argued with Bill [respondent] about how his precision might read, how the robotic time markers might make him look bad' (Horowitz 1993: 141).

In some situations, we may use respondents' narratives in a relatively straightforward way to describe their experience. In other situations, however, we are inclined to search for significance in the seemingly unproblematic and this is, perhaps one of the hallmarks or 'occupational traits' (Barbour 1987) of the sociologist. Nevertheless – and, perhaps, as a result of our concern to engage dialogically with those whom we research – we have recently had to be reminded of the need to avoid taking respondents' accounts at face value (Atkinson 1996). Although we may no longer be dwelling on the specifics of our respondent's life and experiences in this venture, we are now taking his/her confidences and treating them not as a story which is interesting in its own right, but as an example

of a specific (sociological or anthropological) phenomenon in which we are interested. It is perhaps not surprising that our respondents may be offended and feel
that we have breached the contract they believe us to have made with them
whereby we have promised to 'tell their story'; for now, what we are telling is our
own story. Strathern argues:

> However much multiple authorship is acknowledged, using people's experi-
> ences to make statements about matters of anthropological interest in the end
> subordinates them to the uses of the discipline.
>
> (Strathern 1987: 289)

ENGAGING WITH THE 'OTHER'

Ethnographies are written with particular audiences in mind and reflect the
presumptions carried by authors regarding the attitudes, expectations and back-
grounds of their intended readers (van Maanen 1988: 5). These expectations are
thrown into sharp focus when our reports are read, or accessed, by others for
whom they were not originally intended. In the course of my research I gave
presentations at AIDS conferences (attended by a wide range of interested
parties, including health and social care workers, representatives of voluntary
organisations, pressure groups, individuals with HIV/AIDS, service planners,
managers and academic researchers), medical sociology conferences, seminars
organised by the Medical Research Council (who had funded my research),and
dissemination sessions (attended mainly by my respondents, other workers whom
I had not interviewed, policy-makers and other interested parties). Although
these different fora provided a challenge in terms of pitching my material, I had
not considered some of the wider implications for the social construction of
knowledge, agency and representation.

I was forced to confront some of these issues, however, when I was presenting
a paper at a medical sociology conference and realised, with a sense of generalised rather than focused unease, that Hugh Masters was amongst my audience.
By this stage, Hugh was studying for an M.Phil. at Edinburgh University. As he
explains (in Chapter 5) his research interests had grown out of his involvement as
a practitioner and he was now a member of my own professional peer group.
However, he was also one of my respondents and it was this identity which was
uppermost in my mind, as I hurriedly considered how he was likely to receive
my presentation.

Marcus and Fischer (1986) have highlighted the importance of our native and
potentially critical readership. Indigenous or native scholars are often our
harshest critics: 'The number of so-called native or indigenous anthropologists is
increasing and, aside from the ethnographic work that they produce, they are
writing about their particular problems and perspectives on fieldwork in their
own society and of their relationship with the larger global anthropological
community' (Brettell 1993: 14).

I did not read the above book until some time after the encounter which I describe here, and I doubt whether these comments would have comforted me at the time. With the benefit of hindsight, both Hugh and I consider that we have learnt something from this chance event. As Clandinin and Connelly (1994) have observed, life and method are inextricably intertwined.

Looking back, Hugh tells me that it had not occurred to him at the time that attending my conference presentation presented any problems and he had come along purely out of interest – and for a 9.30am slot on a Sunday morning at that! He does recall, however, that he was late in arriving and that, as I looked across the room at him, he did sense that I was uncomfortable about his presence.

Although I had presented my findings to Hugh on a previous occasion, this had been at one of the dissemination sessions which formed part of my project. My intention, on this occasion, however, was rather different and I wanted to use this short presentation and the ensuing discussion as an opportunity for trying out emergent ideas. My paper for the medical sociology conference was rather grandly entitled 'The discourse of disclosure in AIDS work'. I was claiming academic credibility through using a shared sociological vocabulary (Richardson 1994) whilst simultaneously looking for help to illuminate the concepts with which I was still wrestling. The paper built on an earlier paper I had written (Barbour 1994) – and presented at an AIDS conference – on confidentiality, which showed that, although it was held up as a ideal, it was quite difficult to put into practice, given certain structural and organisational features of AIDS-related work. The 'new' paper compared lay and professional views of confidentiality and pointed out that the receipt of confidences from clients may be a source of considerable professional pride for workers. Clients may, in turn, exploit this 'professional vanity', embellishing and contradicting their stories, with the result of exacerbating professional and interpersonal rivalries. (Indeed, as Guro Huby, Chapter 10, suggests, they may also do this to researchers.) I then went on to point out that confidentiality is, by its very nature, largely invisible, being in the eye of the 'withholder'. The part of the paper which still needed a lot of work was the section on the rewards which staff derived from their 'confidence work'. I quoted an interviewee who told me:

> . . . it's changed me in a way that nothing I've ever known in the past [has]. People trust you with their most incredible confidences – part of themselves.
>
> (Charge nurse – specialist AIDS unit)

I also began to explore the possible potential for illuminating my data by looking at parallels between 'confidences' and 'secrets', suggesting that a comment made by Georg Simmel about secrets might also shed light on the satisfaction that AIDS workers derived from the trust placed in them by clients:

> Since the others are excluded from the possession, the converse suggests itself psychologically, namely, that what is denied to many must have special value.
>
> (Simmel 1969: 332)

I was not, of course, suggesting that confidentiality and secrecy were synonymous, but felt rather uncomfortable about my suggestions that AIDS workers derived pleasure from the often upsetting revelations made by clients. In my previous AIDS conference presentations and in the dissemination sessions I had tried to locate myself, if not as an insider, then at least as someone who was sympathetic to the concerns of staff and who wanted to contribute towards arguing a case for better support provision, and greater recognition of the difficulties caused by particular organisational structures. Patricia Hill Collins (1990, cited by Denzin 1994: 503) comments on the use of the pronoun 'we' to embed rather than distance oneself from the subjects of one's study. On occasion, I had done so myself in earlier presentations, in order to soften some of the apparent criticisms I made of the way in which AIDS organisations were structured and in order to denote sympathy for the difficulties involved in addressing these issues. This time, though, my own professional peer group were the implicit 'we' of my text and my respondents had become the explicit 'they'. If I had previously been granted permission to make critical comments and poke mild fun at some of the workers' comments as a member – albeit it, a marginal one – of the group I was studying and reporting back to, I was now no longer laughing *with* respondents, but laughing *at* them.

During the discussion which followed my paper Hugh was quick to point out that I should beware of conflating confidentiality and secrecy and that AIDS workers were very clear about the difference between the two. He was, of course, quite right, although his tone at the time suggested to me that he was perhaps a little offended by my observations and I felt that, as I had feared, he had possibly not accepted my comments in the spirit in which they were intended. Subsequent conversations with Hugh about this occurrence have confirmed that he remembers making this comment and that he thought he reacted to it because the staff at Milestone House 'had a bee in our bonnets about being clear about the difference between confidentiality and secrecy' at that time. Had Hugh and I not been engaged in the collaborative venture of the current collection, however, I doubt whether these conversations would ever have taken place.

CONCLUSION

Students are trained to observe, listen, question and participate. Yet they are trained to conceptualize writing as 'writing up' the research, rather than as a method of discovery. Almost unthinkingly, qualitative research training validates the mechanistic model of writing, even though that model shuts down the creativity and sensibilities of the individual researcher.

(Richardson 1994: 517)

In this chapter I have argued that we need to engage analytically with the assumptions and conventions which structure both our written work and oral presentations. Employing reflexivity as a method of discovery affords valuable insights into the social processes through which the products of the research enterprise are constructed. I have shown that such an approach allows us to explore both the politics and the practicalities of the research bargains which we strike with respondents; the reciprocities involved in these exchanges; the sharing of insights and interpretations; the social construction of the subjects and themes of our study; the selection and presentation of material; and our engagement with those who participate in our research.

With Richardson (1994), I would argue that we must take pains to ensure that we do not shut down our 'creativity and sensibility'. However, there is a danger that we will be immobilised by the myriad possibilities and implications of extending reflexivity in the ways advocated here. Notwithstanding the spiralling of interpretations which may result from directing our 'gaze' at our own academic products, we must ensure that we are not discouraged from making a start in terms of trying to make sense of the data we have elicited. We can always return to our texts and rework them later.

> Analysing interviews [and, I would add, data collected using other methods] presents a critical methodological challenge. . . . However, if we allow all possible objections to cause us to doubt the status and utility of the data, the chances are that we would not undertake research at all. Notwithstanding the philosophical debates from Wittgenstein to the post-moderns, if we are going to tell a story, we have to be less epistemologically squeamish and get on with it.
>
> (Melia 1997: 30)

ACKNOWLEDGEMENTS

I am grateful to the Medical Research Council for providing funding for the study which is discussed here and to my co-grantholder, Sally Macintyre, and other colleagues at the MRC Medical Sociology Unit in Glasgow for many stimulating discussions about doing AIDS research.

REFERENCES

Aldridge, J. (1993) 'The textual disembodiment of knowledge in research account writing', *Sociology (Special Issue: Auto/Biography in Sociology)*, 27(1): 53–66.

Atkinson, P. (1990) *The Ethnographic Imagination: Textual Constructions of Reality*, London: Routledge.

—— (1996) 'Narrative turn or blind alley? Reflections on narrative and qualitative health research', plenary paper presented at the Third International Interdisciplinary Qualitative Health Research Conference, University of Bournemouth, 30 October–1 November.

Barbour, R.S. (1987) 'The irritating sociologist: notes towards defining an occupational stereotype', in N.P. McKeganey and S. Cunningham-Burley (eds) *Enter the Sociologist*, Aldershot: Avebury.

—— (1993) '"I don't sleep with my patients – Do you sleep with yours?": Dealing with staff tensions and conflicts in AIDS-related work', in P. Aggleton, P. Davies and G. Hart (eds) *AIDS: Facing the Second Decade*, London: Falmer.

—— (1994) 'A telling tale: AIDS workers and confidentiality', in P. Aggleton, P. Davies and G. Hart (eds) *AIDS: Foundations for the Future*, London: Taylor & Francis.

—— (1995) 'The implications of HIV/AIDS for a range of workers in the Scottish context', *AIDS Care*, 7(4): 521–5.

Bloor, M. (1983) 'Notes on member validation', in R.M. Emerson (ed.) *Contemporary Field Research: A Collection of Readings*, Boston: Little, Brown.

—— (1997) 'Techniques of validation in qualitative research: a critical commentary', in G. Miller and R. Dingwall (eds) *Context and Method in Qualitative Research*, London: Sage.

Brettell, C.B. (1993) 'Introduction: Fieldwork, text and audience', in C.B. Brettell (ed.) *When They Read What We Write: The Politics of Ethnography*, Westport, CT and London: Bergin & Garvey.

Clandinin, D.J. and Connelly, F.M. (1994) 'Personal experience methods', in N.K. Denzin and Y.S. Lincoln (eds) *Handbook of Qualitative Research*, London: Sage.

Collins, P.H. (1990) *Black Feminist Thought, Knowledge, Consciousness and the Politics of Empowerment*, New York: Routledge.

Davis, M.S. (1971) 'That's interesting! Towards a phenomenology of sociology and a sociology of phenomenology', *Philosophy of the Social Sciences*, 1: 309–44.

Denzin, N.K. (1994) 'The art and politics of interpretation', in N.K. Denzin and Y.S. Lincoln (eds) *Handbook of Qualitative Research*, London: Sage.

Edmondson, R. (1984) *Rhetoric in Sociology*, London: Macmillan.

Emerson, R.M. and Pollner, M. (1988) 'On the uses of members' responses to researchers' accounts', *Human Organization*, 47(3): 189–98.

Horowitz, R.P. (1993) 'Just stories of ethnographic authority', in C.B. Brettell (ed.) *When They Read What We Write: The Politics of Ethnography*, Westport, CT and London: Bergin & Garvey.

Hughes, C.C. (1992) '"Ethnography": What's in a word – process? product? promise?', *Qualitative Health Research*, 2(4): 439–50.

Johnson, A. (1996) '"It's good to talk": The focus group and the sociological imagination', *Sociological Review*, 44(3): 517–38.

McBeth, S. (1993) 'Myths of objectivity and the collaborative process in life history research', in C.B. Brettell (ed.) *When They Read What We Write: The Politics of Ethnography*, Westport, CT and London: Bergin & Garvey.

Marcus, G.E. and Fischer, M.M.J. (1986) *Anthropology as Cultural Critique: An Experimental Moment in the Human Sciences*, Chicago: University of Chicago Press.

Melia, K.M. (1997) 'Producing "plausible stories": Interviewing student nurses', in G. Miller and R. Dingwall (eds) *Context and Method in Qualitative Research*, London: Sage.

Morse, J.M. (ed.) (1994) *Critical Issues in Qualitative Research Methods*, London: Sage.

Munhall, P. (1988) 'Ethical considerations in qualitative research', *Western Journal of Nursing Research*, 10(2): 150–62.

Richardson, L. (1994) 'Writing: a method of inquiry', in N.K. Denzin and Y.S. Lincoln (eds) *Handbook of Qualitative Research*, London: Sage.

Rock, P. (1979) *The Making of Symbolic Interactionism*, London: Macmillan.

Schutz, A. (1972) *The Phenomenology of the Social World*, London: Heineman.

Sheehan, E.A. (1993) 'The student of culture and the ethnography of Irish intellectuals', in C.B. Brettell (ed.) *When They Read What We Write: The Politics of Ethnography*, Westport, CT and London: Bergin & Garvey.

Simmel, G. (1969) *The Sociology of Georg Simmel*, K.H. Wolff (trans. and ed.), New York: Free Press.

Strathern, M. (1987) 'An awkward relationship: the case of feminism and anthropology', *SIGNS: Journal of Women in Culture and Society*, 12(2): 276–92.

Tierney, W.G. (1995) '(Re)presentation and voice', *Qualitative Inquiry*, 1(4): 379–90.

van Maanen, J. (1988) *Tales of the Field: On Writing Ethnography*, Chicago: University of Chicago Press.

Whyte, W.F. (1958) 'Editorial', *Human Organization*, 17(2): 1–2.

Chapter 12

Carrying out HIV-related research in an area of low prevalence
Issues for researcher and researched

Cathy Stark

INTRODUCTION

This chapter is based on experiences of carrying out research for my Ph.D. thesis. The research focused on the experiences of seventeen informal carers who were looking after a family member with HIV-related illness in the north of England. This simple statement belies the immense difficulties inherent in bringing that sample together and belittles the issues that arose for myself, in the role of interviewer, and the carers, in the role of interviewees. Some of the problems experienced in 1990 at the time when the interviews were being set up were a product of that time and the situation may have changed since then.

The chapter begins by examining the problems I experienced in gaining access into the field and collecting a sample in an area of low prevalence. It then looks at issues which are pertinent to both the interviewer and interviewees – the interview itself, interpretation of what is recorded, and confidentiality.

COLLECTING THE SAMPLE: ACCESS TO THE FIELD

The north of England is an area of low prevalence as far as AIDS diagnoses are concerned. In 1990 when the interviews were being set up there were 83 people in the North East living with AIDS[1] and 357 were known to have HIV. These figures compare quite dramatically to regions such as North West Thames, where 1544 people were living with AIDS in 1990 and 4682 were known to have the HIV virus. How many of these people were in contact with organisations and therefore 'contactable' remains unknown.

Low prevalence was associated with problems I had in recruiting a sample and also impacted on the material I collected. It probably contributed to practitioners' and professionals' concerns about confidentiality and exposure of clients. Moreover, if carers felt they might be identified, this might have prevented them from reporting negative feelings about the organisations to which they were attached. Low prevalence also exacerbated problems of clients being 'over-researched' and staff complaining of 'research fatigue'.

The low prevalence and high visibility of HIV contrasted sharply with the high number of carers for chronically ill people and the invisibility of their plight. The General Household Survey of 1985 (Green 1988) revealed that there were 6 million people in this country who provided varying amounts of informal care to disabled, ill or elderly relatives and friends. For many of them life as a carer is a long hard 'daily grind' (Bayley 1973). Carers are a largely hidden population. They are attached to the confines of the home by virtue of their caring role and many will have neither the time nor the energy to question their circumstances. They remain thus an invisible, unrecognised and undervalued resource. This research was attempting to contact carers of people with HIV so I was aware of the difficulties this would entail.

It is well acknowledged that HIV-related illness is a condition that attracts prejudice, stigma and blame and it is not surprising that many people with HIV are cautious about disclosing their antibody status. Carers of people with HIV can sometimes be put in a difficult position fearing the consequences of disclosure for themselves, their loved ones and their families. The result is a group of people who are extremely difficult to contact. The secrecy about the seropositive status of dependants maintained by some of the carers interviewed for this study bears witness to these worries (Stark, 1995).

The following three carers held back from telling the neighbours in their respective villages about their dependants' AIDS diagnosis:

> To be honest I don't want to say anything because I'd be worried about the backlash. This is one of the reasons we haven't really got involved . . . people here know he's seriously ill but probably think its leukaemia. But I've no problem telling other folk because the more its out the closet the easier it becomes.
>
> (Stark 1995: 71)

> We live in a village and it's a bit like a goldfish bowl and we want [him] to come and people to accept him. He would tell people if they asked but I'd rather it came from him, not me. One friend asked if he was HIV but I wouldn't tell her because it wasn't really my place to say.
>
> (Stark 1995: 71)

> Friends and family know [about HIV] but people in the village don't. If people don't understand then that's their problem. But it's for [Paul's] sake. He's well known in the village. It gives him somewhere safe to come home too. He's suffered enough.
>
> (Stark 1995: 71)

The following quote illustrates the carer's philosophy that it is better to say as little as possible, although such an approach raises questions about isolation and lack of support for carers.

> I think I've protected myself because there's very few people who know.
>
> (Stark 1995: 71)

CONTACTING CARERS

Apart from the problems occasioned by carers of someone with HIV-related illness deliberately concealing their status, a number of other factors made contact difficult. Firstly, all the carers who were eventually contacted were attached to some type of organisation. This inevitably makes for a biased sample as there was no way of contacting more isolated carers, whose experiences may have differed from those recruited. The workers at these places were anxious to protect their clients. In light of the stigma associated with AIDS it is not surprising that staff were extremely cautious and their primary concern was to protect already vulnerable people from further upset and strain.

Secondly, the response of organisations to my request for help in recruiting my sample was clearly affected by other things which were going on at the time. A social worker at one of the organisations approached stated that the organisation was suffering from 'research fatigue' and they were disinclined to become involved in any other research projects. Whilst staff are clearly concerned about clients, and demands on their own time, such reasoning may also serve to protect themselves and their organisations which are frequently engaged in territorial disputes with other agencies.

At the time when the sample was being collected, the local AIDS organisations seemed very territorial and competitive and their relatively short history had been turbulent. Individuals becoming disillusioned with one organisation would set up or form allegiances with another. Being associated with one organisation could mean being looked upon with suspicion by another. Teething problems in voluntary organisations are nothing new. It seems that the growth of an organisation can result in changes at all levels and the necessity to change as the organisation grows may be seen by some as losing its *raison d'être*. The mid- to late 1980s to early 1990s were a time of flux for local AIDS organisations in the north of England and the research was in some ways caught up in those transitions.

However, a number of ways were explored in the attempt to contact carers, some of which proved blind, others of which were successful to varying degrees. The three main routes through which contact with carers was attempted are explored below.

Through contacts with a voluntary organisation, support for the research was found via the Family Support Group Co-ordinator, who initially approached members of the group on my behalf. This proved very successful. I was already involved in a voluntary capacity with this organisation and this greatly facilitated accessing carers. However, this may also have worked against me whilst trying to access carers from another local organisation.

The north of England is fortunate in having a well-established haemophilia centre. People with haemophilia were hit hard by the rise of HIV and staff at the centre have lost a great number of patients through AIDS.

Members of staff in Haemophilia Centres will have known their patients for many years, and many have been present at the births and marriages of people now dying from AIDS.

(Jones 1989: 19)

Because of the close relationship of patients and staff in the centre, losing people to AIDS has obviously had a great impact on them. There is the additional problem that the treatment given by the staff was the route of their HIV infection. However, Jones describes the continuation of good staff–patient relationships in one haemophilia centre:

> It is salutary to find that it is the sense of humour and friendship of those who have lost relatives because of contamination of their treatment that helps support staff who prescribed it.

(Jones 1989: 119)

Staff at the centre were extremely wary about volunteering carers for the research until they were convinced that the interviews would be handled well and that the carers would not be caused any unnecessary upset. Their paramount concern was, quite rightly, to protect already vulnerable people and, because of this, negotiations with the haemophilia centre demanded far more time and sensitivity than any of the other routes. Eventually carers were recruited through the centre's Bereavement Support Group.

The situation at another local hospital was very different. Having contacted the appropriate doctor at this hospital, a meeting was arranged to discuss the project. However, the means of contacting the carers suggested by the hospital proved too indirect and oblique a route and ultimately proved unsuccessful. The need to protect the confidentiality of the patients was the main stumbling block and one which was again difficult to overcome.

Despite the problems involved in collecting this sample, it is personally reassuring to know that no one who took part in the interviews was pressurised into doing so.

These practical issues in gaining access to participants highlight a number of other concerns around research in this area: firstly, the ethics of eliciting data on sensitive topics from individuals who may well be vulnerable; secondly, how to ensure that the data elicited are an accurate reflection of the interviewees' experiences; thirdly, representation and interpretation of the interviewees' perspective; fourthly, the confidentiality of respondents. In all these areas the contrast between the highly 'visible' concerns around stigma and confidentiality with regard to HIV and the 'invisibility' of the day-to-day work of carers was an issue.

ETHICS

There has been a growing interest in recent years around the area of 'sensitive research' (for example, the edited collection by Renzetti and Lee [1993]) and the ethics of carrying out research into such areas. HIV is one such 'sensitive' research area and it is a topic charged with emotion, loaded with moral meanings and carrying a burden of stigma. The question of whether sensitive research should be carried out may be answered in terms of the benefits of doing the research. However, as MacIntyre (1982) points out, there is no consensus among social scientists about what counts as a benefit. Researchers generally have greater power than those researched to define the costs and benefits. For MacIntyre,

> The study of taboos by anthropologists and of privacy by sociologists show how important it is for a culture that certain areas of personal and social life should be specially protected. Intimacy cannot exist where everything is disclosed, sanctuary cannot be sought where no place is inviolate, integrity cannot be seen to be maintained – and therefore in certain cases be maintained – without protection from illegitimate pressures.
>
> (MacIntyre 1982: 188)

Renzetti and Lee (1993) point out that empirical studies of researchers' ethical decision-making are surprisingly lacking and suspect that relatively few researchers desist from research because the costs involved outweigh the benefits, or because, as MacIntyre states, it is not morally acceptable to do wrong to anyone through infringing on privacy. However, areas of social life are 'hidden' for a variety of reasons and the pros and cons must be carefully considered in each case where one contemplates attempting to increase knowledge through research. In defence of researching sensitive topics, Sieber and Stanley have argued:

> Sensitive research addresses some of society's most pressing social issues and policy questions. Although ignoring the ethical issues in sensitive research is not a responsible approach to science, shying away from controversial topics, simply because they are controversial, is also an avoidance of responsibility.
>
> (Sieber and Stanley 1988: 55)

Renzetti and Lee also point out that permitting research into the private sphere might reveal

> that in many instances, particularly in sensitive areas, research participants desire catharsis rather than sanctuary. That is, research on sensitive topics may produce not only gains in knowledge but also effects that are directly beneficial to research participants.
>
> (Renzetti and Lee 1993: 9)

Indeed, it is easy in an emotive topic such as HIV and AIDS to overlook the mundane, taken-for-granted aspects of the carers' life. These everyday aspects of carers' lives turned out to be equally deserving of research attention as are the more 'sensationalist' topics of HIV and stigma. In amongst all the concern with stigma, contagion and unpredictability of the new disease, the carers of someone with HIV were also dealing with the everyday work of shopping, housework and juggling of responsibilities. Often it was these routine and therefore 'invisible' aspects of caring which made it a 'daily grind' (Bayley 1973). A woman caring for her friend with HIV recounts:

> I gave up an awful lot, I also gave up my family's time too. I'd spend hours there on a weekend and then come home and have piles and piles of washing to do.

> (Stark 1995: 134)

James (1993) has suggested that academic research may be inherently exploitative because it transgresses feelings. This may be the case if the research is not set up or handled well, but the counter-argument to this is that the interview process can become a form of counselling because it allows people to talk about their experiences (see Jill Bourne, Chapter 6, and Neil Small, Chapter 8). It was clear that the carers I interviewed welcomed the opportunity to talk about these aspects of their caring role.

Counselling – a much misused term in itself – suggests a relationship to which both the counsellor and the client bring certain expectations and enter into a type of 'contract' to ensure that these expectations will be realised. An interview seeks out information, and an interview for the purposes of research does not have the overt goal of helping the interviewee. If some good does come out of an interview, perhaps in the form of an advisory report that informs policy, then this is an added bonus but purely secondary to the interview's primary purpose. The role of an interview itself is not to help, change or counsel. Neil Small (in this volume) discusses why people may agree to take part in research and what they may get out of it.

Some carers – most notably those who were isolated or who felt uncomfortable talking in a group situation – did say they found the interview helpful. However, carers need proper support and not the feeling of help which a one-off research interview might provide.

One possible suggestion would be to get the carers to do their own research, to broadcast their own situation and tell their own story. But, in view of carers' heavy and time-consuming workload, this is not a realistic solution to the problem either. A compromise would seem to be to handle interviews as sensitively as possible and to try to ensure that the person is no worse off for having shared their experiences. This necessitates careful management of and reflection upon the interview situation.

ELICITING DATA

It is necessary to have some basic premises from which to work; otherwise an interview would be impossible. The question of preconceived ideas is important here. Because of a person's common-sense assumptions and intellectual agenda, preconceived ideas are inevitable. For me, the question loomed as to whether a focus on certain topics, for example stigma and social support, would influence what the interviewees said about certain aspects of their caring role to the exclusion of others. As Tait (1988) wonders, are the interviewees in some ways 'set up'? The question of whether the experiences of the respondent are accurately interpreted by the researcher is both important and difficult. On a purely practical level, the interview consisted of a schedule of 'areas to be covered', but once the interview was under way it was very much carer-led and carers talked about issues which were important to them. This gave rise to a great deal of information which was not anticipated. One of the strengths of semi-structured in-depth interviewing is that it does allow for the carer to raise issues which were not included in the research schedule.

The interviews were initially designed on the assumption that the stigma of HIV was a main concern for carers and I have questioned whether the interviewees were in some ways 'set up' by my desire to cover certain topics. The respondents, likewise, brought their assumptions to bear on the interview, and they too have some authority to affect what is produced – whether they are aware of this or not. Samuel and Thompson (1990) question where 'myth' comes into the research process. They suggest that 'myth' is vital to understanding social realities because they include feelings and sentiments that drive action and thought. Any recollection of an event will be selective and this is an important 'fact' to note. In this way, the relationship between 'myth' and what are seen as 'factual accounts' becomes a topic of interest. Tonkin suggests that

> Histories are arguments created by people in particular conditions. These conditions include the very social worlds in which they live, and which, by their telling, they model and sometimes seek to alter.
>
> (Tonkin 1990: 29)

Some of the interviews carried out were retrospective in that the carer had lost the person they were caring for to AIDS before the interview. The time the carers had been bereaved varied from five years in the longest case to two or three months for the most recently bereaved. How the carers perceived their role as carers and how they felt about it will doubtless have changed over time.

Taking a 'life history' from the carer may have helped fill in some of these types of gaps, but interest (because of practical constraints) had to be limited to these people's experience of AIDS. Interestingly, however, in the case of the mothers of sons with haemophilia, their stories began with the birth of their sons and their discovery of the condition. Thus quite a detailed picture of life with haemophilia, even before the advent of AIDS, was able to be built up, giving a much more complete picture of where caring and HIV fitted into the lives of the interviewees. That the mothers of sons with haemophilia began their accounts of caring long before the rise of HIV illustrates that for them HIV may represent a continuation of a caring role, rather than the development of a new identity as a carer.

Peneff (1990) suggests that when recounting their life stories (especially rags to riches stories) people are often selective in their telling, let themselves off lightly (shameful behaviour is seldom recalled) and sometimes 'fantasy' and 'reality' become mixed up. It becomes appropriate to suggest that in recounting their experiences of caring, the carers may have been themselves unconsciously affected by 'myths' surrounding HIV and that these had had an impact on their response to their situation. *All* the carers had guarded against backlash by being careful to whom and how they disclosed their situation. However, very few of the carers had experienced any actual stigma. Those who had not were surprised (and relieved) that this was the case.

A young carer who looked after her brother had initially been extremely careful about whom she told. She explained that at the time that her brother disclosed his diagnosis, she had heard many stories of discrimination against people with AIDS and did not wish her brother to experience this. She was also anxious about how the family might react to news of her brother's illness. However, as time passed and the close family learnt of her brother's diagnosis and were supportive of him, she became less anxious about possible backlash and re-evaluated her opinions about potential discrimination

> I don't think people are as bad as most of the world think they are these days. I don't think they'd take it as bad as some people think.
>
> (Stark 1995: 181)

None the less, they were all aware that it was possible and that they should take precautions to prevent it. It is impossible to say how widespread stigma against carers, their families and their dependants would be because no one would expect the carers to put themselves out on a limb to find out. There are plenty of anecdotes that suggest AIDS and stigma go hand in hand and this is enough to cause people to act accordingly.

In my study, one carer recounted the story of another carer, also interviewed for the study, with whom she had become acquainted through visiting the haemophilia centre. Whilst recounting the story of the other carer, the woman explained how relieved she was that she had not been hounded by the press and how sorry she felt that her acquaintance had been. The carer who had been 'hounded' by the press described to me how this felt and how she had been afraid to leave her house in case of backlash. However, when she did venture out of the house she had been relieved by how understanding people were.

> When I did go out I'd meet people and they'd say 'It's awful.' So they were sympathetic and I had no qualms. I've had no trouble and the people still talk about how good [my husband] was.
>
> (Stark 1995: 175)

Despite her experience of being pestered by the press, she felt herself 'lucky' that she had not experienced backlash from villagers. However, her comments suggested that 'others' would not have been so fortunate.

I've had no trouble at all. Not like some people.

(Stark 1995: 175)

Another carer who had lost a loved one to HIV illness compared herself to others who were 'worse off':

It must be crucifying when it's in the family. One lad had it and passed it on to his wife. And they were worried if they died what the bairns would do and I just thought 'God, you don't realise how lucky you are.'

(Stark 1995: 279)

Some of the problems that carers faced and their responses were very much a product of the social climate of the time. In an area of low prevalence of HIV at a time when misunderstandings about the disease abounded, the question of a person's reaction to stigma, whether real or perceived, takes on added importance. The carers' perception and remembering of events will be affected by these matters. The ever-changing autobiography of the carer is important when considering what is produced.

INTERPRETATION AND REPRESENTATION

Tait (1988), in her study of the experiences of women who had undergone a mastectomy, used her experiences of interviewing one particular woman to look at the mechanisms by which she came to understand the interviewee. She suggests that there are multiple realities inherent in the transcripts.

She goes on to explore how one factor in feeling distanced from the text is in the temporal separation as time has passed since the interviews were carried out and so the immediacy of the transcript has gone, relegated to history. During the analysis the interviewer is always one step removed from it – by writing it *now* one is already removed from the *there and then* – and the researcher is ready with concepts, theories and analysis to 'understand' the data. There is a danger that transcripts could be seen as a 'docile text' (Garfinkel 1967) where they would be used simply as a transcription of what went on, without taking into account the context in which the transcript was 'produced' by the interviewer and interviewee. In order to guard against this it is important – and happily possible – to try to remember how one felt at the time and to try to use those feelings when working at 'understanding' the interviewee's experience. Retrospective reconstruction (or re-presentation of someone else's re-presentation) will, of course, include many factors, feelings from then and now and all those in between. An account was kept of comments on all the interviews, including feelings on them at the time. In some cases a considerable distance was travelled on public transport to visit the carers and, because of the infrequency of the bus services, some time was often spent with the carers after the interview. In all cases the carers were extremely hospitable and the researcher helped them with household tasks or shopping until the bus was due. Often the conversation would come back round to their caring experiences and I wondered whether these extra comments should remain strictly 'off the record' or whether they could be included as part of the interview. Even the most formal of structured interviews generate a great deal of observational data, although these tend to be filtered out as irrelevant. However, from the moment a researcher enters a house to carry out an interview, he or she is seeing as well as listening.

Learning more about a person's circumstances undoubtedly affected the understanding of the taped interview – some comments cast a slightly different light on the way the data were interpreted. For example, one carer spoke about marital difficulties and this illuminated why she was unsupported in her caring role. It also suggested that her role as a carer exacerbated some of the problems at home, and at the same time some problems at home made the caring role more demanding. It gave a fuller context from which to understand what was being said.

The fact that the writing up of the findings is then read by a third party removes them yet again further from its original state. What the researcher believes the carers meant was informed by common-sense assumptions, personal biography and intellectual agenda. In the same way, how a third party, uninvolved in the actual data collection process, responds to the presented interpretation of the data depends in turn on that person's intellectual agenda and common-sense assumptions.

With the passing of time and the growth of one's life experience, one's view of the world changes, as does the way one believes one felt during the interview. Oakley (1981) argues that it is important for the interviewer to invest his or her personal identity in the research. If this is so, then a researcher's own personal biography becomes significant in understanding an interpretation of the data. However, many researchers, including for example Rosaldo (1989), have hesitated to move down this path for a number of reasons.

> Introducing myself into this account requires a certain hesitation both because of the discipline's taboo and because of its frequent violation by essays laced with trendy amalgams of continental philosophy and autobiographical snippets. If classic ethnography's vice was the slippage from the ideal of detachment to actual indifference, that of present day reflexivity is the tendency for the self-absorbed Self to lose sight altogether of the culturally different other.
>
> (Rosaldo 1989: 7)

However, in order to explain how he finally came to understand how rage in grief can impel the Ilongot men to headhunt, Rosaldo felt he had to mention his own experiences. Before losing his wife, he could not fully understand the force of anger possible in bereavement. The death of his wife released in him feelings which he then came to recognise as those experienced by the Ilongot. He then felt in a position to revise his earlier understandings of Ilongot headhunting and focus on the anger and rage that grief provoked.

Rosaldo's 'personal biography' was extremely pertinent to his study of the Ilongot headhunting. My own 'personal biography' is no doubt important in order to understand how the particular knowledge I presented was produced. Shortly after completing the interviews for the Ph.D., I became a mother and then struggled through a long, life-threatening illness. These two events have no doubt influenced how I reinterpreted the stories I was told by the carers. The accounts the mothers told me of bringing up sons with haemophilia and caring for a loved one with a chronic illness featured strongly in my thesis. It was not until I later reflected on this in the methodology chapter that I realised how my own personal biography had influenced what was selected, and this in turn became part of the discussion about presentation and representation of the data.

Many people have debated whether or not the researcher really should invest his/her biography in their research. Geertz (1988), in his book *Works and Lives: The Anthropologist as Author*, argues that it is important to take note of how ethnographic texts are constructed, the role that the anthropologist plays in their construction, and how we, as readers, become convinced of their validity. Geertz suggests that because anthropologists have the ability to convince us that they have actually 'been there' and have penetrated (or been penetrated by) another way of living, we are inclined to accept what (eminent) ethnographers say. When two reputable scholars seem to be contradicting each other, the tendency is to 'regard the problem as stemming from different sorts of minds taking hold of different parts of the elephant'. This emphasises the impact that the researcher can have upon the text which is produced and it is important to document this as a *social* phenomenon rather than an individual experience.

Reflexivity is often dismissed as 'navel gazing' or self-indulgence, but an increasing number of authors have come to recognise that the race, gender, age and personality of the researcher are significant. When returning to the same place and people after months or years, the passage of time will have led to changes in both the researcher and the researched and changing experiences can lead to reinterpretations (see, for example, Okeley and Callaway 1992). Cohen notes that 'interpretation cannot begin from a *tabula rasa*. Rather it must use all the resources of sense making that are available to us' (Cohen 1992: 223). Each person's 'sense making' will be different and dependent on his or her own set of experiences.

As Rosaldo, drawing on the work of Clyde Kluckhohn, noted

> ... eclectic book knowledge and a range of life experiences, along with edifying reading and a self-awareness, supposedly vanquish the twin vices of ignorance and insensitivity.
>
> (Rosaldo 1989: 8)

However, at what point can people say that they have completed their learning or their life experience? Rosaldo draws attention to

> the relative youth of field workers, who, for the most part, have not suffered serious losses and could have, for example, no personal knowledge of how

devastating a loss of a long-term partner can be for the survivor.

(Rosaldo 1989: 9)

Therefore, in my own case, the researcher's remembered understanding of how she felt at the time of interview had no doubt been changed by experiences during the period which had elapsed between interview and analysis.

There are many layers involved in the construction of an account. It is impossible to say that a researcher has reached a 'truth' about something because the truth of one researcher would differ from the truth of another. That in turn would differ from the interviewee's experience and the interpretation made of the account by the reader. In conclusion, then, perhaps Tait's (1988: 37) suggestion that 'What all of us who write produce simply stands as the version of "what went on here"' could be amended to 'What all of us who write produce simply stands as *one* version of "what went on here."'

There are many factors such as time and personal biographies which subconsciously affect what is presented in research writings. However, in the case of HIV where research is carried out in an area of low prevalence, I discovered that additional – and pressing – concerns affected and changed what was produced. Measures had to be taken in order to protect the identity of the interviewees.

RESPECTING CONFIDENTIALITY: PRESENTATION OF THE DATA

In the case of HIV and AIDS, especially in an area of low prevalence, the problem of confidentiality is one which must be taken seriously. An example of the problems arising when matters of confidentiality are not properly addressed is given in a case study by Kimmel (1988). Kimmel recounted the problems of a study carried out by Vidich and Bensman (1958) where the authors failed to disguise the identities of individual participants. The study intended 'to explore the foundations and social life in a community which lacks the power to control the institutions that regulate and determine its existence' (Vidich and Bensman 1958: vii). Before the study was begun, the town's residents were assured by research staff that no individuals would be identified in reports. Prior to its publication some concern was expressed that, whilst individuals had been given fictitious names, certain persons were identifiable by the townsfolk and described in ways that would be damaging to them. This assessment turned out to be prophetic and publication of the study embarrassed members of the town who strongly objected to the descriptions of their leaders despite the attempts to disguise their identities. Indeed the townsfolk's hostility towards the research led them not only to question academic rigour but also to reject the possibility of a follow-up study to redress inaccuracies.

This study was of great interest because, whilst writing up the findings of the research on carers of someone with HIV illness, it was realised that certain measures were necessary in order to avoid similar problems in the present small-scale study of carers in a particular region with low prevalence.

Since the research relied upon key gatekeepers in identifying carers, those individuals, be they staff at the haemophilia centre or workers at a local AIDS organisation, know which people participated in the study. Also, the 'AIDS field' in the north of England was at that time a small closely knit one and those involved in the field tend to know or know of others working in the same field. In some ways it is a case of 'everyone knows everyone else' and so issues surrounding confidentiality become acute.

Confidentiality is a term which is socially constructed and whose meaning is context-dependent (see also Barbour 1994). At one end of the spectrum it may be regarded as synonymous with secrecy. At the other end it may be deemed in the best interest of the person or persons concerned if the information is made available to certain significant others. 'Confidentiality' can mean different things in different contexts. It could mean anonymity in society at large; anonymity in AIDS circles; or in what respondents tell the researcher. 'Confidentiality' will likely mean different things to a Catholic priest in the confessional, a social worker concerned with child protection, and a rape crisis counsellor. In the context of research, findings could never be entirely 'secret' or there would be little point in carrying out the research in the first place.

The problem I had was to be able to use the data in such a way that the carers' identity remained protected. The normal precautions are of course taken – using fictitious names, changing place of residence – and these measures are sufficient to ensure anonymity amongst people outside the AIDS field. However, the majority of people would still be recognisable to colleagues within the AIDS field in this area by virtue of their particular circumstances. Those involved in working with people with HIV-related illness tend to come across the same people. An example will illustrate this. The researcher was expressing concern to a colleague about the problem of anonymity and stated that, for example, the place of residence of an unnamed carer could be changed from Cumbria to Northumberland in order to protect her identity. The colleague's reply was that this particular carer would not pose a problem as she had spoken to the press. He knew who was being referred to because of his own work in the AIDS field and because he knew the person who helped assemble the sample! The second point here is that regardless of whether the carer has spoken to the media since the interview was carried out, at the time of interview she was told that the project was confidential so there was a duty to honour that part of that bargain. However, interviewees may have different understandings of the term.

There were a number of choices which could have been made. Firstly the carers could have been recontacted where possible and the dilemma explained to them. However, at the time I was still working through the problem myself and did not wish to cause them any undue concern. It did not seem appropriate to 'offload' my dilemma on to them. Moreover, because there was a large time lapse between interview and writing up, it did not seem appropriate to recontact them 'out of the blue'. It was also felt that a number of appropriate measures had been taken which would certainly ensure confidentiality to those readers outside the local AIDS field. In retrospect the difficulty of working in an area of low prevalence should have been anticipated and the problems foreseen. However, at the time, it was not anticipated that the particularity of each carer's experiences could lead to identification.

A second option would have been to embargo the thesis, but this seemed a rather extreme measure to take and one which would not allow for the circulation of findings – confidentiality at the expense of representation. The third option was to acknowledge that those people who might be able to identify the carers were people who would be supportive of them. If any identification occurred it would do so within a safe haven and would matter less – the people most likely to recognise a carer would be the negotiators from the haemophilia centre or the AIDS organisations who helped find the carers in the first place. However, this last option was not entirely satisfactory as the carers had been told that the interviews were 'confidential'.

With hindsight, what was actually meant by that term and what the carers actually understood by it appears rather ambiguous. The carers were informed of the intention to feed back the results to interested agencies in report form and no one had objected to the data being used in this way.

The following account illustrates measures taken to anonymise carers' experiences so that the individuals become unidentifiable. A carer expressed dissatisfaction over the handling of HIV test results. However, as this person was very happy with other aspects of the service and did not wish to be seen to be 'ungrateful', it was stressed that it would be preferable if these views remained anonymous. It was important to honour these wishes and so it was necessary to devise a way of 'anonymising' the data.

One way forward was to strip carers of identifying factors, as in the example given above: it was not stated whether the carer was male or female or his/her dependant someone with haemophilia or a gay man. This approach may also mean pulling the issue from its context and losing some 'human interest' value but leaving the facts (as the researcher understood and interpreted them) unchanged.

Having acknowledged that context is important in research, and particularly in qualitative research, the problem of sometimes sacrificing context for the sake of confidentiality loomed large. In some instances the relationship of carer–cared for was deliberately changed if this could leave to immediate identification. For example, there was only one grandmother in the sample who was the main carer and describing her as such would make her immediately identifiable to some workers in the HIV field. More anonymous terms such as 'she' or 'female carer' could be used so that her experiences became difficult to separate out from those of the other female carers.

In some discussions it was not mentioned whether a dependant had haemophilia or was gay unless it had a direct bearing on what was being discussed: for example, when discussing the social support available for an individual and his or her carer. People attached to the haemophilia centre had a ready-made support mechanism already in place when HIV arose. In sharp contrast, those carers travelling down to the south to 'care at a distance' for a gay son who had made a life for himself in London had to seek out support for themselves and were often extremely isolated when they returned to the north of England.

Stigma is another issue where it is important to look at the carer's experience within its social context. It is often assumed that the stigma associated with haemophilia and HIV would be less than that associated with homosexuality and HIV and therefore knowing how a person became infected would help in under-standing more fully experience of stigma. On another level, however, being gay or having haemophilia was largely irrelevant to some issues discussed: for example, both carers of gay men and people with haemophilia described their loved ones as fiercely independent and talked about the problems this caused. Thus the 'context' in terms of the route of HIV infection did not need to be mentioned when the data relating to the desire for independence were presented.

Another mechanism which was utilised involved using a number of fictitious names for the same carer and cared for so that their whole circumstances could not be knitted together, thus leading to identification. For example, if it was recounted that Mr and Mrs X cared for their son in London, and that the same couple faced backlash from neighbours, and that they also were unhappy about certain aspects of their dependant's hospital treatment, any one of these factors, or certainly a combination of them, may lead workers in the HIV field to iden-tify Mr and Mrs X. However, if the same couple are referred to by different names each time they are mentioned then their circumstances cannot be knitted together as readily, thus avoiding identification and protecting confidentiality. The drawback of this is that it is not possible to give long, integrated accounts of each carer's circumstances which give a clearer picture of caring for someone with HIV in an area of low prevalence. Thus confidentiality is protected at the expense of detailed sketches of carers' experience.

This strategy involved deliberately misleading in order to protect identities. Descriptions were reconstructed, in that the total picture was different by virtue of details being changed. However, only details extraneous to the issue under discussion were changed so as to protect identities and confidentiality. The expe-rience of caring for someone with HIV (as the researcher understood and interpreted it and as it was recounted) has remained unchanged.

CONCLUSION

This chapter has discussed issues which are important to the researcher and the research participants throughout the research process. These issues take on added significance when a study looks at an emotive issue such as HIV and AIDS in an area of low prevalence.

Accessing carers of people with HIV is difficult as carers are a largely 'hidden' population and carers of people with HIV have to consider the added burden of potential stigma, making them cautious about disclosing their role. Negotiating with local AIDS organisations proved demanding as their decisions to allow research access was influenced by the climate of the time and the territorial and political considerations which this involved.

There are ethical questions to be considered when carrying out sensitive research and means of accessing the population is but one of these. It is extremely important to achieve a balance between protecting the interviewees from upset or worry and being able to do justice to important research.

How data are transformed from the stories of carers to the pages of written research findings is a complex one. It involves questioning what is being produced at a number of levels and at various stages of the research process. A number of questions have to be addressed: Are the interviews in some way 'set up' by the researcher? How much authority do the respondents have in affecting what is produced? How does it inform and affect the research process? The carers' perception and memories of events will be affected by these matters, and the ever-changing autobiography of the carer and the researcher is important when considering what is produced.

In an area of low prevalence, many of the factors mentioned above take on added significance. It was a continual struggle to present the data in ways which protected the identities of the carers whilst at the same time representing the research findings. The fact that 'confidentiality' is context-dependent became apparent. Some readers may be able to work out who some carers are because their cases are unique. It is this uniqueness that has made them interesting and deserving of research in the first place. Their experiences are important and in order to document and learn from them it is important to take the risk and say something, rather than err on the side of caution and end up saying nothing. With respect to the final product I hope and believe that what needed to be said has been said without jeopardising the carers' well-being, and that the research achieved a delicate balance between the two extremes of disregarding confidentiality for the sake of research findings and disregarding research findings for the sake of confidentiality.

NOTE

1   These figures are taken from the Central Statistical Office publication *Regional Trends*. They are based on data from the Public Health Laboratory Service, the Communicable Disease Surveillance Centre and the Communicable Disease (Scotland) Unit. Figures for 1990 represent the cumulative total of people reported with AIDS or HIV-1 antibody positive reports up to 31 December 1990 and 1991 figures are based on reports up to 31 December 1991. Comparable figures (cumulative totals) for the UK during 1990 were 3961 people reported with AIDS and 15,166 reports of HIV. By the next year numbers had risen to 5451 reports of AIDS and 16,828 people diagnosed with HIV. By the end of the first quarter of 1995 the number of AIDS cases in the Northern and Yorkshire Region had risen to 418 and 1028 people had been given a positive antibody test.

REFERENCES

Barbour, R.S. (1994) 'A telling tale: AIDS workers and confidentiality', in P. Aggleton, P. Davies and G. Hart (eds) *AIDS: Foundations for the Future*, London: Taylor and Francis.

Bayley, M.J. (1973) *Mental Handicap and Community Care*, London: Routledge & Kegan Paul.

Cohen, S. (1992) 'Self-conscious anthropology', in J. Okely and H. Callaway (eds) *Anthropology and Autobiography*, ASA Monograph No. 29, London: Routledge.

Garfinkel, H. (1967) *Studies in Ethnomethodology*, Englewood Cliffs, NJ: Prentice Hall.

Geertz, C. (1988) *Works and Lives: The Anthropologist as Author*, Cambridge: Polity.

Green, H. (1988) *Informal Carers*, Supplement A, General Household Survey 1985, London: HMSO.

James, N. (1993) 'Divisions of emotional labour: disclosure and cancer', paper presented at the British Sociological Association Medical Sociology Conference, University of York, September.

Jones, P. (1989) 'The counselling of HIV antibody positive haemophiliacs', in J. Green and A. McCreaner (eds) *Counselling in HIV Infection and AIDS*, Oxford and London: Blackwell Scientific Publications.

Kimmel, A.J. (1988) *Ethics and Values in Applied Social Research*, Applied Social Research Methods Series Vol. 12, Newbury Park, CA: Sage.

MacIntyre, A. (1982) 'Rise, harm and benefit assessment as instruments of moral evaluation', in T.L. Beauchamp, R.R. Faden, R J. Wallace and L. Waters (eds) *Ethical Issues in Social Science Research*, Baltimore: Johns Hopkins University Press.

Oakley, A. (1981) 'Interviewing women: a contradiction in terms', in H. Roberts (ed.) *Doing Feminist Research*, London: Routledge & Kegan Paul.

Okely, J. and Callaway, H. (eds) (1992) *Anthropology and Autobiography*, ASA Monograph No. 29, London: Routledge.

Peneff, J. (1990) 'Myths in life stories', in R. Samuel and P. Thompson (eds) *The Myths We Live By*, London: Routledge.

Renzetti, C.M. and Lee, R.M. (eds) (1993) *Researching Sensitive Topics*, London: Sage.

Rosaldo, R. (1989) *Culture and Truth: The Remaking of Social Analysis*, London: Routledge.

Samuel, R. and Thompson, P. (eds) (1990) *The Myths We Live By*, London: Routledge.

Sieber, J.E. and Stanley, B. (1988) 'Ethical and professional dimensions of socially sensitive research', *American Psychologist*, 43: 49–55.

Stark, C.M. (1995) Caring for Someone with HIV-Related Illness: The Experiences of Family Carers, unpublished Ph.D. thesis, University of Newcastle Upon Tyne.

Tait, A. (1988) *The Mastectomy Experience: Two Interviews Examined*, Studies in Sexual Politics No. 10, Department of Sociology, University of Manchester.

Tonkin, E. (1990) 'History and the myth of realism', in R. Samuel and P. Thompson (eds) *The Myths We Live By*, London: Routledge.

Vidich, A.J. and Bensman, J. (1958) *Small Town in Mass Society: Class, Power and Religion in a Rural Community*, Princeton, NJ: Princeton University Press.

Chapter 13

Evaluation within a policy-making and contracting culture
Reflections on practice

Edwin van Teijlingen and Guro Huby

INTRODUCTION

This chapter is based primarily on one of the author's (Edwin van Teijlingen's) experiences as a researcher evaluating over ten different organisations and projects concerned with HIV/AIDS prevention and care, together with organisations involved in prevention of drugs, alcohol and tobacco abuse in Scotland in the ten-year period from 1987 to 1997. At the Department of Sociology, University of Aberdeen, Edwin was involved in the evaluation of Grampian Smokebusters and an alcohol rehabilitation centre funded by the Church of Scotland. In the early 1990s, as a researcher with Lothian Health Board's Centre for HIV/AIDS and Drug Studies (CHADS), he participated in a number of evaluations of statutory and voluntary organisations in the HIV/AIDS and drug field in Lothian. In the mid-1990s he returned to Aberdeen where he participated in an evaluation of the Ayrshire and Arran's Smokebusters Project and a drug agency in Shetland. Together, we carried out an action-research project which involved the evaluation of co-ordination of services for people with HIV in Lothian (Huby *et al.* 1995), although this chapter does not draw directly on this material. Our experience has provided us with insights into the social processes around evaluation and the links between evaluation and policy-making. Our aim in this chapter is to critically examine assumptions and realities around these links.

In an ideal world, evaluation involves collecting information about interventions and services in order that effect and cost-effectiveness may be independently and objectively assessed. However, 'facts are not given, but constructed by the questions we ask' (Lather 1991: 105) and evaluation involves a negotiation about the questions to be asked and interpretation of the findings produced. Evaluation is not simply a process of collecting data which are summarised and digested for consumption by management. Rather, evaluation may be seen as the outcome of a combination of 'hard' and 'soft' data and a process of political negotiation at several levels about the data to be collected and the interpretation of findings. To the more cynical observer evaluation may be seen as a 'cover up' for problems and issues in service provision, while, to others, evaluation research can be said to be 'invented to solve social problems' which cannot easily be addressed by direct action. In this paper we will outline a more realistic view of evaluation through a consideration of the day-to-day informal and invisible negotiations which take place in the course of particular projects. We describe an example of evaluation where it was excluded from the process of information exchange where 'facts' were constructed on the basis of which decisions were made and we argue for a realistic view of the relationship between evaluation and decision-making.

POLICY-MAKING, EVALUATION AND THE CONTRACTING CULTURE: THE HIV/AIDS AND DRUG EVALUATION INDUSTRY

In Britain in the 1970s and 1980s evaluation seemed to have grown parallel with the expanding voluntary (non-statutory) sector in health and social work care. In addition, a more general development in the organisation of health care occurred with the introduction of the NHS and Community Care Act in 1990. The Act marked a fundamental shift in the organisation of health and social care (Pettigrew et al. 1992) which resulted in an 'internal' or 'quasi-'market mechanism (as distinct from a 'commercial marketisation' [Laing and Cotton 1996: 719]) regulating relationships between supply and demand in health and social care. The split between purchasers and providers in both sectors, together with the drive towards 'evidence-based' practice, has increased the need to evaluate those services 'bought' by local health authorities (health boards in Scotland) and local authorities on behalf of taxpayers. As a consequence, 'evaluation has increased with legislative changes to the health, community care and family support fields and, since 1990, new arrangements for purchasing and providing services' (Everitt 1995: 56).

Evaluation, then, is seen as an aid to policy formulation by providing feedback on the impact and cost-effectiveness of policy and/or funding decisions. Evaluation has become 'a growth industry' based on certain assumptions about research as context- and value-free. The concept of 'evidence-based' practice implies that criteria of quantity, quality and cost of service are a matter of scientific objectivity rather than political value and negotiation. However, this view belies the complexity of everyday practicalities and decision-making which an evaluation entails. The 'evaluation industry' in the Lothian and Scotland HIV/AIDS and drugs care and prevention field offers several examples of this complexity.

In 1983 government money especially targeted for community-based drug projects became available for the first time (Allsop and Slavin 1992: 127). From 1986, all health authorities and health boards were expected to make formal arrangements for dealing with HIV/AIDS (Bennett 1993b: 25). Lothian was one of the Scottish health boards which responded relatively quickly to the growing number of people living with HIV/AIDS in the region. In the early 1990s Lothian

Health Board stressed the need to work together with other statutory bodies, especially the Regional Council's Social Work Department.

> Joint Planning is a fundamental requirement for HIV/AIDS activity in Lothian. The epidemic is too pervasive for it to be the predominant responsibility of a single sector. The extent and balance of infection also has been such that no particular population has been able to claim sole ownership of the epidemic. It is likely that this contributed to the quality of joint work that has been undertaken by statutory and non-statutory bodies alike.
>
> (Lothian Health 1993: 1)

At the same time the Scottish Office reported that

> comparatively little detailed evaluation has been undertaken of local HIV-related campaigns and associated material . . . the time is now ripe for boards to identify which types of presentation have been most effective. This should help lead to the fine tuning of existing approaches and materials.
>
> (Forsyth 1992: 34–5)

Against this background an evaluation programme was developed for the HIV and drug agencies receiving funding from the Health Board.

There are a number of reasons why evaluation is regarded as more important in the area of HIV and/or drug services than in many other health and social care areas. Firstly, both HIV infection and drug use are heavily stigmatised and, therefore, there is a need to prove that money spent on people living with HIV and/or with a drug problem has not been 'wasted'. This need for evaluation of service provision to drug users 'has been increasingly felt in Europe during the last 5 years', according to Vara and Llivina (1994: 77), but probably nowhere was this so strongly felt as in Britain at a time when its health and social services moved to an internal market approach, as outlined above.

Secondly, proof of cost-effectiveness was crucial at a time when both the health and social services were in a funding crisis and many charities had difficulty in fund-raising, with 'the HIV/AIDS ring-fenced allocation representing just about the only growth area' (Bennett 1993b: 27). One can understand the jealousy and scepticism from professionals, carers and patients coping with other long-term limiting illnesses, especially at a time when reports appeared suggesting that the incidence and prevalence of HIV and AIDS was not increasing as rapidly as previously had been feared or claimed (Public Health Laboratory Service 1990).

Thirdly, it has been noted that proposed solutions to the drug problem are more 'finance-led' than, for example, measures to prevent and treat alcohol problems, which tend to be embedded in and a part of general forms of health and social care (Allsop and Slavin 1992: 127). It is the visible and clearly defined financial input which makes the funders require evaluations to be conducted.

At the level of individual agencies, the reason for conducting an evaluation will vary. For some, it is simply a contractual obligation. Some may also feel the pressure from funders and policy-makers to 'prove' that a project or intervention is worthwhile, or wish to show politicians and the mass media how taxpayers' money is spent and that it is well spent. Weiss (1972: 11) suggests that evaluation might be a delaying tactic in times of political conflict or impasse and a way to shift responsibility or to get positive publicity for the intervention. Yet others might conduct an evaluation because it is the 'in' thing to do or to keep the users of the services happy.

A decision to proceed with an evaluation often involves a mixture of reasons. More often than not, a prominent motivation will be an agency's genuine wish to improve the quality of their services and to ensure that a maximum number of potential users of their services is reached and benefit from their work. However, agencies operate in a political context where the links between evaluation and funding decisions are by no means straightforward and have to manage the evaluation accordingly.

EVALUATION OPERATIONALISED: ASSUMPTIONS AND PRACTICALITIES

Evaluation is not 'really a different method of doing research, usually it is research done for a specific *purpose*' (Baker 1994: 289). Evaluation is a process of bringing together relevant 'factual' information in a way which allows measurement, comparison and a critical assessment of costs and benefits of a particular programme, intervention or action. This definition of evaluation implies that there is a 'reality' out there waiting to be measured and assessed. In the Lothian HIV and drug field this quantitative approach was dominant. The HIV/AIDS strategy for Lothian, authored jointly by the Health Board and the local authority, stated: 'quality implications for service provision are straightforward despite the epidemic's complexity and continued evolution' (Lothian Health and Lothian Regional Council 1992: 8–9). These 'quality implications for service provision' were seen to be: (a) care and treatment; (b) prevention; (c) public attitudes; and (d) safety and hygiene (Lothian Health and Lothian Regional Council 1992). However, this clear picture of both purpose and method of evaluation was somewhat muddied by the details of implementation and operationalisation of evaluation in this particular setting.

The evaluation of voluntary and statutory organisations funded from the Scottish Office HIV allocation was conducted by the Centre for HIV/AIDS and Drug Studies in Edinburgh. This research centre formed part of the Health Board's planning structure. The evaluation of agencies was based on the existing funding so that only those organisations receiving money through the HIV allocation were evaluated, while other organisations performing similar tasks without this kind of funding were not evaluated. Furthermore, resources allowed only a limited number of organisations contracted by the Health Board to be evaluated at any one time – some agencies had to wait between one and two years for an evaluation. CHADS worked on a three-year evaluation cycle, but some of the agencies worked on a one-year funding cycle. The decision as to the order in which organisations were to be evaluated was a political as much as a practical one. The choice had to be made between, on the one hand, evaluating those organisations first which were perceived to have problems and/or were performing below expectation and, on the other, randomly allocating the agencies to different years.

HIV/AIDS, drugs and alcohol services for care and prevention are provided by a multiplicity of voluntary and statutory organisations, some operating in the health field, some in the social service field, and some crossing that boundary. These agencies often receive funding from a number of different sources, such as, for example, the health board, the regional social work department, national government grants (Urban Aid) and/or voluntary donations. This has implications for policy and for allocation of roles, responsibility and accountability (Bennett and Ferlie 1994: 117). It also has implications for evaluation.

Bennett (1993a: 38–9) lists the following boundaries for collaborative working in the HIV field: (1) disciplinary; (2) geographical; (3) practice; (4) ideological; (5) status; (6) political; and (7) experiential. Boundaries imply potential for both co-operation and competition and the CHADS' evaluation programme ran the risk of becoming entangled in the latter. Evaluation of one specific service or organisation by one funder can easily be seen as a threat by another funder or another organisation providing similar services.

Issues arose when it became clear that the evaluation of an agency is not the same as the evaluation of a particular service provided by that agency. For example, the Health Board, as purchaser, may have contracted for one particular service, for example counselling from a non-statutory drug agency, or patient transport from an HIV support agency. These agencies, by their nature, offer a range of services of which the service purchased by the Health Board was only one. The question then arose what exactly to evaluate. The agency could, and often would, argue that the evaluator from the purchaser should evaluate only those services purchased. However, most evaluators would argue that it is very difficult to pick out one aspect of an agency's total service provision. The separation of services provided by one organisation became even more difficult when it was forced to spend considerable time and effort on fund-raising to finance the support services needed to sustain the main service bought by the purchaser.

The potential for blurring of roles and functions extended to the boundary between evaluation and policy-making. For example, the director of CHADS, the research unit, was personally involved in strategic planning committees which helped shape future service provision. This arrangement made sense as it allowed a close relationship between evaluation and planning. However, the policy-making role was sometimes hard to separate from the role as independent research co-ordinator. Even without this role blurring there was ample scope for policy and evaluation to intermingle in ways contrary to the explicit purpose of evaluation as assessing cost-effectiveness and user needs. At the time of the evaluation the Health Board was also drafting the service specifications for the

statutory and non-statutory services. It was difficult to maintain that the evaluation reports would not be used in any way to inform the Health Board in their
first attempt to set up commissioned services.

One purpose of deregulation of services according to market principles is to
let user choice, rather than predetermined specifications, inform provision.
However, the relationship between evaluation and planning perpetuated the
tendency for existing services to determine what 'needs' were to be met. The
problem often lay in different interpretations of the word 'evaluation'. For
example, in Lothian self-evaluation reports were requested from all agencies
which did not receive an in-depth (or external) evaluation. According to the
researchers who designed and implemented self-evaluation for HIV agencies, it
'proved to be an effective system' (Williamson *et al.* 1995: 237). However, 'self-
evaluation' can be defined and operationalised in different ways. For example
Sapsford and Abbott (1992: 127–35) see 'self-evaluation' as an exercise in reflection and advise prospective participant observers of the workplace to

> Spend a good period of time trying to describe your own life and values on
> paper, from before you ever joined the given line of work to the present day,
> covering what you think the job is for, what you want out of it (not necessarily
> the same question), where you would like to go next, what you think others
> bring into the job, what you think motivates them, whether it motivates
> you . . .
>
> (Sapsford and Abbot 1992: 133)

For the drug and HIV agencies in Lothian, however, self-evaluation meant
primarily completing open-ended questionnaires asking for information on a
number of key inputs (for example, funding, staffing) and outputs (activities
organised and clients seen). The evaluators were then asked for advice on how to
fill in these forms, not simply in terms of how to do it but also on what approach
to take, or which services to highlight and which to play down.

The self-evaluation reports were used for policy-making as well as for
assessing the individual agency. For example, they provided the bulk of material
for the 1994 confidential report by Lothian Health *Drug Misuse Services in Lothian*
(Lothian Health 1994).

Being evaluated is, of course, a very real experience for those at the receiving
end. We are all a bit wary if someone comes along to assess our work, be it
providing an HIV service, a drug service or teaching medical students. To the
interested outsider, evaluation often appears to be a rather mechanical retrospective activity focusing on decisions already made, processes in place, and impacts
already felt (Vanderplaat 1995: 82). However, to many workers in non-statutory
agencies, evaluation by a researcher connected to the funding body might seem
like a mechanism of control and surveillance or plain interference with the
running of the agency. To some of the people evaluated in the project with
which this chapter is concerned, the exercise must have seemed like a political
activity only thinly covered with a gloss of 'research'.

However, detailed understanding of the evaluation process can also be used creatively by agencies, who are not completely at the mercy of evaluators and funders. An example is provided by the competition for Health Board funding between two Edinburgh organisations providing information, support and HIV risk reduction advice to sex workers, and the events which led to one of them being successful in acquiring this funding.

In Edinburgh female sex workers can be roughly divided into two groups: those working on the streets and in bars; and those working in saunas or massage parlours or through escort agencies (Morgan Thomas 1993: 91). In the early 1990s two voluntary organisations providing care and HIV prevention for sex workers had emerged which targeted their service at these two different groups. The Centenary Project, an agency established by the Church of Scotland, focused on street working women. It received substantial Health Board funding. Scot-PEP (Scottish Prostitutes Education Project) targeted its services at sex workers based in saunas. Scot-PEP had emerged out of an Edinburgh University research project on HIV and sex work. This organisation received only small amounts of funding from the Health Board. Both organisations provided a medical outreach clinic, free condoms and counselling. There was little co-operation and much antagonism between Scot-PEP and Centenary and both the Health Board and other stakeholders were drawn into, and took sides in, the contest between the two organisations. In 1992, it became clear that Lothian Health was moving to a system of tendering and contracting services from voluntary organisations. The Church of Scotland's requirements for staff at Centenary did not fit the Joint Regional AIDS Strategy for Lothian. The Church insisted that Centenary staff had a 'life church connection' and the Church's guidelines on the provision of condoms were felt to be restrictive. A new agency was established called Shiva which developed out of Centenary and had the kind of professional organisation previously only seen in Scot-PEP.

In 1994 Shiva and Scot-PEP both tendered for funding from the Health Board. Neither of the agencies had been evaluated, although both were, in effect, well known to the Health Board. In the end, Shiva won the tender, not least because of a well-formulated section on evaluation and monitoring of output in the tender document. The following year, 1995, Scot-PEP obtained Health Board funding for three years (Scott 1995: 3).

The requirements of evaluation also shape in significant ways what is to be provided. As part of an evaluation certain questions are likely to be asked because the answers are quantifiable. Other questions are not asked because the answers cannot easily be measured. To some extent this is a matter of methods and parallels the debate about the relative strengths and weaknesses of qualitative and quantitative methods. However, it is also a practical question about the discrepancy between, on the one hand, the complexities to be considered and, on the other, limited time and budget for evaluation. Whatever reason, quantitative methods in evaluation can easily lead to service providers deciding to provide those services that can be quantified and spend less resources on interventions whose outcomes are less measurable. According to Vanderplaat: 'It is not often recognised that the need to evaluate, in and of itself, plays a major role in how social interventions are mentally constructed and technically designed' (Vanderplaat 1995: 82). However, around these constructions of objective measures of service outcomes, political manoeuvring takes place which compels a qualitative assessment of the evaluation process and outcomes.

NEGOTIATING EVALUATION

The negotiations around the evaluation take place during all stages of data collection, analysis, interpretation and report writing. For example, during the evaluation of the Lothian HIV/AIDS and drugs agencies, the researcher was repeatedly told by one agency that the previous researcher, who conducted the evaluation the year before, did not understand that particular agency's approach and philosophy. Implicitly and explicitly, it was made clear that this year the evaluation would be better and fairer because the new researcher would be more 'open-minded', and therefore write a more favourable evaluation. This put considerable pressure on the evaluator both before and during the research process. This pressure was more subtle and less visible than the pressure which can be exerted after the evaluation has been conducted and the findings made available. At this stage, the agencies and workers evaluated, together with other stakeholders, often engage in negotiations about the interpretations made by the evaluators, together with the interpretations of findings and even the use of language. This leaves scope for all involved to question and dispute the findings.

This process can be an explicit and agreed part of the evaluation process. In Lothian each evaluated agency was provided with a draft copy, and comments and criticisms were requested from them. Factual mistakes would be automatically changed and disagreements about interpretation of the effect of the intervention were either solved through discussion and the final report amended accordingly or, if no agreement was reached, a section was added entitled 'agency's reply to this evaluation report'.

The process can be more *ad hoc* and informal, particularly if findings from the evaluation are unexpected. For example, an evaluation of the Smokebusters clubs in Grampian suggested that the initiative had, in effect, little impact on the smoking careers of young people targeted by the clubs. In an attempt to keep those evaluated involved, the researchers on the evaluation of Grampian Smokebusters took their draft report to Smokebusters Scotland to discuss the findings and their implications for the Smokebusters clubs and also to warn them about possible publicity given to the publication of the report. The Scottish Smokebusters co-ordinators were worried about negative mass media publicity if the publication of the report was accompanied by a press release. The researchers received a letter from the organisers of Scottish Smokebusters clubs (Van Teijlingen *et al.* 1995: 363). The letter made a number of fair and unfair points criticising the methodology and methods employed in the evaluation, finishing off with the statement: 'If published, the research could potentially be damaging professionally to . . . and the researchers. If published, . . . co-ordinators would be in a position where they would have to openly criticise and question the research's aims, methodology and findings.'

In order to discuss the way forward and find a balance between the interests of the evaluators, the wider research community, the funders and the Smokebusters clubs, a seminar was organised in Edinburgh. A range of researchers involved in the field of children and smoking in Britain were invited to the seminar plus a representative from (1) the funder (the Cancer Research Campaign); (2) the Health Education Board for Scotland; (3) Action on Smoking & Health (Scotland); (4) Grampian Smokebusters Campaign; and (5) Smokebusters Scotland. The seminar was held at the Department of General Practice at the University of Edinburgh.

One of the thank-you letters summed up the evaluator's own (Edwin's) feelings at the time: 'I enjoyed the meeting last week very much, although I am not sure that you are left any the wiser about how to proceed with dissemination of the findings!'

However, another participant wrote: 'I felt that the meeting . . . was extremely useful and that the major issues were aired fully and fairly. At the meeting it was agreed that, while an academic paper should certainly be prepared giving details of the second stage of the evaluation, there would be no accompanying publicity to the press.' This participant added: 'The academic paper will be of interest only to the academic community and . . . is most unlikely to draw any press attention.'

One of the outcomes of the meeting was that the transcribed tapes were used as the basis for a document on evaluation for Smokebusters clubs. The idea originated from the facilitator of Smokebusters Scotland and was embraced by the majority of the co-ordinators of Scottish Smokebusters clubs. Although Edwin was later told that one or two were not certain, allegedly 'because of the sensitivity of the evaluation subject', the Cancer Research Campaign as the funder of the evaluation informed the evaluators that it was very keen 'to see the issues brought to the attention of health promoters so that the planning of future programmes may benefit from the findings [of our evaluation]'. Consequently a report with the title *Scope and Limitation of Evaluation: Lessons Learnt from a Smokebusters' Club* was published by the Cancer Research Campaign (Van Teijlingen *et al.* 1994).

The evaluators went ahead with the submission of the academic paper, but decided not to send out a press release announcing the completion of the final report or the publication of the journal papers. Findings from the evaluation have since been accepted for publication by peer-reviewed journals, without any further repercussions from the anti-smoking campaigners. In this case, negotiation had resolved a potentially difficult situation.

The evaluation process thus intertwines with other overtly or covertly political processes. This also goes for the use of evaluation outcomes. Ostensibly, evaluation results are to inform funding decisions, but there is room for other considerations and events to impinge on decisions to continue funding. For example, as funding in Lothian for HIV/AIDS became tighter, purchasers had less money available to buy services from the non-statutory sector. This affected the contracting negotiations and in 1995 and 1996 two agencies closed down. However, there were several factors which contributed to this and the outcome of the evaluation seems to have played only a small part. The closing down of the Lothian branch of SAM (Scottish AIDS Monitor) in spring of 1996 affords one example. As a recipient of health board funding, SAM had been evaluated and the evaluation showed that the organisation complied with the contract specifications concerning both service provision and return of evaluation data. The closure of SAM was a long process, which was entangled in local politics around the organisation. The conflict, in turn, affected SAM's internal management and running and changed funders' confidence concerning strategic direction and management styles. In a similar vein, the closure of SAFE (Support on Addiction for Families in Edinburgh) between 1995 and 1996 illustrates the situation of a small organisation trying to survive in an increasingly competitive environment of the welfare marketplace and had little to do with the quality of their service to clients as described in its overall favourable evaluation report. SAFE's befriending service, run since 1989, had to close in 1995 (Hooton 1995: 13), while the workshop providing recycled furniture and household appliances to people with drug problems and people living with HIV continued until spring 1996. SAFE was by 1994 identifying a number of options which would help cut down administration costs and provide a more secure base for continued existence. Merger with a larger organisation was identified as one way forward. Negotiations were initiated with an organisation which was willing to take on SAFE provided Lothian Social Services provided service-level agreements to which the organisation could work. However, these agreements were not produced in time. The exact and full reasons are not clear, but lack of stability and clarity around the new contracting process, together with bureaucratic inertia, both seem to have played a part.

RULES OF EVALUATION: FORMAL AND INFORMAL INFORMATION EXCHANGE

The complexity of evaluation and the formal and informal pressures exerted on the process impinge significantly on the evaluation workers. Ideally, evaluators are outside of and impartial to political issues and conflicts of interest which inevitably arise between people and organisations affected in various ways by a service or an intervention. However, doing evaluations involves managing many and conflicting loyalties, and it is extremely difficult for researchers to remain impartial players in the game. In political disputes, a researcher becomes a potential resource for any faction in its attempts to discredit each other. Katie Deverell (Chapter 7) describes evaluation as a 'balancing act'. Formal and informal rules and guidelines of practice are often drawn up to address issues arising from this. There is, however, an informal element of information exchange which cannot easily be regulated. As Cathy Stark (Chapter 12) points out, the meanings of, for example, 'confidentiality' and 'accountability' are context-dependent and have to be determined and negotiated anew with each project.

The process of gathering information in evaluation involves 'official' data-collection methods and techniques, such as face-to-face interviews, administration of questionnaires and observation. However, there is also an element of 'unofficial' data gathering through gossip and storytelling. In the Lothian HIV field in particular, policy-making, service provision and social research occupy more or less the same universe of gossip. The researchers were both compelled and expected to use information collected through informal 'gossip', which, although invaluable for research purposes, had to be used with considerable caution. The dividing line between, on the one hand, 'contextual information' and, on the other, 'gossip' had to be drawn with great care (cf. Guro Huby, Chapter 10). In the evaluation of Lothian HIV/AIDS and drugs agencies, rules were established to regulate the relationships between evaluators and the settings in which they worked and to keep the evaluation outside of and neutral with regard to the overly political negotiations which were taking place. However, in this particular setting, where information exchange was a vital part of social interaction, the formal rules concerning evaluator neutrality hindered, rather than helped, the evaluators' effectiveness. We will mention two types of rules: one concerned dissemination of information; the other evaluator partiality.

The exchange of information, whether formal or informal, raised issues of confidentiality and the careful management of sensitive information. For example, as part of the evaluation and because of the need to plan services, Lothian drug and HIV agencies were asked about amount and sources of funding. The agencies were reluctant to provide financial information for a number of reasons. First and foremost, they were afraid that successful fund-raising from charitable organisations might lead to a reduction in funding from the statutory sector. A second issue, especially for those agencies that were more successful in fund-raising, was that they did not want everybody to know their sources of charitable funding. If they had found a specific charitable trust willing to fund them for a year or for a specific project, they did not want other HIV or drug agencies to find out and apply for funding from that same source the following year, thus reducing their own chances of repeat funding. In addition, as one chair of an HIV agency's management committee pointed out: 'Some donors would like to stay anonymous.' This referred mainly to donations from private individuals and largely because of the stigma attached to supporting drug and/or HIV services.

There are, of course formal criteria for the ownership of data, accountability for its use and methods of dissemination and these issues were addressed early on in the research. Reports from the evaluations were not freely circulated but kept and censored by the funders of the evaluation. This had a number of implications for both respondents and researchers. Researchers could not supply the products of their research to interested people and this made it difficult to maintain and cultivate relationships. Also, because the reports were not 'for public consumption', they could not be worked up for academic papers. Edwin came away from the job as evaluator with CHADS without any publications directly based on this work, at a time when publications are becoming more and more essential for careers and job prospects.

Issues concerning evaluators' impartiality were also complex. The evaluator's first loyalty is to the funders of the evaluation. If the researcher is on the pay-roll of one of the factions in a possible conflict of interest, be it the policy-makers, the funders or the agency, he or she is not impartial. On the other hand, regardless of source of funding, researchers can become closely involved in the agencies which they evaluate. For example, by the nature of the evaluations of HIV/AID agencies in Lothian, the researchers (of whom there were three at the time) spent considerable time in each agency and asked in-depth questions about the staff and service users, their own performance, their relationship with colleagues within and outwith the agency, management committees, clients, and funders and policy-makers. Consequently, the different researchers tended to claim a special relationship to 'their' agency in discussions about the evaluation. In a similar fashion, anthropologists tend to become obsessed about 'their hill tribe'.

The possibilities of blurring of responsibilities and roles were acknowledged, and measures were taken to prevent this. Several non-statutory agencies asked Edwin as a researcher to join their management committee. By the statutes each agency needs to have a management committee, which often consists of a mix of local dignitaries, representatives of the staff and service users, and members of other agencies in the same field. Management committees are, among other things, involved in policy-making, long-term planning of the agency's activities and fund-raising. Having a researcher with special knowledge and connections on the management committee can be in the agency's interest, especially if the researcher is employed by the funding body. However, these invitations were declined by Edwin. In order to avoid a conflict of interest, evaluators should not get formally involved in the field they are researching. Despite being aware of the dangers of overidentification with agencies and seeking to formalise relationships and accountability, blurring of roles and functions did occur.

The rules did not address the informal exchange of information which was integral to interaction in this particular setting. In the Lothian HIV/AIDS and drugs agency evaluation, the researchers in the field themselves became sources of information for the practitioners. By the nature of their work the researchers were acquiring information about the intricacies of the way in which HIV/AIDS and drugs services were run and managed. Staff and members of management committees of voluntary agencies were always keen to find out what was going on in the statutory sector, in Health Board planning circles, in the joint work between health and social services, and between other (competing) voluntary organisations and the Lothian Health Board. The evaluators were actively involved in trading one piece of information for another. Some staff in the HIV and drug agencies 'used' the evaluators to get their opinion heard at the Health Board. Some even tried to mislead the researchers about their agency's performance.

Similar considerations arose in the question of dissemination of information. Because of the evaluators' position in the networks through which gossip circulated, the day-to-day evaluation process was a vehicle for dissemination as well as collection of information.

There was thus a marked discrepancy between, on the one hand, the vague, pliable and implicit rules for the circulation of 'informal' information and, on the other, the rigid restriction of 'formal' information in the form of, for example, reports. This discrepancy had implications for the work of individual evaluators.

LOOKING AND ACTING INFORMED

In anthropological and sociological research it is sometimes both acceptable and advisable to act as the ignorant interested outsider or the naive stranger. Thus Jackson, having interviewed seventy fieldworkers, almost all of them anthropologists, suggested that 'Often the anthropologist's non-native status, his or her being neither fish nor fowl, can aid the research' (Jackson 1990: 14). This outsider status generally worked for both of us when interviewing users of drug misuse or HIV services, where our foreign origin (Dutch and Norwegian) was a great help. However, it did not aid Edwin in the research among staff and management of drug and HIV agencies. Because he was employed by the Health Board, he was clearly a 'native' to those working in these agencies and he was regarded to some extent as associated with one of the stakeholders. However, the rules by which the evaluation programme operated excluded evaluators from important information.

Sometimes researchers on their visits to the agencies they evaluate were told informally what was going on at a policy-making level, since some of the more senior people involved in non-statutory agencies were members of joint advisory board or policy-making bodies. Within CHADS the policy was that the researchers would not be involved in policy-making and therefore were kept away from these advisory bodies. However, some of the evaluation material made its way to these advisory bodies, where it was seen by people involved in the voluntary sector. Thus a member representing the drug agencies might be shown a document reporting on his or her own or a competing drug agency. The researchers were not always aware who in the hierarchy might cast eyes on their evaluation reports. This made claims by the evaluators that their evaluations were confidential hard to sustain. If they did not even know what was happening with the results of their work, how could they be trusted by an agency under investigation? The fact that evaluators were not aware of progress and process of policy-making in the region also meant that they sometimes came across as uninformed.

As an evaluator, that is, someone who is going to make an assessment, it is important to be regarded by the evaluated as competent and able to do a good job. It is the job of a researcher to collect information, that is, to be informed, and when the evaluator comes across as uninformed about certain policy issues he or she can be taken at best for a junior and unimportant researcher, or, at worst, a very poor one. The lack of knowledge becomes a source of insecurity in the researcher also and a nagging feeling that 'perhaps I should have known'.

Perhaps more importantly, the formal exclusion of evaluators from the informal exchange of information and stories, together with the narrow definition of 'facts' which underpinned the evaluation, meant that the evaluation was less than effective in informing perceptions and decision-making.

EVALUATION AND MYTH MAKING

Guro Huby (Chapter 10) describes how the informal exchange of stories in the Lothian HIV/AIDS field created and sustained perceptions of service provision and service use which informed decisions concerning care. Some of the stories formed a part of inter-agency rivalry. For example, one hospital-based practitioner commented on a community-based HIV agency in Edinburgh that

> They deal with people who won't have real . . . problems. I know because we share some clients. . . . They hang on to patients and create dependency. They are too much a buddy for too many people, ferrying them around, and so forth. They are too overpaid for that.

Policy-makers, many of whom were also involved in service provision, took part in these exchanges, both in formal meetings and at social events. 'Facts' about service provision were constructed in these exchanges which impinged on policy decisions concerning funding and development of services. These 'facts' were often impervious to counter-information produced by evaluation.

For example, one particular voluntary organisation provided a befriending service to people with HIV together with practical help such as home decorating and, importantly, transport to and from hospital, for shopping trips and to take children to and fetch them from school. The service was provided by volunteers. In Health Board circles it was sometimes referred to as 'just a taxi service' which was 'too expensive per lift delivered'. In-depth evaluation by the researchers explained to a large extent why the service cost so much per lift. The explanation included trips cancelled at the last minute by either patients or clinic staff, a limited availability of trained volunteers (with their own car) and the long waiting time at the outpatient clinic. Moreover, the transport service was only a small part of what the organisation offered, although many of these were not included in calculations of 'cost-effectiveness.' However, no matter how often these findings from the evaluation were repeated, the discussions never moved beyond confirmations of 'the myth' about the expensive service.

The evaluation was defined by narrow and formal criteria concerning the status of data, and the role of the evaluators and the informality and complexity of the evaluation process were screened out of the official view. The evaluation was, in fact, excluded from the information exchange where the perceptions and 'facts' were constructed which drove the decision-making process.

CONCLUDING REMARKS: PUTTING 'VALUE' BACK IN 'EVALUATION'

In the current health and social care environment evaluation is rapidly becoming a popular management tool, since evaluation provides feedback to management, funders and policy-makers which helps in the process of policy formulation and allocation of resources. Evaluation is being used to study current practice as well as planned and unplanned change in a variety of organisational settings.

From a positivist perspective, many of our actions and processes are quantifiable and the evaluator can go out and, using the correct methodologies and methods, assess the quality of the work conducted by, for example, an alcohol agency, a drug worker or an HIV counsellor. However, one should bear in mind that evaluation always involves making an assessment about what is to be quantified and studied, and this is a qualitative question. Moreover, qualitative methods might be more useful to answer certain questions, for example why an agency provides one particular service rather than another. However, qualitative methods are often seen to be more difficult to incorporate in an evaluation. Qualitative methods and information are also often seen as difficult to defend from criticism from stakeholders.

However, the qualitative aspects of evaluation need to be made visible, understood and utilised. Evaluation is never free of the 'human' factor and it rapidly becomes embedded in the particular channels of information exchange and the systems of knowledge production which operate in any particular setting. Evaluation becomes part of the world evaluated. This has a number of implications.

First of all, the notion of the independent and objective researchers conducting an evaluation needs to be revised so that adequate measures of support and supervision may be put in place. Secondly, a more realistic view of the role of evaluation in policy-making and practice is needed to make maximum use of such research. Thirdly, a detailed understanding of the role of the evaluator is theoretically interesting in terms of the political contexts of production of knowledge. In short, it is time to put 'value' back in 'evaluation'.

REFERENCES

Allsop, D. and Slavin, W. (1992) 'Scottish voluntary alcohol and drug services', in M. Plant, B. Ritson and R. Robertson (eds) *Alcohol and Drugs: The Scottish Experience*, Edinburgh: Edinburgh University Press.
Baker, T.L. (1994) *Doing Social Research* (2nd edn), New York: McGraw-Hill.
Bennett, C. (1993a) 'DHPCs and collaborative working: issues for the future?', in B. Evans, S. Sandberg and S. Watson (eds) *Healthy Alliances in HIV Prevention*, London: HEA.

—— (1993b), 'HIV/AIDS: some organizational and managerial issues', *Health Manpower Management*, 19: 25–8.
—— (1996) 'The crucial role of professional change: the development of services for HIV/AIDS', in J. Leopold, I. Glover and M. Hughes (eds) *Beyond Reason? The National Health Service and the Limits of Management*, Aldershot: Avebury.
Bennett, C. and Ferlie, E. (1994) 'HIV/AIDS: the influence of ideologies', in *Managing Crisis and Change in Health Care*, Buckingham: Open University Press.
Everitt, A. (1995) 'Values and evidence in evaluating community health projects', *Critical Public Health*, 6: 56–65.
Forsyth, M. (1992) *HIV and AIDS in Scotland: Prevention the Key (Report of Ministerial Task Force*, Edinburgh: Scottish Office Home and Health Department.
Hooton, A. (1995) 'Losing a buddy', *The Scotsman Weekend*, 25 November: 12–13.
Huby, G., Porter, A.M.D. and Bury, J. (1995) *Quality of Care for People with HIV/AIDS in Lothian: Final Report*, Edinburgh: Department of General Practice, University of Edinburgh.
Jackson, J.E. (1990) '"Deja entendu": the liminal qualities of anthropological fieldnotes', *Journal of Contemporary Ethnography*, 19(1): 8–43.
Laing, A.W. and Cotton, S. (1996) 'Purchasing health care services: information sources and decisional criteria', *Journal of Marketing Management*, 12: 719–34.
Lather, P. (1991) *Getting Smart: Feminist Research and Pedagogy within the Postmodern*, New York: Routledge.
Lothian Health (1993) *HIV/AIDS in Lothian: Changing Times and Shifting Targets* (A report in response to the AIDS (Control) Act 1997), Edinburgh: Lothian Health.
—— (1994) *Drug Misuse Services in Lothian: A Report. The National Services Division of the NHS Management Executive*, Edinburgh: Lothian Health, Centre for HIV/AIDS and Drug Studies.
Lothian Health and Lothian Regional Council (1992) *An HIV/AIDS Strategy for Lothian*, Edinburgh: Lothian Health and Lothian Regional Council.
Morgan Thomas, R. (1993) 'AIDS risks, alcohol, drugs, and the sex industry: a Scottish study', in M.A. Plant (ed.) *AIDS, Drugs and Prostitution*, London: Routledge.
Pettigrew, A., Ferlie, E. and McKee, L. (1992) *Shaping Strategic Change in the NHS*, London: Sage.
Public Health Laboratory Service (1990) 'AIDS in England and Wales to end 1993: projections using data to end September 1989', *Communicable Disease Report* (The Day Report).
Sapsford, R. and Abbott, P. (1992) *Research Methods for Nurses and the Caring Professions*, Buckingham: Open University Press.
Scott, G.R. (1995) 'Medical services for female prostitutes in Lothian', *ANSWER 26 May*, Glasgow: Scottish Centre for Infection and Health.
Teijlingen, E.R. van, Friend, J.A.R. and Twine, F.E. (1994) *Scope and Limitation of Evaluation: Lessons Learnt from a Smokebusters' Club*, London: Cancer Research Campaign.
—— (1995) 'Problems of evaluation: lessons from a Smokebusters campaign', *Health Education Journal*, 54: 357–66.
Vanderplaat, M. (1995) 'Beyond technique: issues in evaluating for empowerment', *Evaluation*, 1: 81–96.
Vara, C.A. and Llivina T.S. (1994) 'Evaluation: a challenge for the 1990s', *Drugs: Education, Prevention and Policy*, 1: 75–9.
Weiss, C. (1972) *Evaluation Research: Methods of Assessing Program Effectiveness*, Englewood Cliffs, NJ: Prentice Hall.
Williamson, L., McPhail, K. and Lewis, R. (1995) 'HIV agencies: can they evaluate their own services?', *AIDS Care*, 7: 237–42.

Part V

A tribute to Phil Strong and an overview

Introduction to Chapter 14

Anne Murcott

Although 'The pestilential apocalypse: modern, postmodern and early modern observations' addresses one of the main themes of this book, the chapter itself makes no mention of the matter. Nor, indeed, does it refer to its own inclusion here. For, as the editors record (Rosaline Barbour and Guro Huby, Chapter 1), its publication is posthumous. In order, then, to provide a little explanation, this introduction seeks to indicate the manner in which the piece takes its place in such a collection. As will be proposed, its provenance casts the chapter as not only a representation of, but also a commentary on, elements of the intellectual heritage available to those attempting to grasp the import of HIV/AIDS – a simultaneity that is inalienably reflexive.

Before enlarging on this proposal, some comment on the mode of proceeding is needed. A conservative stance has been adopted both in this introduction and in the preparation of the manuscript for publication. This is partly because of the form in which the chapter survives, and partly because a closely related piece, written some four months later, is now publicly available (Strong 1997). As noted (Rosaline Barbour and Guro Huby, Chapter 1), a whole paper was submitted to the editors very early on. Despite being marked 'draft', it had already been worked up for (small-scale) public consumption at the invitation of the London History of the Present Group.[1] That first draft was circulated to the Group's members and duly presented at its meeting on 9 November 1994. The original intention, of course, had been to elaborate the draft with an eye to developing common themes set to emerge once the *Meddling with Mythology* collection as a whole began to take shape. Although that more focused elaboration never took place, the piece was still revised to clarify some of the points that had been particularly compressed in the November 1994 draft. It is this later version (stored in a computer file dated 6 December 1994) that, with only minor editing, appears here.

The chapter forms part of a much larger, unfinished, project one of whose main, if implicit, preoccupations was the dynamic between the nature of the phenomena under investigation and the manner in which they may best be analysed. By far the greater part of the project was to come. But there is sufficient in print (and thereby accessible to the reader to judge for him- or herself rather than rely solely on the gloss presented here) to be able to suggest the manner in which attention to this dynamic was evolving in a reflexive, even recursive fashion – thus making 'The pestilential apocalypse' an apt contribution to reflections on knowledge 'post- AIDS'.

Among the items available in print, four are generally material to the discussion here (Strong and Berridge 1990; Strong 1990, 1994, 1997). But, unsurprisingly, since the evolution of the thinking is at issue, comparison of just the earliest and the most recently published pieces serves the present purpose tidily enough. The first, 'No one knew anything: some issues in British AIDS policy' (Strong and Berridge 1990), is one of a pair of preliminary papers arising from the initial, pilot phase of a longer study of the history of the social impact of AIDS in Britain. It sought to identify the beginnings of 'a sociological perspective', while its companion (Berridge and Strong 1991) argued, through a chronology of the development of Britain's AIDS policies, for the relevance of 'contemporary history'. The other item, 'One branch of moral science: an early modern approach to public policy' (Strong 1997), referred to above, is also published posthumously.

Though neither 'No one knew anything' nor 'One branch of moral science' poses the questions in quite this paired form, both may be read as seeking answers to two unexceptionable, but vital, types of query. What are the phenomena to be investigated? What theory is to be deployed for their satisfactory analysis? The core of this Introduction's discussion lies in the proposal that it is the dynamic relation, the interrelation, between these two types which constitutes the reflexive mainspring of 'The pestilential apocalypse'. This proposal is sketched, predictably enough, via brief exposition and summary of each of the other two articles in turn, beginning with the earlier.

From the present vantage point, the poignancy of the title 'No one knew anything' bites that much deeper. It derived from a 1988/9 interview with a senior civil servant who was reflecting on the early part of the decade when AIDS was so startling a novelty. Poignant enough at the time, the remark captured the initial shock engendered by AIDS, and served as the article's point of departure. For almost none of the small amount of sociological literature just starting to become available made anything of that extraordinary initial shock, albeit making due mention of it. Yet,

> for us . . . the initial shock is worth exploring in depth, because, though obvious enough, it seems closely linked to key aspects of the wider impact of AIDS and the ensuing policy response; aspects which are less than adequately characterized in the accounts that we have so far considered.
>
> (Strong and Berridge 1990: 235)

But as the article went on to indicate, the novelty of AIDS was shocking to *all* concerned. Certainly it is an appalling shock to anyone diagnosed with the condition, but 'what sets it apart from other fatal conditions is the way in which so many others were shaken too' (Strong and Berridge 1990: 236). Placing this point about the extent of the shock in the centre of the field of investigative vision allowed questions to be raised about how that initial impact was to be analysed. Treating AIDS as just another health policy topic was judged unduly narrow and failed to grasp the extent of the impact of, the 'great ravages' (Strong and Berridge 1990: 237) wreaked by, AIDS in the policy world, and beyond.

Analyses appealing to 'moral panics' were likewise deemed unhelpful in conflating far too many disparate phenomena. Four of these were separated out: 'stigmatization, moral debate, panic and fear – *each of which needs its own analysis*' (Strong and Berridge 1990: 245; emphasis added). Of course, this declaration that separate analyses are needed unavoidably also characterises the phenomena to be analysed – and does so with arguably that much more specificity than dependence on theorising in terms of 'moral panic' *tout court*. Further, as the article later rather sharply observes, 'panic' needs unpacking, for, in the case of AIDS it includes an anxiety that is wholly *rational*.

Still casting about for a suitable means of capturing the first few years of AIDS, 'No one knew anything' turned to contemplate a phenomenon which too many know only too much about. Comparing the initial impact of AIDS with war may be inappropriate or in dubious taste, 'yet one may invoke the image of war, not in a spirit of militarism, but to make the analytic point that both are emergencies of a closely related kind' (Strong and Berridge 1990: 248). Though, of course, not exactly identical, the 'parallels are real and worthy of much closer examination' (Strong and Berridge 1990: 249). So it was fitting in more ways than one that the article concluded with a section entitled 'The end of the beginning'. Thus it not only signalled that at the time of writing there was a great deal further to go in understanding the epidemic, in developing policies, in putting them into practice, and more; but it also implied that there was as far to go in devising suitable sociological approaches to the complex panoply involved.

The choice of heading for that last section echoes the poignancy of the whole article's title not solely when it was written, but, with redoubled effect now, some eight years later. It had opened with the observation that through much of the relatively limited amount of work available ran a core question: 'how did governments respond to AIDS, given its initial identification with gay men?' (Strong and Berridge 1990: 233). The question, it was held, invited considering 'a common set of political and scientific concerns: the nature of deviance, élites, expertise, morality, the masses, minorities, the media, policy, sexuality, the state, science and stigma' (Strong and Berridge 1990: 233). The invitation was accepted, but left trailing. So, while not exactly mirroring the manner in which shocked patients, doctors, policy-makers and all the others involved in the early days were so bereft, the added poignancy underscores the present proposal that 'No one knew anything' may be read as the start of a continuing and sustained effort both to describe the object under scrutiny and to settle on a satisfactory analytic approach. In other words, the suggestion here is that it was not so much 'not knowing anything' as casting about to identify both what it was to know and how to know it.

To take this suggestion further, the present discussion now moves to the latest published stage in this effort (Strong 1997). Appearing in a volume devoted to the problems and possibilities in qualitative sociological research, 'One branch of moral science' does not, at first sight, seem to be much concerned with phenomena most particularly associated with the social import of AIDS/HIV. It opens with reference to the limited and uneasy connection between sociological research and public policy. The latter is left unspecified in the body of the text, but the chapter's acknowledgement is more precise, explaining that its substance grew 'out of a study of the British public debate over AIDS policy and what that, in turn, reveals about policy formation in a liberal society' (Strong 1997: 195).[2]

The chapter itself does not delineate any particular policy or set of public policy concerns. Instead, the object of study is discussed via presentation of 'a model of the contemporary policy arena in liberal societies' (Strong 1997: 185). The insistence on liberal society is significant. There is a 'crucial difference between policy formation in liberal and authoritarian societies' (Strong 1997: 189). And, by implication, science and scientific research (whether in qualitative sociology or quantum physics), together with their public representations, are also critically different between liberal and authoritarian societies. Science, the diffusion of scientific knowledge, the social networks involved, all are part of the complex mix comprising the policy arena of liberal society. In this sense, that is, as science, sociological research is to be understood as part of the object of study. The reflexivity – what, in the early 1970s, was known as the sociology of sociology – is almost too obvious to need noting . . .

Science may be a feature of the contemporary policy arena, but there is a key distinction to be drawn between the place of modern natural science within it and that of social science. The history of the latter familiarly indicates that it stands in a different relation to public policy from the natural sciences. That same history also, but rather less familiarly, indicates that, like it or not, social science continues to bear the marks of its origins as a 'moral science': 'social science remains an integral branch of politics and of ethics . . . attempt[ing] to create an ethically justifiable public policy on a secular and materialist basis' (Strong 1997: 189).

Whether regarded a moral science or not, in a context where public policy is to be subjected to investigative scrutiny, it is thus cast as *integral to* the object of study. But at the same time of course, social science research, the effort made by those named as sociological researchers, is also to *reveal* the object of study. In the process, that effort helps mark out the evolution of what is involved in achieving the designation of its object of inquiry. Put another way, the effort is to comment on its own path at the same time as travelling along it. Social science, moral science, is simultaneously the object of investigation and the means whereby it shall be investigated.

At this point, 'One branch of moral science' turns back on itself not simply to examine the theorising of the version of moral science with which the social sciences began, but, very precisely, to announce that this version now needs to be embraced by modern sociology. What requires resurrection, it insists, is the version of liberalism enshrined in moral science of the early modern period when writers such as Hobbes first propounded it. 'This was a secular, chastened, pluralist, materialist and experimental morality which, breaking with the dominant classical and medieval ideals of consensus and virtue, set its sights a good deal lower' (Strong 1997: 190). It was a policy doctrine which required, matter-of-fact, due acknowledgement of the worst as well as the best of human nature, and required realising that the worst may serve as the basis for collective mutual advantage. Policy should not, in other words, aim impossibly high. Given human fallibility it cannot work. Instead, much more modest, achievable aims should be adopted, selecting those where there is a tolerable chance of getting some collective assent.

> Our public policy goal should therefore be, not the *summum bonum*, the greatest good, but the more pragmatic avoidance of the *summum malum*, the systematic circumvention of the greatest human evils such as tyranny, famine and civil war. The provision of liberty, food and security might not be everything but this was, still, a fundamental framework within which many other things might flourish.
>
> (Strong 1997: 190)

In effect, this statement represents the climax of 'One branch of moral science'. Indeed, it might be said to encapsulate the version of social science, the early modern moral science, with which the chapter urges sociology to be reconciled. And it is the statement which succinctly summarises one of the absolutely essential elements of the intellectual position reached in the published work.

'The pestilential apocalypse', which appears in this volume can, it is hoped, now be seen in context. The ground was already cleared in 'No one knew anything'. It meant that with tolerable intellectual safety, AIDS/HIV, despite its terrible particularities, could later be characterised as one of the same class of potentially devastating events as war, stock market crashes and political crises. In this sense, AIDS had to be identified as a phenomenon which threatens social collapse.[3] So, quite straightforwardly, 'The pestilential apocalypse' may be thought of as a later stage in fashioning a suitable characterisation. It may also, incidentally, be seen as exhibiting the method of moving toward achieving that characterisation. Certainly, it pursues the usual academic procedure of taking existing literature seriously – in this instance subjecting Rosenberg's arresting exposition to a close examination and applauding, though only in part. But it does so with a certain twist. In practice, it is saying that what is needed to secure an adequate delineation of the object of study is, in Goffmanesque fashion (cf. Bloor 1996), perpetual comparison with more and less like phenomena, in more and less like historical eras, identified in a moderately eclectic set of sources.

If, however, that is all 'The pestilential apocalypse' is taken to be doing, its final section risks being rendered mysterious, mystical maybe, possibly even redundant.[4] It is important not to be deceived. The chapter's apparently single-minded emphasis on achieving an adequate characterisation is a product, quite simply, of the difficulty of doing more than one thing at a time. Yet, in key respects, it is as much concerned to propose the manner in which the phenomena under investigation are to be analysed as to designate what they are held to be. It is merely that it only refers to, rather than provides an exposition of, the mode in which the analysis is urged. A good part of that exposition is to be found in 'One branch of moral science'. Though creating greater labour for the reader, detecting quite how well 'The pestilential apocalypse' sits with the aims of this volume is, it is proposed, best achieved as sketched here, that is, by studying it alongside scrutiny of its companions.

ACKNOWLEDGEMENTS

I am grateful to the Nuffield Trust (formerly the Nuffield Provincial Hospitals Trust) and to the grantholder, Nick Black, for their readiness to see posthumous publication of the work. I should also like to thank Rose Barbour and Guro Huby for their invitation to provide this introduction. In undertaking so unfamiliar a professional assignment I am deeply indebted to an even larger circle of friends and colleagues than usual. So, with apology only to those who could not be listed too, I particularly wish to thank: Gerry Bernbaum, Joy Lowe, Cathy Pope and Hilary Rose for, one way or another, their unstinting moral support; Basiro Davey, Jerome Fletcher, Hilly Janes and Virginia Olesen for discussions about the general business of editing; Graham Burchell, Alastair Gray, Colin Gordon, Robert Dingwall, Ali McGuire, Elizabeth Murphy, David Oldman, Teresa Rees and Tony Wootton for conversations about the academic import of Phil Strong's work. Naturally, only I am to be held responsible for the chapter's introduction and its editing.

NOTES

1   Grateful acknowledgement is due to the organisers, and especially Nikolas Rose, for that invitation.
2   It is an important aside to note the style in which those same acknowledgements thank the Nuffield Trust not just for their funding but also for 'the intellectual openness' which permitted the development of more general reflections.
3   So saying, of course, is still much condensed. The designation AIDS is a shorthand not just for the phenomena listed in 'No one knew anything' or the specifics of moral science. It is also to encompass the substantive concerns inspected in 'The pestilential apocalypse' – including the emergence of a liberal public sphere's creation of the possibilities for 'spiralling reflexivity' that, with near banal archness, become available as the object of yet further, reflexive commentary.
4   The undeveloped observations about the neglect of Hobbes, and about the promise that the macro–micro split might be dissolved in a sociology reconciled with early modern moral science, are to be understood, of course, as theses due to be developed in the larger, unfinished project. There may have been time before this chapter's

delivery date to have elaborated satisfactorily for publication. But, equally, the advice may have been taken to remove them in order to avoid the sin of beginning the next piece of work in lieu of concluding the one in hand. The editorial decision to risk a bathetic effect is taken in part to make available for the reader a sense, no matter how sketchy, of the direction the thinking was taking, and in part, to remain as faithful as possible to the extant text.

REFERENCES

Berridge, V. and Strong, P. (1991) 'AIDS in the UK: contemporary history and the study of policy', *Twentieth Century British History*, 2(2): 150–74.

Bloor, M. (1996) 'Review essay: Philip Strong (1945–1995) an appreciation of an essayist', *Sociology of Health & Illness*, 18(4): 551–64.

—— (1990) 'Epidemic psychology: a model', *Sociology of Health & Illness*, 12(3): 249–59.

—— (1994) 'Two types of ceremonial order', in S.O. Lauritzen and L. Sachs (eds) *Health Care Encounters and Culture: Interdisciplinary Perspectives*, Botkyrka, Sweden: Multicultural Centre.

—— (1997) 'One branch of moral science: an early modern approach to public policy', in G. Miller and R. Dingwall (eds) *Context and Method in Qualitative Research*, London: Sage.

Strong, P. and Berridge, V. (1990) 'No one knew anything: some issues in British AIDS policy', in P. Aggleton, P. Davies and G. Hart (eds) *AIDS: Individual, Cultural and Policy Dimensions*, London: Falmer.

Chapter 14

The pestilential apocalypse
Modern, postmodern and early modern observations

Philip Strong

> I shall now speak of what caused so many deaths in so short a period of time, many
> more than has been witnessed in any other epidemic. I am convinced that the Devil
> was responsible. . . . Everything was permitted, even though it frightens me to say it.
> There was no end to the selfishness of everyone against everyone else, as a lack of
> charity unleashed our evil nature. . . . The shamelessness was such that it is impossible
> to tell of it. . . . [There were] many small children in the streets whose parents had
> died, and lacking help they went about looking for food, and if anyone gave them
> something it was by throwing it to them like dogs. They could be found near the city
> gates, where they died either from hunger or disease.
>
> (Andres de la Vega, a Seville shopkeeper, writing of the plague of 1649).[1]

INTRODUCTION

On Tuesday 27 September 1994, the front page of *The Independent* listed, as it
does every day, a short summary of various stories alongside its main leads.
Among them was the following: 'Plague Spreads: panic gripped Bombay as the
number of pneumonic plague cases exceeded 50'. The reader was invited to
turn to page 16, to a longer story about the city of Surat where the epidemic had
started:

> Over the past five days plague has . . . caused the flight of over 400,000 poor
> labourers from the industrial city's teeming slums. . . . On Sunday, mobs
> fought to board the [Bombay] train. . . . In Pakistan, newspapers urged a ban
> on flights from India. . . . In Canada, airport workers refused to unload a
> cargo plane from Bombay.

The Surat story and its wider consequences are familiar enough to a modern
audience which has heard something of the terrifying plague of the later
medieval and early modern periods, and personally experienced both the initial
social impact of AIDS and the much shorter, more recent frisson over necro-
tising fasciitis. My chapter explores two angles on this striking class of events.
One portrays it as a product of microbiology now increasingly mediated by
modern forms of mass communication; the other as a sub-type of a more

general, indeed omnipresent social phenomenon. In both cases I want to put forward an early modern perspective.

THE PESTILENTIAL DRAMA

My first argument is taken from the work of the leading American medical historian, Charles Rosenberg, author of a major study of nineteenth-century cholera and, more recently, of a comparative essay on the general societal experience of large-scale, fatal epidemic disease; an analysis which, to my mind, is much the best of the attempts at analysing the social impact of AIDS (Rosenberg 1992). Although Rosenberg's argument contains some very powerful points, much of it is also highly condensed. It needs elaboration in some places and serious qualification in others.[2]

His argument begins by considering a standard form of inter-species biological process: the population explosion typical of a successful micro-parasite as it finds, invades, then feeds off ever more numbers of its host population. Such an explosion cannot continue indefinitely. The host species is limited in numbers and not all its members are accessible or vulnerable. After a time, therefore, the process winds down. With fewer susceptible hosts on which to feed, there is a slow but steady decline in morbidity and mortality within the affected species. Such epidemics end with a whimper, not a bang.[3]

In human beings, and where there is no effective cure or prophylaxis, this standard biological sequence can generate a parallel and highly distinctive societal trajectory. For an epidemic of this kind is an infectious disease so immediate, so visible, so patently fateful, at least potentially, for large numbers within the affected human society that, though there is sometimes a period of denial at its onset (when its effects are too little known about to be taken seriously, or too economically and socially devastating to be acted upon unless there is overwhelming evidence of its presence), there comes a time when the potential implications of the biological process can no longer be denied. At this point, there is a striking switch in public attention. Far from being ignored, the disease and its progress now become the object of urgent, increasingly systematic observation and action, of a potentially gigantic mobilisation and reorientation (both individual and collective) as members of the affected population withdraw from their workaday routines and focus instead on the pestilence within their midst.

This pattern of increasing, and increasingly compelled, involvement, followed eventually, as the disease declines, by diminishing attention and a switch to other, more pressing matters, has one further, important aspect. Some of the core features of the sequence can be analysed in very similar terms to those which we use when describing our engagement with a play or a film. For, just like the classic epidemic, genres such as the tragedy, the thriller and the melodrama create the same intense collective involvement and much the same sequence by which their spectators become involved: firstly, engrossing their audience's attention through steadily increasing terror and tension, then letting them down, gently or other-wise, at the end.[4]

Rosenberg, in fact, describes four main acts in the pestilential drama: 'Act I: Progressive Revelation'; 'Act II: Managing Randomness'; 'Act III: Negotiating Public Response'; and 'Act IV: Subsidence and Retrospection' (Rosenberg 1992: 281–7). Of course, different societies produce the same drama in very different ways: the collective management of randomness, for example, has taken a rather different form with AIDS in the secular late twentieth century from that which it took with bubonic plague in the fourteenth century. None the less, at a more fundamental level, the basic problems posed to any collectivity – and the sequence in which they occur – remain the same. Thus much the same Acts can be identified regardless of the type of society in which the pestilential drama is played.

If, however, the classic pestilential drama has several distinct, biologically shaped acts, many of the more modern versions of the play have developed a new, socially shaped beginning. From the nineteenth century onwards, so Rosenberg goes on, the immediate societal consequences of the micro-parasitic dynamic have been mediated, and thus partially reshaped, by science and by new technology. The development of global reporting systems, some of them catering to mass markets, has meant that some acts in the social drama are no longer geographically tied to the immediate unfolding of the biological form. Local productions of an epidemic drama which began elsewhere in the globe now start with an increasingly elaborate warm-up act: 'A sort of prologue takes place "off-stage", as particular communities follow the gradual spread of a pandemic and anticipate its arrival' (Rosenberg 1992: 281).[5] Finally, though only in the period of AIDS, the enormously increased rapidity, intensity and scale of such reporting has produced a qualitative transformation in our overall percep-tion of, and involvement in, the pestilential drama. AIDS may, thus, be called 'postmodern', given 'the self-conscious, reflexive, bureaucratically structured detachment with which we regard it. Countless social scientists and journalists watch us as we watch ourselves; that reflexive process has become a character-istic aspect of America's experience with AIDS'. AIDS in the West has been a 'media reality, both exaggerated and diminished as it is articulated in forms suit-able for mass consumption. The great majority of Americans have been spectators, *in* but not *of* the epidemic' (Rosenberg 1992: 290).

BIOLOGICAL REDUCTIONISM AND REFLEXIVITY IN THE PUBLIC SPHERE

How much weight should we place on Rosenberg's analysis? I want first to deal with the sharp dichotomy contained in his thesis: the claim that up until the nineteenth century microbiology alone determined the epidemic drama but that by the late twentieth century public perception of, and participation in, such tragedies had been fundamentally modified by the mass media. Though I think his account captures a central part of the pestilential dynamic, both points need serious qualification.

Take first the microbiological determination of the drama. Rosenberg's account of this is primarily based on a large corpus of research into epidemics in late eighteenth- and early nineteenth-century Europe and the United States, though a similar social trajectory can, I think, be found in many other periods and places (Bell [1924] 1951; Ziegler 1969; Thucydides 1972; Wols 1977; Evans 1987; Berridge and Strong 1991; Parets 1991). Of course, no pestilence is quite the same as any other, for times and human circumstances change. None the less, where there is no effective protection against a sudden, major outbreak of fatal, infectious disease, or where such protection exists but is not used, such differences may no longer matter. As AIDS has shown, the disease becomes once more a pestilence; an epidemic with the same compulsive collective involvement, the same basic drama and plot-line, in societies separated by great gulfs in time and by profound differences in knowledge, belief and technology.

But, having said this, I think we need to make a careful distinction between, on the one hand, the plot-line of the pestilential drama and, on the other, the extent to which a society becomes transfixed by a particular performance of the play. Rosenberg's microbiological reductionism applies exclusively to the first point: that, behind the diverse ways in which local companies may play the epidemic drama, the fundamental plot remains the same. Here the historical evidence seems very strong. But once we turn to consider the occasion and degree of collective involvement, then matters look rather different. At one extreme, the plague drama may be performed even where there are, in fact, no actual cases of plague. At the other extreme, there may be plague but no plague drama. Some circumstances make Death dramatically manifest, even where little or no dying is actually done; others may blanket the corpses and muffle the groans.

The public visibility of an epidemic – and thus the extent to which the pestilential drama is unleashed – seems to be mediated by a range of factors. Not all of that mediation affects the microbiological hypothesis. The ease and mode of transmission of the micro-organism, the incubation period of the disease, the proportion of the population affected in a particular disease outbreak, and the fatality rate (the proportion of those infected who subsequently die from the disease) are all matters that are heavily shaped by biology and all factors which can powerfully affect the intensity and duration of the pestilential drama.

Consider the most dramatic epidemic in European history, the Black Death of 1348–9; an epidemic where all these biological variables came together to produce a novel, sudden, violent and fateful eruption – it is estimated that some-where between one third and one half of the European population died. Those who did so died between three and six days after being infected, while the disease itself, probably a mixture of bubonic and pneumonic plague (different versions of infection by *Yersinnia Pestis*), moved with great speed through the affected populations. In some small villages and hamlets almost everyone seems to have died. In such circumstances, the epidemic was not only accompanied by the pestilential drama but it also became plausible to give that drama in apocalyptic terms. Here, for instance, are what seem to be among the last words of Friar John Clyn of Kilkenny:

> : . . . being myself as it were among the dead, waiting for death to visit me, [I] have put into writing truthfully all the things that I have heard. And, lest the writing should perish with the writer of the work and fail with the labourer, I leave parchments to continue this work, if perchance any may survive and any of the race of Adam escape this pestilence to carry on the work I have begun.
>
> (Open University 1985: 46).[6]

Some *biological circumstances* may thus enhance or, in other cases, diminish the production of the pestilential drama. Exactly the same is true of the *social circumstances* in which an epidemic occurs. Consider the great plague of Athens of 430 BC, the first major epidemic in European history of which we possess a detailed record. The collective drama here seems to have been considerably amplified by the presence within the city of large numbers of refugees from the surrounding countryside; refugees who had fled to Athens to escape from an invading Spartan-led army and now found themselves in the midst of a pestilence:

> A factor which made matters much worse than they were already was the removal of people from the country into the city. . . . There were no houses for them, and, living as they did during the hot season in badly ventilated huts, they died like flies. The bodies of the dying were heaped one on top of the other, and half-dead creatures could be seen staggering about in the streets or flocking round the fountains in their desire for water. The temples in which they took up their quarters were full of the dead bodies of people who had died inside them.
>
> (Thucydides 1972: 154–5)

The occurrence and intensity of the pestilential drama may also, it seems, be shaped by the relative novelty or familiarity of the disease, by the existence, or otherwise, of other more compelling social dramas, by precisely whom the disease does and does not affect, and by a wide range of social, political and economic forces; all of which may lead, on the one hand, to increasing amplification or, on the other, to continuing denial.

Disentangling the individual effects of each social factor under different circumstances, and carefully separating each from the particular impact of the range of biological variables, are tasks well beyond the scope of this essay. However, the more fundamental point about the significant effect of social as well as biological factors in the production of the pestilential drama is much more readily made. Having seen some suggestive evidence from Thucydides' account of the plague of Athens, I want now to consider two striking contrasts, two 'natural experiments', both of which occurred in much more recent and better documented times. The first concerns the contrasting social impact of the Spanish Flu pandemic of 1918; possibly the greatest killer of them all. Across sub-Saharan Africa, a terrain massively disrupted by colonialism and where flu was a new and terrifying disease, it had an impact somewhat akin to the flagellant movements associated with the Black Death, giving birth to charismatic forms of Christianity which continue to this day (Ranger 1988). But in a United States gripped by its entry into the First World War and where flu was a familiar disease – if not quite in this devastating form – there is no sign whatsoever of the conventional pestilential drama. Spanish Flu here was a private not a public tragedy (Crosby 1989).

Rosenberg's second argument, however, seems much weaker. He argues that in the late twentieth century scientific and mass media commentary have fundamentally altered our sense of involvement in the pestilential drama; that we are caught up instead in an ever-increasing reflexive spiral as mere spectators rather than participants. This clearly ignores the obvious examples of mass fear of modern epidemics – the behaviour of the Canadian baggage handlers faced with luggage from Bombay and the well-documented initial response to AIDS (McKie 1986). It also seems surprisingly ahistorical. The mediation of our perception of pestilence is nothing new. Indeed, it has roots deep in the past and cannot be understood without considering the evolution of that past. One may note, to begin with, that the way plague was perceived in the medieval and early modern period was shaped in a much more powerful fashion than press or television can accomplish with any modern pestilence. For then there was only one mass medium:

> The preaching parson was the great link between the illiterate mass and the political, technical and educated world. Sitting in the 10,000 parish churches of England every Sunday morning, in groups of 20, 50, 100 or 200, the illiterate mass of the people were not only taking part in the single group activity which they ordinarily shared with others outside their own families. They were also informing themselves, in the only way open to them, of what went on in England, Europe and the world as a whole. The priesthood was indispensable to the religious activity of the old world, at a time when religion was still of primary interest and importance. But the priesthood was also indispensable because of its functions in social communication.
>
> (Laslett 1983: 9)

Given this monopoly, the early modern state, as it developed new policies on pestilence, made certain that it controlled just what was said in those 10,000 pulpits.

In 1603, for example, new plague prayers were issued by the state-controlled Church of England. The old prayers had stressed the need for religious submission to fate. Now a long and vehement 'Exhortation' insisted instead on the natural causes of plague, on their infectious rather than miasmatic nature, and on the religious duty of quarantine. Those who had 'thought that they were not "bound in conscience to shun and avoid the persons and places that are infected"' now, so it turned out, 'tempted God with their presumption and brought about "a public and manifest detriment to the state"' (Slack 1985: 230). Not everyone agreed. A Calvinist pamphlet published that year continued to insist that plague was due to divine providence. Its author, the preacher Henoch Clapham, was imprisoned and his release made dependent on signing this statement:

> That howsoever, there is no mortality but by and from a supernatural power, so yet it is not without concurrence of natural causes also, for the most part. . . . And I clearly and expressly hold the plague to be infectious and that it is most expedient for the parties infected to be severed and shut up (they having things necessary and convenient provided for them). . . . That a faithful Christian man, whether magistrate or minister, may in such times hide or withdraw himself, as well corporeally as spiritually, and use local flight to a more healthful place (taking sufficient order for the discharge of his function).
>
> (Cited in Slack 1985: 235)[7]

The only mass medium available at this point, thus, allowed space for only the most limited version of reflexivity. The state itself held the mirror up to nature and prescribed what the mirror was to reflect. Multiple commentary, spiralling reflexivity, could, therefore, not readily occur until there was a more liberal public sphere.[8] One hundred years later, however, there was. Here, for instance, are some observations from the journalist Richard Steele writing in 1709 in *The Tatler*, one of the most influential of the middle-class periodicals that rapidly sprang up after the abolition of most English state censorship with the Licensing Act of 1695. Steele comments in an ironic and reflexive fashion on some of the habits of his fellow-hacks, on, for example, the early career of 'the judicious and wary Mr I. Dawks', who was now a rabid and unreliable war-journalist but who had first 'got himself a reputation from plagues and famines; by which in those days, he destroyed as great multitudes as he has lately done by the sword. In every dearth of great news, Grand Cairo was sure to be unpeopled.' [9]

Another such example, even more postmodern in its spiralling reflexivity of commentary upon commentary upon commentary, occurs in James Boswell's *London Journal* in the entry for Christmas Day 1762. Two gentlemen in Child's coffee-house had been examining the latest London *Bill of Mortality*, the weekly mortality report compiled regularly from the seventeenth century onwards to monitor epidemic trends; a document that in a pestilence-ridden society was regularly checked by those who could read. Boswell, who had dropped in to Child's on his way back from church, heard his neighbours talking and, using the technique that later produced his classic biography of Samuel Johnson, recorded the following:

> *Citizen 1:*   Why here is the bill of mortality. Is it right doctor?
> *Physician:*   Why, I don't know.
> *Citizen 1:*   I'm sure it is not. Sixteen only died of cholics. I dare say you have killed as many yourself.

Citizen 2:   Ay, and hanged but three! O Lord, ha! ha!

(Pottle 1982: 114)

Having considered the tale of Henoch Clapham and the Exhortation and heard, a century later, from Steele and Boswell, let me sum up, very rapidly, the point of this section. The mediation of our perception of plague – along with many other things – is nothing new. Moreover, publicly available, reflexive commentary is a product not of postmodernism, but of early modernism, of that combination of modern science, journalism and a liberal public sphere which dates back to the seventeenth and eighteenth centuries. [10]

TWIN WORLDS, PARALLEL APOCALYPSES

So far I have taken Rosenberg's analysis of the pestilential drama on its own terms. I want now to set it in comparative perspective and view it simply as a sub-type, if an unusual one, of a universal class of phenomena. From this angle, a great pestilence cannot be interpreted solely in microbiological terms but has something in common with many other more conventional social crises. The classic epidemic is merely an outlier, a natural experiment, which, because it takes an unusually dramatic form, throws a penetrating and disturbing light on the rest of our lives. [11]

To show this, I want to go back to the point at which this essay began, to the front page of *The Independent* on 27 September 1994. I began by focusing on just one small detail: the news about the epidemic of pneumonic plague. Now consider the stories on the rest of the page. The five lead stories and the other three summary stories had the following headlines, listed in order of the priority given to them by the paper: (1) 'Labour Party Still Not Trusted On Economy' (a story based on an opinion poll); (2) 'Rail Talks Go On Today Amid Hopes Of Settlement' (a national strike); (3) 'Abuse Homes: Video Equipment Found' (allegations of rape and assault by staff in a home for the mentally handi-capped); (4) 'Haiti Killers Denied Promised Amnesty' (the American government had gone back on part of an agreement reached with the Haitian military rulers once the UN-sponsored invasion had proved successful); (5) 'All British Athletes Using Drugs To Be Named' (a story which followed threats to the participation of British athletes in international competition; (6) 'Death Of A Well-Known Lawyer From Cancer'; (7) 'Cheaper Telephone Calls'; and (8) 'Tennis Star' ('reveals that the strains of success brought her near suicide').

No less than seven of these stories touch on threats to diminish, or opportuni-ties to increase, what might be termed national integrity. Four deal with inner integrity – of the economy, of the rail and telephone network, of health and social care institutions – while the remaining three look outwards: to the interna-tional reputation of the nation's sporting representatives, to the military invasion of another country conducted under the auspices of an international body, and to the possible threat from pandemic disease. In addition, three of the stories concern death or possible death, a fourth is about assault and rape, while five deal with a cluster of issues surrounding trust, negotiation, disputes, cheating and panic. Finally, despite this overall focus on degradation, distrust and disaster, there is evidence of another, rather different perspective in several of the stories, of the possibility of concerted, effective human action: of giving justice to the handicapped and the Haitians, of settling disputes, of integrating the nation through one means or another.

From this wider perspective, the Surat drama was merely one drama among many. Indeed, most of the previous day's public life, as revealed through *The Independent*, consisted of drama in one form or another. The reason for that seems to be not so much cheap sensationalism, but that there is plenty to be sensational about, for the kind of social collapse that took place in Surat, far from being unique, is endemic in all human institutions. Of course, these data are taken from just one page of a single day's newspaper and the Surat story is the only instance of actual collapse. Can one really generalise from this to the whole of human experience?

It may, therefore, be helpful to consider the very wide range of forms of collapse that can readily be discovered once we turn beyond plague and beyond one day's news. Take some of the more important instances of major and minor social apocalypse: those recurrent crises, for instance, in economic credit which were so formative of early modern institutions and the political and social thought of the period,[12] and which still shape both realms today;[13] or the equally dramatic crises of political credit which range all the way from the extraordinary events of the French Revolution (Schama 1989) to the 'Westland affair' which first undermined Mrs Thatcher's standing within her cabinet (Young 1990: 431–41); [14] or, apparently more trivial, but in fact no less important, there are the perennial crises in the little world of the face to face encounter (Goffman 1959, 1961, 1967; Garfinkel 1967; Heritage 1984) – a world whose centrality to our lives was so accurately captured by Spencer:

> If disregarding conduct that is entirely private, we consider only that species of conduct which involves direct relations with other persons; and if under the name government we include all control of such conduct however arising; then we must say that the earliest kind of government, and the government which is ever spontaneously recommencing, is the government of ceremonial observance. More may be said. This kind of government, besides preceding other kinds, and besides having in all times and places approached nearer to universality of influence, has ever had, and continues to have, the largest share in regulating men's lives.
>
> (Herbert Spencer, cited in Goffman 1971: ix)

Of course, complete social collapse, the vision of hell witnessed by Andres de la Vega in Seville in 1649, may be relatively uncommon, but the threat of some sort of apocalypse remains a permanent possibility in every human encounter and institution. What, therefore, needs analysing when we consider 'society' is not one world but two; twin worlds of association and dislocation which each have their own distinctive form but yet revolve around, and are penetrated by, the other; mirror-image worlds of community and collapse which together comprise the ordinary social worlds in which we live. Of course, the experience of pestilence is unusual. Just because it is so it reveals, in a readily analysable way, the dark star, the hidden planet, whose orbit regularly crosses the more congenial, collective forms of social life.

What might explain the existence of these twin worlds and parallel apocalypses – assuming that we reject, even if we can sympathise with, de la Vega's assumption of Satanic intervention? I want to finish by arguing that the pestilential apocalypse – what was seen in embryo in Surat in 1994 and in terrifying maturity in Seville in 1649 – is simply one instance of that 'war of all against all' which Thomas Hobbes, the sage of Malmesbury, famously defined as 'the state of nature', saw as a perennial possibility in human society, and, as such, urged the necessity for the force and authority of a Leviathan to try to hold it at bay (Hobbes [1651] 1962: 100).

Obviously, such a claim is very far from new in twentieth-century social theory. *The Structure of Social Action* by Talcott Parsons, first published in 1937, is premised on the need to find some social mechanism which might satisfactorily explain why the Hobbesian state of nature is not a permanent state of affairs (Parsons [1937] 1949).[15] And since then, the 'problem of social order', as Parsons rechristened it, has been a permanent, if normally minor, fixture in conventional sociological theory courses. [16] For although Hobbes is normally referenced, he is rarely read and even less frequently understood. The enormous growth of Hobbes studies in political theory and the history of thought over the last few decades has had little or no impact on social theory.[17] As a result, his powerful analysis of the 'causes of quarrel' is simply ignored (Hobbes [1651] 1962: 99). His fundamental argument insists not so much on some innately aggressive or acquisitive properties of the human character – though both are certainly given due attention – as on the central importance of knowledge, certainty and trust if association rather than dissociation is to be constructed. As we have seen, a large, fatal epidemic with no hope of prophylaxis or cure provides a striking, if unusual, example of the state of nature that can ensue when these basic constituents of peaceful human interaction are missing. And, as we have also noted, states of nature – of various degrees of intensity – may also result from collapses in economic, political and interactional faith, from social as well as microbiological causes. The pestilential apocalypses at Seville in the seventeenth century or Surat in our own era cast a cold light on a much more general societal phenomenon.

But if this is granted, why does Hobbes play such a small part within conventional social theory, at least in its sociological form? Several possible answers spring to mind. One relates to the strange periodisation still current within the discipline. Just like psychologists (also members of a discipline given academic form in the nineteenth century), sociologists seem to find it hard to imagine that people could have had serious thoughts in their area before the period in which their subject received its contemporary name. Most introductions to sociological thought simply ignore all previous ideas in the area, or pass over them in a few pages before getting on to the real meat of Marx, Weber and Durkheim.[18]

This rather sad form of condescension is linked to two other striking failings. The first concerns the noticeable tendency in so much nineteenth- and twentieth-century social theory to impose some form of metaphysical human meaning upon the world. Kant and Hegel and, through them, Marx, Durkheim and Parsons, all seem to lie within the Augustinian tradition of Christian apocalyptics – if in a secularised version rather than that of Henoch Clapham.[19] Though they accept some version of the Hobbesian state of nature, they subsume such potential horrors under an account of necessary or managed human progress. The problem of order is apparently 'solved' by this or that means. What they really proclaim, therefore, is their solution, rather than the condition.[20] Thus, the sceptical or, more accurately, post-sceptical approach of Hobbes remains as uncomfortable to most of us now as it did to most of his contemporaries.[21]

Finally, there is the strange and relatively recent separation of the micro from the macro social realm; a sure means to hinder human self-understanding. Until the end of the eighteenth century, moral science, including of course Hobbes, based itself firmly on propositions from both arenas (Burns 1992: 19–20). [22] Social theory is now trying, painfully enough, to put the two together again (for example, Knorr-Cetina and Cicourel 1981; Giddens 1984; Alexander 1987; Mouzelis 1994). As we do so, we need to learn from some of the more successful practitioners of the past.

ACKNOWLEDGEMENTS

I would like to thank the Nuffield Trust for the generous funding which made possible the research into AIDS' social impact on which this chapter is based.

NOTES

1 Cited in Parets 1991: 99–100.
2 The main part that I have elaborated a little concerns the relationship between the underlying microbiology and the form of the pestilential drama.
3 For an introductory exposition from a modern biological exposition see Halliday 1994.
4 Charles Morgan, a British theatre critic, describes this as follows: 'The great impact of the theatre is neither the persuasion of the intellect nor a beguiling of the senses. . . . It is the enveloping movement of the whole drama on the soul of man. We surrender and are changed' (cited in Geertz 1983: 28).
5 Thus, AIDS produced a collective crisis in Japan at a time when only two cases had actually been identified in the country (Ohi *et al.* 1988).
6 At the end of this account, Clyn wrote the words 'great hardship' and then appears to have died.
7 Clapham refused and stayed in prison for eighteen months.
8 Habermas's (1992) account is the fundamental theoretical treatment of this sphere,

despite its obvious limitations, particularly a Whig optimism about the early public sphere and a Frankfurtian pessimism about its later manifestations. See, in particular Schudson 1992 on the former point and, on the latter, Dayan and Katz 1988. For the possibilities for public reflexivity in the arts before the creation of that sphere and during the transition to it see Patterson 1984.

9 'Painful position of the news-writers if peace should come' (Steele 1968: 17).

10 Boswell was not a one-off. Robert Burns gave his fellow-Scots a famous warning about this sort of thing, commenting on a study of Scotland undertaken, this time, by an English spectator: 'If there's a hole in a' your coats, I rede you tent it [mend it], A chield's amang you takin' notes, And faith he'll prent it' ('On the late Captain Grose's peregrinations in Scotland', 1789). Likewise, it is hard to imagine a more dazzlingly reflexive novel than Laurence Sterne's *Tristram Shandy* (1759–67). The belief that postmodernism is modern is a striking, contemporary example of what Pitirim Sorokin called the 'obsessive discoverer's complex' and wrote about, some-what intemperately, in a case-study of 'Amnesia and new Columbuses' (Sorokin 1956). This complex seems endemic in human society.

11 On the role of illuminating incidents in social theory see Garfinkel 1956 on Goffman's use of metaphor and Runciman 1983, particularly Chapter 4, 'Descript-ion in social theory'.

12 See Earle 1989 for an analysis of the effects of credit on early modern life and Pocock 1975 for the effects of credit crises on the political thought of the period.

13 The following was written a week after the Surat story cited earlier: 'Bubonic plague has got nothing on the ability of financial markets to spread fear around the world. Yesterday brought another of those famous Wall Street sneezes prompting heavy falls in bond and equity prices throughout the world's financial sectors.' 'Europe victim of US excess' ('View from City Road'), *The Independent*, 6 October 1994, p. 33.

14 On the fundamental general importance of credit and its maintenance for the careers of individuals, institutions and nations, see also Goode 1978; Sacksteder 1989; Bourdieu 1991.

15 Buxton's (1985) analysis of Parsons' work in the early 1930s argues that his interest in Hobbes stemmed from fears of national social collapse prompted by the great depression in the United States and the rise of fascism in Europe.

16 For contrasting views on its importance see Giddens 1977 – against; and Dawe 1978 and Heritage 1984 – for.

17 See, for example, the reviews in Tuck 1989, 1993a; Minogue 1994.

18 Swingewood 1984 is just one example.

19 See Sullivan 1989 and the essays in Patrides 1984, particularly those by Abrams, Reeves and Tuveson.

20 A related form of belief in successful management can be found in the mainstream liberal economic tradition, which, though it partially originated in Hobbes, became, with the success of capitalism, a good deal more optimistic (Hirschman 1977; Tuck 1993b).

21 Hobbes, of course, also proclaimed a solution: that of Leviathan. But he took good care both to analyse the problem in great detail and to stress that there was no guar-anteed solution, that key aspects of life remained, to use another of his powerful metaphors, a 'race' (Hobbes [1640] 1994: 59–60). Goffman's work has had a similar reception to that of Hobbes and for identical reasons. He too is praised for his bril-liance but attacked for his view of human nature. For like Hobbes, he too has a Janus-faced view of the human condition (Strong 1988).

22 Kant's assault on the ethical status of rhetoric may be partly responsible for this (Minson 1993). A recent analysis of nationalism – apparently another great British

invention – suggests a further possible reason (Newman 1987). The middle-class assault on the international culture of the aristocracy, done in the name of 'patriotism' and with a new stress on 'openness' and 'honesty', seems to have dealt powerful blows to the ancient aristocratic interest in manners and rhetoric; both central subjects of what we now call micro analysis.

REFERENCES

Alexander, J.C., Giesen, B., Munch, R. and Smelser, N.J. (eds) (1987) *The Micro–Macro Link*, Berkeley: University of California Press.
Bell, W.G. ([1924] 1951) *The Great Plague in London, 1665*, London: Bodley Head.
Berridge, V. and Strong, P. (1991) 'AIDS in the UK: contemporary history and the study of policy', *Twentieth Century British History*, 2(2): 150–74.
Bourdieu, P. (1991) *Language and Symbolic Power*, Cambridge: Polity.
Burns, T. (1992) *Erving Goffman*, London: Routledge.
Buxton, W. (1985) *Talcott Parsons and the Capitalist Nation-State: Political Sociology as a Strategic Vocation*, Toronto: Toronto University Press.
Crosby, A.W. (1989) *America's Forgotten Epidemic: The Influenza of 1918*, Cambridge: Cambridge University Press.
Dawe, A. (1978) 'Theories of social action', in T. Bottomore and R. Nisbet (eds) *A History of Sociological Analysis*, London: Heinemann.
Dayan, D. and Katz. E (1988) 'Articulating consensus: the ritual and rhetoric of media events', in J.C. Alexander (eds) *Durkheimian Sociology: Cultural Studies*, Cambridge: Cambridge University Press.
Earle, P. (1989) *The Making of the English Middle Class*, London: Methuen.
Evans, R.J. (1987) *Death in Hamburg: Society and Politics in the Cholera Years, 1830–1910*, Harmondsworth: Penguin.
Garfinkel, H. (1956) 'Some sociological concepts and methods for psychiatrists', *Psychiatric Research Reports*, 6: 181–95.
—— (1967) *Studies in Ethnomethodology*, Englewood Cliffs, NJ: Prentice Hall.
Geertz, C. (1983) *Local Knowledge: Further Essays in Interpretive Anthropology*, New York: Basic Books.
Giddens, A. (1977) *Studies in Social and Political Theory*, London: Hutchinson.
—— (1984) *The Constitution of Society: Outline of the Theory of Structuration*, Cambridge: Polity.
Goffman, E. (1959) *The Presentation of Self in Everyday Life*, New York: Doubleday Anchor.
—— (1961) *Encounters: Two Studies in the Sociology of Interaction*, Indianapolis: Bobbs-Merrill.
—— (1967) *Interaction Ritual*, Harmondsworth: Penguin.
—— (1971) *Relations in Public: Microstudies of the Public Order*, Harmondsworth: Allen Lane.
Goode, W.J. (1978) *The Celebration of Heroes: Prestige as a Control System*, Berkeley: University of California Press.
Habermas, J. (1992) *The Structural Transformation of the Public Sphere*, Cambridge: Polity.
Halliday, T. (1994) 'Living with other species', in B. Davey and T. Halliday (eds) *Human Biology and Health: An Evolutionary Approach*, Buckingham: Open University Press.
Heritage, J. (1984) *Garfinkel and Ethnomethodology*, Cambridge: Cambridge University Press.
Hirschman, A.O. (1977) *The Passions and the Interests: Political Arguments for Capitalism Before Its Triumph*, Princeton, NJ: Princeton University Press.
Hobbes, T. ([1640] 1994) *The Elements of Law Natural and Politic: Part I, Human Nature*, Oxford: Oxford University Press.
—— ([1651] 1962) *Leviathan: or the Matter, Form and Power of a Commonwealth, Ecclesiastical and Civil*, New York: Collier Books.

Knorr-Cetina, K. and Cicourel, A.V. (eds) (1981) *Advances in Social Theory and Methodology: Toward an Integration of Micro and Macro Sociologies*, London: Routledge & Kegan Paul.

Laslett, P. (1983) *The World We Have Lost – Further Explored*, London: Routledge.

McKie, R. (1986) *Panic: The Story of AIDS*, Wellingborough: Thorson's.

Minogue, K. (1994) 'Hobbes and his critics', editor's introduction to T. Hobbes, *Leviathan*, London: Dent.

Minson, J. (1993) *Questions of Conduct: Sexual Harrassment, Citizenship, Government*, London: Macmillan.

Mouzelis, N. (1994) *Sociological Theory: What Went Wrong?*, London: Routledge.

Newman, G. (1987) *The Rise of English Nationalism: A Cultural History*, London: Weidenfeld & Nicolson.

Ohi, G. *et al.* (1988) 'Cost–benefit analysis of AIDS prevention programmes: its limitation in policy-making', in A. Fleming *et al.* (eds) *The Global Impact of AIDS*, New York: Alan R. Liss Inc.

Open University (1985) *Medical Knowledge: Doubt and Certainty*, Milton Keynes: Open University Press.

Parets, M. (1991) *A Journal of the Plague Year: The Diary of the Barcelona Tanner, Miquel Parets, 1651*, J.S. Amelang (trans. and ed.), Oxford: Oxford University Press.

Parsons, T. ([1937] 1949) *The Structure of Social Action: A Study in Social Theory with Special Reference to a Group of Recent European Writers*, New York: Free Press.

Patrides, C. (1984) *The Apocalypse in English Renaissance: Thought and Literature*, Manchester: Manchester University Press.

Patterson, A. (1984) *Censorship and Interpretation: The Conditions of Writing and Reading in Early Modern England*, Madison: University of Wisconsin Press.

Pocock, J.G.A. (1975) *The Machiavellian Moment: Florentine Political Thought and the Atlantic Republican Tradition*, Princeton, NJ: Princeton University Press.

Pottle, F.A. (ed.) (1982) *Boswell's London Journal, 1762–1763*, London: Futura.

Ranger, T. (1988) 'The influenza pandemic in Southern Rhodesia: a crisis of comprehension', in *Imperial Medicine and Indigenous Societies*, Manchester: Manchester University Press.

Rosenberg, C.E. (1992) *Explaining Epidemics and Other Studies in the History of Medicine*, Cambridge: Cambridge University Press.

Runciman, W.G. (1983) *A Treatise on Social Theory: The Methodology of Social Theory*, Cambridge: Cambridge University Press.

Sacksteder, W. (1989) 'Mutually acceptable glory: rating among nations in Hobbes', in P. Caws (ed.) *The Causes of Quarrel: Essays on Peace, War and Thomas Hobbes*, Boston: Beacon Press.

Schama, S. (1989) *Citizens*, London: Viking.

Schudson, M. (1992) 'Was there ever a public sphere? If so, when? Reflections on the American case', in C. Calhoun (ed.) *Habermas and the Public Sphere*, Cambridge, MA: MIT Press.

Slack, P. (1985) *The Impact of Plague in Tudor and Stuart England*, Oxford: Clarendon.

Sorokin, P.A. (1956) *Fads and Foibles in Modern Sociology and Related Sciences*, Chicago: Henry Regnery.

Steele, R. (1968) *The Tatler*, London: Everyman.

Strong, P. (1988) 'Minor courtesies and macro structures', in P. Drew and A. Wootton (eds) *Erving Goffman: Exploring the Interaction Order*, Oxford: Polity.

Strong, P. and Berridge, V. (1990) 'No one knew anything: some issues in British AIDS policy', in P. Aggleton, P. Davies and G. Hart (eds) *AIDS: Individual, Cultural and Policy Dimensions*, London: Falmer.

Sullivan, R.J. (1989) *Immanuel Kant's Moral Theory*, Cambridge: Cambridge University Press.

Swingewood, A. (1984) *A Short History of Sociological Thought*, London: Macmillan.

Thucydides (1972) *History of the Peloponnesian War*, R. Warner (trans.), Harmondsworth: Penguin.

Tuck, R. (1989) *Hobbes*, Oxford: Oxford University Press.

—— (1993a) 'History', in R.E. Goodin and P. Pettit (eds) *A Companion to Contemporary Political Philosophy*, Oxford: Blackwell.

—— (1993b) *Philosophy and Government, 1572–1651*, Cambridge: Cambridge University Press.

Wols, M (1977) *The Black Death in the Middle East*, Princeton, NJ: Princeton University Press.

Young, H. (1990) *One of Us: A Biography of Margaret Thatcher*, London: Pan.

Ziegler, P. (1969) *The Black Death*, Harmondsworth: Pelican.

Chapter 15

Conclusion
From meddling to mastery?

Rosaline S. Barbour and Guro Huby

THE RESEARCH BARGAIN, REFLEXIVITY AND THE SOCIOLOGICAL GAZE

In this volume, the way conventions, expectations and protocols around the research role have shaped and constrained contributors' interactions with respondents is stressed throughout. Using contemporary social theory and ideals of practice we dwell in detail on power, agency and the research bargains we make and sometimes break. For many of us, our contribution amounts to a chase of the elusive 'dialogic ideal' of equal exchange of views and experiences between researcher and the researched and we consider, sometimes agonise over, the possibility that research often means selling our respondents short.

This agonising, although nothing exceptional in social science research, has taken a peculiar shape and intensity in AIDS research. We have taken this 'dialogic ideal' into a field of action where systems of prevention, support and care are often founded on explicit ideals of equity of access and equality of relationships between providers and users of services. Failure to realise our ideals appear perhaps more starkly, and are felt most acutely, in a situation where there seems to be broad agreement about how social relationships should function. These ideals of equality and dialogue often come up against a reality of ambiguous policy contexts where several and contradictory perceptions of 'equality' compete. Dima Abdulrahim (Chapter 3) describes the competing definitions of the terms 'ethnic minority' and 'culture' and the resulting exclusion of ethnic minority clients from services. Moreover, as Katie Deverell (Chapter 7) describes, dialogic ideals are not necessarily seen as applicable to research and evaluation which may be regarded pragmatically as providing a means to an end, whether it be engineering changes in risky behaviour or continuing funding: 'Never mind the methods and the process, just give us the facts.' As Neil Small (Chapter 8) points out and Edwin van Tejlingen and Guro Huby (Chapter 13) elaborate, the maturing trajectory of the academic field of AIDS research clashes with an ever-increasing pressure to produce quantifiable answers to questions of cost-effectiveness of services.

We consider and discuss with considerable candour and honesty our own agency in responding to the structural and political contingency of our work. Deverell describes in detail the 'balancing acts' she had to perform while juggling participation/observation, private/public roles and distance/intimacy in research relationships. Jill Bourne (Chapter 6) and Hugh Masters (Chapter 5) discuss how a lack of protocols concerning the display of researcher emotions affected and sometimes restricted their interactions with respondents and analysis of data. Guro Huby (Chapter 10) rejected the possibility of challenging a drug user's idealisation of the heroin days, and for perhaps less than honourable reasons, namely the need to increase response rates to a survey. Was this a breach of the contract or a pragmatic approach to a difficult situation? What material would have emerged if Brian Heaphy (Chapter 2) had realised the dialogic ideal and challenged his respondents on their use of clinical trials and new treatments? Or if Philip Gatter (Chapter 4) had challenged the counsellor directly rather than through subsequent writing?

We also discuss whether relationships of good faith can be extended to the exchange of results between the researcher and our various audiences. Rosaline Barbour (Chapter 11) discusses the choices we make in selecting quotes and examples from field material to illustrate or develop the points we wish to put across and the potential and limitations in attempting to share these with respondents. Cathy Stark (Chapter 12) and Hugh Masters (Chapter 5) discuss the many ethical concerns and dilemmas which bear on the presentation of research findings in settings where the respondents are known to the audiences of our writing. Getting our message across thus not only depends on the researcher's integrity and honesty, but also on the frame of mind and theoretical reference points from which our audiences judge and interpret what they hear. As Heaphy (quoting Schrijvers 1991) suggests, the researcher can only realise the 'dialogic ideal' through awareness of and active engagement in the particular play of power in the settings under study. Edwin van Teijlingen and Guro Huby (Chapter 13) describe how evaluation research is shaped by the political and practical parameters which frame the research. Neil Small suggests that we may be further away than before from realising 'the dialogic ideal' in an environment where research is driven by concerns of narrowly defined 'cost-efficiency'.

Perhaps Clive Foster (Chapter 9) and Philip Strong (Chapter 14) agonise the least. Foster elegantly sidesteps the issue of 'dialogic ideal' by arguing that exchange of views in the setting he studied is inextricably linked with the creative use of language whereby myths are made. The exchange itself thus shapes the arguments and views exchanged. The exchange is, furthermore, bound up with and embedded in the construction and confirmation of political status and economic interest.

It was ever thus. Phil Strong suggests a fresh look at 'reflexivity' and urges a recognition that attempts to understand and master (wo)man's relationship to a social and physical environment existed before sociology and other branches of the social sciences invented and named themselves as separate professions. For example, reflections similar to our deliberations on the ethics of relationships between researcher and the researched were a central part of early nineteenth-century moral philosophy's debates on man's (*sic*) motivations, free will and ability to transcend social and historical contingency. Strong specifically mentions Hobbes's thinking as being of relevance to our own.

The reflections do, however, appear dressed in different language according to the circumstances, languages and ideologies of the time and they are a by-product of academic and intellectual exchange where, besides reflexive commentary, reputation, recognition and therefore promotion are being traded. The content of the intellectual charges may change but the contested territory of academic reputation remains surprisingly constant. Neil Small (Chapter 8) refers to the debate between Becker and Gouldner about 'whose side we are on'. Here, Gouldner concludes that Becker's motives for casting himself as the spokesperson of people he classed as underdogs – and lacking in the ability and opportunity to speak for themselves – emerged from his position in the academic hierarchies of American sociology at the time. Of course, as Small suggests, Gouldner's position as the defender of a sociology which 'does not take sides' did him no harm either.

In qualitative social sciences,[1] recent trends in 'reflexivity' have produced valuable insights into the nature of the research enterprise and made us aware that history shapes our written products in ways which are beyond both our understanding and control. Ethnography enacts power relations (Clifford and Marcus 1986: 9); it does not merely reflect them. The same goes for other kinds of sociological writing. Paradoxically, however, although we suggested in the Introduction that reflexivity may in some respects have been carried too far, we now suggest that there are still areas of research practice which we can profitably reflect upon.

Some of the factors that shape our research products at any one time are beyond our conscious and intellectual grasp. Others are obvious and immediate to us. A current concern is the pressure to publish in peer-reviewed academic journals in order to stay afloat in an increasingly competitive research environment anxiously looking to the next Research Assessment Exercise. This pressure is over and beyond the personal satisfaction writing may bring and the more worldly rewards associated with academic repute and recognition. Mick Blowfield (1994) suggests that the spiralling in academic papers is happening at a time when academics have less time to read due to increased administrative and bureaucratic responsibilities. More seriously, however, this production does not necessarily help to increase knowledge and awareness of crucial issues among the public at large and in organisations with political leverage to bring about change where change is needed. He describes how he and his colleagues in a project on the international trainer shoe industry in a Third World country worked systematically to organise an awareness-raising campaign through the international press and labour organisations. This was largely successful and brought political pressure on the national government and protection to local labour activists. However, in personal career terms this work paid few rewards.

He himself only got one academic publication out of three years of concerted publishing effort.

There are other ways in which academic reflexivity may not connect constructively with lived realities. Several chapters in this volume suggest that theoretical awareness and sensitivity to power and domination in research encounters does not necessarily translate into techniques which help us address in a practical sense the more messy, uncontrollable and uncomfortable aspects of fieldwork. The reflexivity, in a sense, takes place from the safe distance afforded by academic journals and comes too late, after the damage is done. Many of us will at one time have responded to a colleague or student's confessions of less than competent and sensitive fieldwork with a 'Never mind, dear, there's a paper in this!' rather than helping to confront the pain endured through a constructive discussion of lessons learnt and consideration of the implications for future practice. It is rather like drug prevention workers in London neglecting a detailed scrutiny of their own interactions with 'ethnic minority' drug users and the outcomes of these interactions in pursuit of an abstract but 'politically correct' notion of targeting 'ethnic minorities' (Dima Abdulrahim, Chapter 3). Rosaline Barbour (Chapter 11) urges us to extend our reflexivity to examine the assumptions and conventions which structure our academic products in the form of oral presentations and published papers, arguing that we can use our writing as an analytic tool.

This is not to devalue the many individual examples of good supervision which help and foster reflexive practice, but rather to urge more formal, durable and visible structures of supervision and support within which reflexive research *practice* can take place and develop as a communal professional property (Batchelor and Briggs 1994).

The absence of such structures has consequences for the emotional well-being of individual researchers who may find or feel themselves unsupported. Much damage limitation here takes place in informal encounters where confessions are exchanged, support provided and blame apportioned. However, these sessions rarely go beyond the private and informal. When they do, the balance is not always successfully achieved between, on the one hand, intellectualising painful and conflicting experience and, on the other, making practical and liveable sense of it (cf. Green *et al.* 1993, cited by Jill Bourne, Chapter 6). There are thus areas of practice which lie outside qualitative social science's reflexive gaze upon itself. In thus confining these private deliberations between individual and consenting sociologists (Horobin 1985) and other social scientists to the dark corners of the bar, we might be missing an opportunity to enrich both practice and theory.

'Emotional' issues are marginalised by the academic conventions which structure our writing and also our oral presentations. Although, of late, some researchers have advocated that we experiment with new forms of writing (for example, Richardson 1994) we continue to be constrained by relatively rigid expectations with respect to conference presentations. Whilst an actress is likely to receive plaudits for conveying the poignancy of situations which she describes and re-enacts, academic presentations are characterised by a much flatter style of delivery. It is permissible to become excited by the theoretical perspectives we are outlining, but not, it seems, by the plights of our respondents, and certainly not by the emotions which we ourselves have experienced – and may continue to experience when we revisit our data and analyses. We may not provide the gory slides which are so often a feature of papers given at medical conferences, but we are expected to be equally unflinching in our presentation of potentially disturbing verbal images. Presentational style is all-important in conveying professional competence.

We need to ground our sociological/anthropological 'gaze' in the fleeting here and now of practice. This means recognising the conditions which structure that gaze and its transformations through historic change. Foucault (1973) traces the archaeology of the medical 'gaze' which emerged in eighteenth-century French medicine and which revolutionised medical practice at that time. He analyses 'the clinical gaze' as transformations of clinical discourse through specific constellations of organisational and political change in eighteenth-century French medical institutions. There are clear parallels to be drawn between the medical and a 'sociological' 'gaze'. Like the doctor's 'clinical gaze' in *Birth of the Clinic*, the research 'gaze' in the settings surveyed in this collection helps lay open to scrutiny the 'abnormal' versus the 'normal', the 'sick' versus the 'healthy' and the 'marginal'/'(ethnic) minority' versus 'mainstream' and 'majority' society. It constitutes and defines 'people with HIV/AIDS' as objects of discourses on 'chaos', 'risk', 'danger' 'deviance' – discourses with which we as researchers engage and which we attempt, with varying degrees of success, to deconstruct in pursuit of 'the dialogic ideal'. This ideal remains elusive, of course, because deconstruction carries its own parameters and creates new situations to be deconstructed in turn. Thus, Katie Deverell's (Chapter 7) respondents perceived her invitations for them to become involved in the writing up the results from her research as attempts to control them, rather than offering them control over the final product.

Achieving some degree of mastery over this process requires fine-tuned attention to the details of everyday practice and the shifting contexts in which this occurs. Foucault discusses the changes in epistemological status of 'the eye' as a source of light and ideal knowledge: 'All light has passed into the thin flame of the eye, which now flickers around solid objects and, in so doing, establishes their place and form' (Foucault 1973: xiv).

In the dark spaces 'between the solid objects' apparently insignificant or trivial events and incidents are found which may be the origin of different stories about research and the relationship between researchers and their respondents and in which we can ground a sociological and anthropological reflexivity in the details of practice. We return here to the dark corners of the bar and to the stories which researchers exchange.

THE STORIES RESEARCHERS TELL

Like the stories which circulated among the providers and users of Scottish HIV services (Guro Huby, Chapter 10), the informal stories which researchers exchange serve many functions and touch on diverse aspects of our research endeavour and our experience of doing research. Removed from the stringencies of research contracts, the exigencies of aims and objectives and the pressure in formal paper sessions to score intellectual points off our academic peers and rivals, we can engage in what Herzfeldt (1997) calls 'social poetics': the play with ambiguities, the 'use of metaphor' which 'may . . . unsettle the semiotic illusion of a culture or a moral universe that claims never to change' (Herzfeldt 1997: 22). This is similar to what C. Wright Mills (1959) described as 'a sociological playfulness of mind'. It is an 'intimate' (Herzfeldt 1997) exchange in the sense that (and apart from other forms of intimacy which may develop in the bar at conference time) it draws on a subtle and shared recognition of why we do what we do. This intimacy also implies a distancing from our own action and the possibility that we might (re)act differently.

There are several aspects of the exchange of stories which do not unsettle in this way, of course. A good deal of the exchange consists of 'whingeing' and blaming others for problems and difficulties. Some stories contain an element of ritualised boasting and one-upmanship where status in the formal and informal academic hierachies is challenged or confirmed – rather like the way storytelling on the estate Clive Foster was studying served to uphold dealer hegemony and male power.

Among the more unsettling are stories about the emotional impact of field-work on the researcher (Hugh Masters, Jill Bourne, Cathy Stark – Chapters 5, 6 and 12 respectively) and attempts to elicit emotional support. Along with this emotional work there goes a use of stories to 'structure inchoate situations' (Fernandez 1986 in Clive Foster's chapter). Wilkins argues that our emotional responses aid

> a sophisticated sensibility [which] has an important interpretive function. It is a medium through which intuitive insights and inchoate knowledge arise, and this in turn depends on the availability of similar emotions and/or experience, whether imaginatively, or actually, within our own biography.
>
> (Wilkins 1993: 96)

And, we would add, the biographies of other 'consenting adults' with whom we 'sociologise' (Horobin 1985). Personal biographies are of sociological and analytical interest inasmuch as our own histories are shaped by the very forces which structure the social fields we set out to study (Marcus 1992). Much of the informal exchanges among sociologists, anthropologists and other qualitative social scientists involves a 'trying out' of emergent analyses based on a collective experience of the dynamic interplay of personal biographies and current theory. The stories we as social researchers tell informally often capture the subtlety of these dynamics better than our formal products, and awareness of them may help us produce work which is visibly connected to lived practice – both our own and others'.

There is, though, a danger in feeling or intellectualising too much and theorising too little. A way forward is to engage in an irreverent and self-ironic play with our own contingency from what Tsing (1994) terms 'marginality as a structural position'. The irony and distance with which some of our respondents engage with their own marginality is an example to us all. We as social researchers engage in similar play, of course, but the products of our banter seldom reach the pages of formal papers or reports. Horobin says that only the most secure or arrogant of us treat our experience as data in public. Perhaps it is time to take this risk.

Staying attuned to our own practice also holds the potential of change. We suggest, with Herzfeldt (1997), that it is particularly in the informal and 'culturally intimate' exchange of stories and tales that boundaries lose their rigidity and the seeds for change are sown. We need therefore to acknowledge and pay heed to the more obscure parts of our sociologising as a way of linking theory to practice and stay abreast of the shifting nature of both entities and the way they interrelate. The stories we exchange in the bar are an extremely important part of the craft of sociology and anthropology (as if we didn't know) and can be put to even better use.

According to Brooks (1984) stories always chase the elusive. In Lacan's (1977, referenced in Brooks 1984) terms, there is always slippage between past experience as signified and the story as signifier bringing the story back – hence the universal passion for stories, the quest for the word or saying that will articulate experience, making it whole and real again, but never quite succeeding, always leaving something unsaid. In this slippage, experience is re-enacted and changed and boundaries are challenged and redrawn. In chasing elusive ideals of research practice, however, we need to stay tuned to and rooted in the limitations and conditions of our work.

REFLEXIVITY AND THE ELUSIVE: CHASING THE LAST VISIBLE DOG

The very act of reflexivity sets up new situations to be reflexively scrutinised in turn in what Strong (Chapter 14) terms a 'spiralling reflexivity' (fuelled, we would suggest, by the political and economic pressures which produce a spiralling of academic publications). Ultimately, however, the usefulness of such infinite scrutiny is questionable: as Murcott suggests, reflexive commentary can be pursued with 'near banal archness'. It is rather like 'the last visible dog' on the tin can stumbled upon by the Mouse and his Child of Russell Hoban's story:

bonzo Dog Food said the white letters on the orange label, and below the name was a picture of a little black-and-white spotted dog, walking on his hind legs and wearing a chef's cap and an apron. The dog carried a tray on which there was another can of bonzo Dog Food on the label of which another little black-and-white spotted dog, exactly the same but much smaller, was walking on his hind legs and carrying a tray on which there was another can of BONZO Dog Food, on the label of which another little black-and-white spotted dog, exactly the same, but much smaller, was walking on his hind legs and carrying a tray on which there was another can of BONZO Dog Food, and so on until the dogs became too small for the eye to follow.

(Hoban 1986: 30)

Having imagined themselves the only creatures with privileged access to this deep, but essentially elusive statement, the two characters are later startled to encounter 'The Caws of Art Experimental Theatre Group' performing 'The Last Visible Dog' as a play. The actors too appear to find the message compelling, if somewhat hard to pin down and use:

'Are you absolutely sure you want to do The Last Visible Dog tonight?', said Mrs. Crow.
'Sure, I'm sure', said Crow. It's the hottest thing we've got. It's new. It's far out. It's a play with a message.'
'What's the message?', said Mrs. Crow.
'I don't know', said Crow. 'But I know it's there, and that's what counts.'

(Hoban 1986: 66)

[The performance begins and builds to a climax:]
'BEYOND THE LAST VISIBLE DOG!' shouted Crow.
'There!' he said to his wife. 'See how it pays off? Up and up and up and then Zonk! 'BEYOND THE LAST VISIBLE DOG!'
'It's getting me now', said Mrs. Crow. 'But what does it mean?'
Crow flung wide his broad wings like a black cloak.
'What doesn't it mean?' he said. 'There's no end to it – it just goes on and on until it means anything and everything, depending on who you are and what your last visible dog is.'

(Hoban 1986: 68)

AIDS so clearly reveals the ever-changing context in which research takes place. As Phil Strong suggests, this also goes for the content of our debates: today we are reinventing reflexivity, tomorrow something else will capture our imagination. We have to guard against our reflexivity resembling the Last Visible Dog perpetually chasing its own tail.

Philip Strong is concerned that social theory tends to lie within traditions of Christian apocalyptics looking to some ultimate metaphysical order and urges a re-examination of both the epistemological and moral basis of our work as social scientists. This echoes Neil Small (Chapter 8), who, referring to Bauman (1992), urges a modest research enterprise where we focus on the details of 'our practice as interpreters' rather than on a role as 'umpire of truth'.

Strong suggests we go back to the 'pre-critical' approaches of, for example, Hobbes in order to found our practice on a view of ourselves and our research respondents which accords with such a modesty. The Hobbesian view posits us as complex human beings needing both space and a well-thought-out institutional framework in order to function as ethical creative beings. According to Anne Murcott, Strong's chapter also urges us as social scientists to explain and illuminate the complexities of the particular and let the universals take care of themselves. Like the Mouse and his Child in Russell Hoban's story we can safely settle and make our home with the 'Last Visible Dog'.

NOTE

1 We include under this rubric sociology, social anthropology and other social scientific work which draws on critical political and feminist theory.

REFERENCES

Batchelor, J.A. and Briggs, C.M. (1994) 'Subject, project or self? Thoughts on ethical dilemmas for social and medical researchers', *Social Science and Medicine*, 39(7): 949–54.

Bauman, Z. (1992) *Intimations of Postmodernism*, London: Routledge.

Blowfield, M. (1994) 'Publish or perish', *Anthropology in Action*, 1(1): 23–5.

Brooks, P. (1984) *Reading for the Plot: Design and Intention in Narrative*, New York: Vintage.

Clifford, J. and Marcus, G. (eds) (1986) *Writing Culture: The Poetics and Politics of Ethnography*, Berkeley: University of California Press.

Fernandez, J. (1986) *Persuasions and Performances: The Play of Tropes in Culture*, Bloomington: Indiana University Press.

Foucault, M. (1973) *Birth of the Clinic*, London: Tavistock.

Green, G., Barbour, R.S., Barnard, M. and Kitzinger, J. (1993) 'Who wears the trousers? Sexual harrasment in research settings', *Women's Studies International Forum*, 16(6): 627–37.

Herzfeldt, M. (1997) *Cultural Intimacy: Social Poetics in the Nation-State*, New York and London: Routledge.

Hoban, R. (1986) *The Mouse and His Child*, Harmondsworth: Puffin.

Horobin, G. (1985) 'Review essay – Medical sociology in Britain: true confessions of an empiricist', *Sociology of Health and Illness*, 7(1): 94–107.

Lacan, J. (1977) 'L'instance de la lettre', in *Écrits*, E. Sheridan (trans.), New York: Norton.

Marcus, J. (1992) 'Racism, terror and the production of Australian auto/biographies', in J. Okely and H. Callaway (eds) *Anthropology and Autobiography*, ASA Monograph No. 29, London: Routledge.

Mills, C.W. (1959) *The Sociological Imagination*, London: Oxford University Press.

Richardson, L. (1994) 'Writing: a method of inquiry', in N.K. Denzin and Y.S. Lincoln (eds) *Handbook of Qualitative Research*, London: Sage.

Schrijvers, J. (1991) 'Dialectics of a dialogical ideal: studying down, studying sideways, studying up', in L. Nencel and P. Pels (eds) *Constructing Knowledge: Authority and Critique in Social Science*, London: Sage.

Tsing, A.L. (1994) 'From the margins', *Cultural Anthropology*, 9: 279–97.

Wilkins, R. (1993) 'Taking it personally: a note on emotion and autobiography', *Sociology*, 27(1): 93–100.

Name index

Abbot, P. 223
Abdulrahim, D. 34, 38, 40, 43, 44, 47
Adam, B.D. 9
Adams, J. 79
Adler, P. 86, 87
Aggleton, P. 39, 104, 108, 114
Aldridge, J. 13, 184
Alexander, J.C. 254
Allsop, D. 219, 220
Anderson, K. 29
Armstrong, D. 3
Atkinson, P. 13, 25, 26, 109, 119, 139, 141, 191, 194
Awaiah, J. 40

Bailey, C. 132
Baker, T.L. 221
Barbour, R.S. 1, 2, 8, 11, 17, 40, 78, 99, 100, 111, 129, 187, 194, 196, 213, 262
Barnard, M. 99, 100, 111, 262
Barnes, J.A. 140
Barthes, R. 146, 148, 155
Batchelor, J.A. 262
Baum, F. 107–8, 109, 118
Baum, M. 134
Bauman, Z. 141–2, 143, 266
Baumann, G. 40,41
Bayley, M.J. 202, 206
Bebbington, A. 65
Becker, H. 82, 139, 142, 163
Bell, J. 111
Bell, W.G. 247
Benner, P. 78, 81
Bennet, C. 8, 219, 220, 222
Bensman, J. 212
Berck, R. 79
Berridge, V. 6, 8, 238–9, 247
Bhopal, R.S. 117, 118

Blaxter, M. 81
Bloor, M. 2, 9, 12, 13, 40, 83, 188, 189–90, 241
Blowfield, M. 261
Bluebond-Langer, M. 80
Born, G. 55, 56
Boulton, M. 8, 40, 139
Bourne, J. 77
Boyd, G. 38, 40, 47
Brah, A. 110, 113
Brettell, C.B. 183, 185, 189, 191, 194, 195
Brettle, R.P. 165
Brewer, J.D. 25
Briggs, C.M. 262
Brooks, P. 265
Brown, L. 78
Bruner, E.M. 149, 150, 151, 154, 156, 160
Bucknall, A. 165
Bulkin, W. 78
Burck, H.D. 59
Burns, T. 254
Burroughs, W. 175
Burton, F. 80, 81
Bury, J. 167, 218
Bury, M. 25, 135
Butt, S. 40
Bynum, W.F. 67

Callaway, H. 163, 211
Cameron, J.T. 59
Cannon, S. 140
Carr-Hill, R. 138
Carroll, M. 40
Cicourel, A.V. 254
Cixous, H. 135–6
Clandinin, D.J. 196
Clare, A. 56, 63
Clark, D. 134

Clifford, J. 119, 261
Cohen, A. 55–6
Cohen, S. 163, 211
Collins, P.H. 197
Colvard, R. 86
Connellly, F.M. 196
Cook, J. 22
Copp, A. 91
Corbin, J. 78, 79, 90, 101
Cornwell, J. 77, 140
Costain Schou, K. 141
Cottam, C.M. 117
Cottingham, H.F. 59
Cotton, S. 219
Cousins, M. 55
Craven, B.M. 138
Crosby, A.W. 249

Daniel, T. 40
Davis, M.S. 186
Day, S. 10, 39
de la Vega, A. 244
Deluz, A. 56
Denzin, K. 147, 160
Denzin, N. 25, 26, 162, 197
Derrida, J. 129, 135
Des Jarlais, D. 38
Deverell, K. 111, 113, 118, 120
Donoghoe, M. 37
Donovan, C. 34
Dorn, N. 40
Downes, D. 165
Doyal, L. 138
Duncan, B. 76
Duncombe, J. 26

Edmondson, R. 193
Elston, M.A. 135
Emerson, R.M. 190, 191
European Collaborative Study 82
Evans, R.J. 247
Evans-Pritchard, E.E. 56
Everitt, A. 219

Fallowfield, L.J. 134
Fardon, R. 10
Feldman, A. 151
Feldman, R. 65
Ferlie, E. 219, 222
Fernandez, J. 152, 156
Field, D. 138

Finch, J. 77, 140
Finne, H. 118
Firth, R. 130
Fischer, M.M.J. 195
Fitzpatrick, R. 40
Fonow, M. 22
Forsyth, M. 220
Foster, C. 191
Foucault, M. 7, 10, 11, 23, 25, 35, 54, 67,
    151, 158–9, 173, 263
Fox, N. 133, 135, 136
Frankenberg, R. 9, 39, 163
Fraoili, D. 78
Freirson, R. 95
Friend, J.A.R. 225, 226

Gans, H.J. 108, 110
Garfinkel, H. 209, 251
Gatter, P. 65, 110
Geertz, C. 147, 211
Gelsthorpe, L. 26
Giacquinta, B. 99
Gibson, N. 40, 50
Giddens, A. 135, 254
Giffen, M.B. 59
Gilbert, K.R. 101
Gilroy, P. 41
Gluckman, M. 37
Goffman, E. 251
Good, B.J. 6, 12, 141, 171
Gorfain, P. 149, 151, 154, 156, 160
Gorna, R. 112
Gough, I. 138
Gouldner, A.W. 139, 142
Graham, H. 140
Gramsci, A. 164
Green, G. 99, 100, 111, 262
Green, H. 202
Greenwood, J. 165
Griffen, C. 109–110

Haldane, D. 134
Halliday, M.A.K. 171
Hammersley, M. 25, 26, 109
Hannerz, U. 6, 148, 155, 160
Haraway, D. 113
Harding, S. 22, 26
Hart, G. 40, 139
Heald, S. 56
Heaphy, B. 11, 23, 24, 35
Heritage, J. 251

Herzfeldt, M. 4, 5, 41, 42, 162, 164, 178,
    264, 265
Hoban, R. 265-6
Hobbes, T. 252
Hochschild, A. 92, 93, 110
Holland, J. 77, 101
Hollitscher, W. 56
Hooton, A. 227
Horobin, G. 1, 5, 262, 264
Horowitz, R.P. 185, 194
Huby, G. 3, 11, 17, 33, 167, 172, 174, 218
Hughes, C.C. 184
Hume, D. 137
Hunter, G. 37, 38

Inglis, J.L. 165

Jack, D. 29
Jackson, J.E. 230
Jacobs, J. 77–8
James, N. 206
James, W. 95
Johnson, A. 185
Johnson, J. 80
Johnson, M. 40, 156
Jones, P. 204
Josselson, R. 141

Kahn, T.C. 59
Kapila, M. 108, 114
Kayal, P.M. 133
Kimmel, A.J. 212
King, E. 39, 112
Kitzinger, J. 99, 100, 111, 129, 262
Klee, H. 40, 44
Kleinman, S. 91
Kleinmann, A. 141
Kline, A. 40
Kline, E. 40
Kluckohn, C. 211
Knorr-Cetina, K. 254
Krafft-Ebbing 12
Kubler-Ross, E. 60

Lacan, J. 265
Laing, A.W. 219
Lakoff, G. 156
Laslett, B. 140
Laslett, P. 249
Lather, P. 218
Le Grand, J. 129, 137

LeClair, E.E. 130
Lee, R. 55, 76, 79, 80, 82, 85, 86, 90, 139,
    204, 205
Levi, P. 141
Levin, M. 118
Levi-Strauss, C. 146, 147, 148
Lewis, R. 223
Lieblich, A. 141
Lippman, S. 95
Lipson, J. 77–8, 79, 85
Llivina, T.S. 220
Lofland, J. 80
Lofland, L. 80
Lukes, S. 10
Lutz, C. 91

McBeth, S. 185
McCann, K. 99
McEwan, R. 34, 117, 118
MacIntyre, A. 205
McKee, L. 219
McKevitt, C. 39
McKie, R. 249
McPhail, K. 223
Maguire, G.P. 134
Maitland, S. 112
Malinowski, B.K. 146, 156
Manson, W.C. 56
Marcus, G. 119, 195, 261
Marcus, J. 164, 178, 264
Marsden, D. 26
Marshall, C. 32, 92
Marshall, P. 140
Masters, H. 76, 195
Mauss, M. 137
May, C. 80
Mearns, C. 34
Melia, K.M. 198
Merton, R.K. 138
Merton, V. 140
Mihill, C. 132
Milburn, K. 116
Miller, B. 133
Mills, C.W. 264
Mirza, H. 40
Mitchell, R. 79
Moi, T. 136
Mok, J. 82
Moody, D. 114, 104, 108
Moore, H. 55, 56
Mor, V. 128
Morgan Thomas, R. 224

Morse, J. 78, 79, 81, 183, 184
Mouzelis, N. 254
Munhall, P. 189
Myerhoff, B. 147, 148

Narayan, K. 105
Nencel, L. 25, 26, 31
Nilssen, T. 118

O'Keefe, J. 140
Oakley, A. 26, 33, 77, 94–5, 109, 116, 140
Obeyesekere, G. 56
Okely, J. 96, 163, 211
Oken, E. 40
Olesen, V. 77
Owolabi, O. 40, 44

Paradis, L.F. 133
Parker, D. 113
Parkes, M. 97
Parsinnen, C. 156
Parsons, T. 252
Patton, C. 21, 23, 24–5, 28, 35, 55
Pavis, S. 80
Pearson, G. 40
Peek, P.M. 56
Pels, P. 25, 26, 31
Peneff, J. 208
Perakyla, A. 77
Perera, J. 40, 50
Pettigrew, A. 8, 219
Peutheier, J.F. 165
Philips, K. 38, 40, 47
Phillips, S. 40
Plummer, K. 3, 7, 10, 11, 12, 22–4, 54,
    168
Pocock, D. 131
Polanyi, K. 130
Pollner, M. 190, 191
Porter, A.M.D. 167, 218
Porter, R. 67
Pottle, F.A. 250–1
Power, R. 40, 50
Prior, L. 114
Prout, A. 113, 114, 118, 120
Punch, M. 86, 87
Pye, M. 108, 114

Quimby, E. 39, 45

Ramazanoglu, C. 25, 26, 77, 101

Ranger, T. 249
Rapoport, R. 140
Rasmussen, K. 111, 114
Rawls, J. 138
Reardon, R.C. 59
Renzetti, C.M. 55, 204, 205
Rhodes, P.J. 113, 114
Rhodes, T. 139
Richardson, L. 184, 194, 196, 197, 198,
    262
Ricoeur, P. 140–1
Riessman, C.K. 171
Ritches, D. 11
Roberts, J.J.K. 165
Robertson, J.R. 165
Robinson, I. 25
Rock, P. 165, 186
Roman, P.M. 56
Rooney, M. 39
Rosaldo, R. 5, 81, 165, 191, 210, 211–12
Rose, N. 54
Rosenberg, C.E. 245, 246, 247
Ross, M. 78
Rossman, G.B. 32, 92
Runnion, V.M. 133
Rutherford, J. 110

Sahlins, M. 130, 131
Samuel, R. 6, 207
Sapsford, R. 223
Scambler, G. 25
Schama, S. 252
Schmid, K. 101
Schneider, B. 42
Schneider, H.K. 130
Schrijvers, J. 22, 27–8, 260
Schutz, A. 186
Schwartz, B. 132
Schwartz, H 77–8
Schwartzman, H. 153
Scott, C. 77
Scott, G.R. 224
Scott, P. 39
Secker, J. 116
Seeger, V. 78
Shaffir, W. 100–1, 107, 115
Sharma, U. 56
Sheehan, E.A. 186, 188
Shepherd, M. 67
Sieber, J. 76, 87, 205
Silverman, D. 31, 54, 77
Simmel, G. 196

Singer, M. 120
Slack, P. 250
Slavin, W. 219, 220
Small, N. 134, 138
Smith, A. 56
Smith, D.E. 31
Soderqvist, T. 21, 311
Song, M. 113
Sontag, S. 5–6, 7, 9, 55
Spencer, J. 165
Stacey, J. 31–2
Stanley, B. 205
Stanley, L. 140
Star, S.L. 110
Stark, C. 202, 206, 208–9
Stebbins, R. 100–1
Steier, F. 21, 22, 25, 26–7
Stenhouse, L. 104
Stewart, G.T. 138
Stimson, G. 37, 38, 39
Stimson, G. V. 38
Stolke, V. 41
Stott, S. 101
Strang, J. 39
Strathern, M. 195
Strauss, A. 78, 79, 90, 101
Strong, P. 237, 238–9, 240, 241, 247
Sugden, N. 34

Taghavi, M. 138
Taha-Cisse, A. 49
Tait, A. 207, 209, 212
Taussig, M. 163
Taylor, A. 77, 83
Temoshok, L. 81
Thompson, P. 6, 207
Thompson, S. 56, 63
Thornton, R. 149, 150, 160, 158
Thucydides 247, 248
Tierney, W.G. 4, 10, 101, 165, 184
Tilley, S. 81
Titmuss, R.M. 128, 129, 132, 136–7, 142
Tonkin, E. 171, 207
Tonnies, F. 129–30
Treichler, P. 9, 23
Trice, H.M. 56
Tsing, A.L. 162, 163–4, 178, 265

Turner, T. 10
Turowetz, A. 100–1
Twine, F.E. 225, 226

van Gennep 150
van Maanen, J. 109, 195
van Teijlingen, E. 138, 140, 167, 225, 226
Vanderplaat, M. 223, 225
Vara, C.A. 220
Vidich, A.J. 212
Voysey, M. 92, 98

Wadsworth, E. 99
Wallace, E.R. 56
Wallace, R. 87
Wallman, S. 3
Walsh, M.E. 90, 91
Wan, M. 28
Warner, R. 247, 248
Warren, C.A.B. 111, 114
Warren, P. 65
Watney, S. 55, 139
Watson, J. 116
Weeks, J. 28, 39
Weinstein, F. 56
Weiss, C. 221
Welsby, P. 165
White, D. 38, 40, 47
White, G. 91
Whyte, W.F. 189
Wilkins, R. 80, 93, 96, 264
Williams, R. 136
Williamson, L. 223
Wimbush, A. 116
Wise, S. 140
Wols, M. 247
Woodman, D. 138
Wrubel, J. 78, 81

Young, A. 108, 114
Young, H. 251
Young, J. 163
Young, L. 135

Zich, J. 81
Ziegler, P. 247

Subject index

action research 27–8
advocacy: within researcher and
    researched relationship 139
agency 164
aggregating accounts 187
AIDS: imagery of 6; policy responses 8–9,
    239–40; self-presentation of carers
    97–8; symbolism of 5–7
AIDS work: stressors 78
AIDS/HIV: counselling 60; impact on a
    community 147; psychotherapy 60
AIDS/HIV service provision 165–6;
    providers' versus users' perspectives on
    166, 167, 169
AIDS/HIV treatment stories 29–30
altruism: within the gift relationship 132–4
anecdote 4, 5
audience reception 183
AZT 29

behavioural change: drug users 38; gay
    men 38–9
boundaries 150; evaluation and policy
    making 222–3

carers 202
cathartic impact of research: on
    researchers 102; on respondents 97,
    102, 185, 205, 206
changing roles: nurse to researcher 77
chronic illness 25
collaborative relationships of researcher
    and researched 140–1
collaborative writing: researchers and
    respondents 119–20, 190–1
collective identity 148
confidentiality 44, 47, 48–9, 109, 169, 170,
    175, 201–2, 204, 212–15, 228–9;

disclosure and dissemination of 98,
    213–14; publishing and research 86–7
consent: informed 189; process 189
conversations 26–7
counselling: AIDS/HIV 60; definitions of
    58–9
counselling and therapy: similarities
    between 63–4
credibility of researcher 105–7
cultural determinism: risk 39
culture affording protection 43
cynical stories 192–3
Cypriot drug users 37, 44; role of the
    family 48–50; shame 47–8

data collection: impact of researcher's
    persona on 112, 114
death 3, 75
de-bunking 193
dialogical approaches 22, 27–8
disclosure: to children of parents' HIV
    status 83–4
disclosure and dissemination 85–7, 98
discourses: professional 66–8;
    psychotherapeutic 64
disguising respondents 86
displaying emotions 93–4, 95; by
    researchers 94–5, 97, 98
dissemination 111, 116–20; lack of control
    over 230; reactions of respondents to
    118, 186–8, 195–7, 225–6; restrictions
    to 228–9
dissemination and disclosure 85–7, 98
dissemination and stigma 85–6
drug services provision: research 40
drug trials 29–30
drug use: policy responses 38
drug users: construction of as 'chaotic'

173–4, 174–5; Cypriot 37, 44; impact
of harm reduction policies on 148,
159–60; minority ethnic groups,
marginalisation of 41, 42, research on
40; professionals' construction of 171–3
drug workers: ethnocentrism 46, 49
dying 3

economic versus social models of exchange
129–34: within the NHS 131
editing of respondents' accounts 194
emotions: display of 93–4, 95; public
private and personal 91–2; researcher's
display of 94–5, 97, 98; respondents'
hidden 91–2
emotions in research: study of 90
empowering 25–6, 33, 185
epidemics: reactions to 245–6; social
circumstances 248–9
ethical dilemmas 30
ethnic absolutism 41
ethnic groups, research on 40
ethnic minorities see minority ethnic group
drug users
'ethnic non-compliance' 39
ethnocentrism: drug workers 46, 49
evaluation 104; operationalisation 221–5;
purpose of 221; quantitative and
qualitative methods in 218–19, 224–5,
232; researcher's identification of roles
in 104–5
evaluations: tensions in dissemination of
117–19
evidence-based practice 219
expectations: respondents' 33, 109–10
expert knowledge: medical versus PWAs'
24–5

families 75; Cypriot drug users, role of
48–50
feigned feelings 92
female sex workers 10, 39
funders: expectations of research by 170
funding: competition for 224, 227, 228;
HIV 138–9, 219–20; research 31, 138

gender roles in research 110–11
gender variations: narrative 154–5
gift relationship, the 128–9, 132–3;
altruism 132–4; motivations 132–4
grief 94

haemophilia centre staff 203–4
'hard to reach' groups 37, 40
harm minimisation services: barriers to use
of 44–6, by Cypriots 44–6
harm reduction policies: impact on drug
users of 148, 159–60
health services: organisation of 115–16
heroin stories 148–9, 154, 157, 176–7
heterogeneity: minority ethnic groups 37
HIV antibody testing: impact of 63;
impact of positive results 95
HIV funding 138–9, 219–20
HIV status: disclosure to children of
parents' 83–4
HIV/AIDS: counselling 60; impact on a
community 147; psychotherapy 60
horror stories 160, 208
HIV/AIDS service provision 165–6;
providers' versus users' perspectives on
166, 167, 169
HIV/AIDS treatment stories 29–30

imagery: AIDS 6
impact of HIV antibody testing 63;
positive test results 95
impact of HIV/AIDS on a community 147
impact of research on researchers 61–2,
76, 78–9, 80–1, 95–6, 100–1 107–8,
110–11, 172–3, 175; analytic potential
of 95–6, 99; cathartic 102
impact of research on researcher's
sexuality 112
impact of research on respondents 81–4,
86–7, 96–7 134, 141, 191; cathartic 97,
102; direct consequences of 84–5;
focussing on painful issues 84;
therapeutic 134
individuality 55–6
informal networking 1
informed consent 189

key informants 188

life stories 207–8
low prevalence 201–2

marginalisation 41; of minority ethnic
group drug users 41, 42
marginality as an analytic position 162–5
media: coverage by the 244; responses by

the 249–51, 251–2; themes in the 251–3

member validation 188, 189–91

metaphor 146, 156

metonym 146, 150; function of 151–3

minority ethnic group drug users 44–6; marginalisation of 41, 42; research on 40; resistance to mainstream initiatives by 42; non-utilisation of services by 42

mistrust: by respondents 34, 191

models of exchange: economic versus social 129–34, within the NHS 131

moral panic 239

moral science 240–1

motivation: researcher's 31–2, 61; respondent's 184

motivation within the gift relationship 132–4; researcher's 31–2, 61, 106–7; respondent's 127–8, 132, 134–5

myth 146, 207, 231; function of 147–8, 192

mythology 5–8

myths, urban 191–2

narrative 12, 22–5: function of 147–8, 151–3, 155, 157–60; gender variations 154–5

narrative process 149

narratives 167–71; psychotherapeutic 54

networking: informal 1

objective knowledge 31–2

objectivity 32–3

other, the: construction of respondents as 162–4, 191

otherness 43

policy responses: AIDS 8–9

politics of research 112–13

postmodernism 141–2

power 10–11, 23, 41–2

privileging particular accounts 13, 25, 31, 139, 187, 190

problematising: respondents' accounts 30–1, 194–5

process consent 189

processual text 149

professional discourses 66–8

professional gaze, the 171–3

prosessionals' construction of drug users 171–3

protection: culture affording 43

pseudonyms: use of 86

psychotherapeutic accounts: selectivity of 65; selectivity at an institutional level of 65–6

psychotherapeutic narratives 54

psychotherapy: AIDS/HIV 60; definitions 58; theoretical and therapeutic dimensions of 68

psychotherapy as discourse 64

PWAs: accounts of 24–5; as researchers 21–2

quote selecting 193–4

rapport with respondents 78, 84, 105–10, 113–14, 175–6

recruitment 203–4

reductionism: microbiological 247

reflexivity 3–4, 26–7, 68, 80, 81, 91, 120, 139, 140, 165, 184–5, 198, 211; spiralling 250–1; writing 184

relationships: researcher and researched 33, 79, 105–7, 108–10, 135–6, 140, 175–6, 177–8, 177, 229, 230–1, advocacy within 139, collaboration between 140–1; researcher's credibility within 105–7

representation 140, 141

research: drug services provision 40; funders' expectations of 170; and minority ethnic groups 40; politics of 112–13; psychodynamic aspects of 62; respondents' expectations of 114–16, 170; sensitive topics 55, 139–40, 204–5

research findings: respondents use of 185–6

research funding 31, 138

researcher support 80, 99–100

researcher's persona: impact on data collection of 112, 114

researcher's relationship with researched 79, 105–7, 108–10, 135–6, 140, 175–6, 177–8, 229, 230–1; advocacy within the 139; collaboration within the 140–1

researcher's sexuality: impact of research on 112

researchers: analytic potential of emotions of 99, 101–2, 210; cathartic impact of research on 102; collaborative writing with respondents 119–20; credibility of 105–7; display of emotions by 94–5, 97, 98; impact of

research on 61–2, 76, 78–9, 80–1, 95–6,
   100–1, 107–8, 110–11, 172–3, 175,
   implications for analysis of the 99;
   implications of personal experience for
   'theoretical sensitivity' of 79–80, 90, 91,
   92, 210–11, 211–12; 'insiders' as 77–8;
   PWAs as 21–22; personal motivation of
   31–2, 61, 106–7; political motivation of
   31–2, 61, 106–7; and rapport with
   respondents 105–10, 113–14;
   responsibilities of 68–9, 96–7, 205; and
   requests from respondents 84, 109, 225,
   229; responsibilities of 140; revealing of
   22, 109–10; role adoption by 112
respondents: accessing through research
   the hidden emotions of 91–2; cathartic
   impact of research on 97, 102, 185,
   205, 206; collaborative writing with
   researchers 119–20, 190–1;
   construction of as 'the other' 162–5,
   191; direct consequences of research
   for 84–5; disguising of 86; focussing on
   painful issues with 84; impact of
   research on 81–4, 86–7, 134, 141, 191;
   and knowledge of research 82, 206–7;
   mistrust by 34, 191; motivations of
   81–2, 127–8, 132, 134–5, 184;
   payment of 174; rapport with 78, 84,
   105–10, 113–14, 175–6; reaction to
   dissemination by 118,186–8, 195–7,
   225–6; and requests from researcher
   84, 109, 225, 229; strategies of
   resistance by 33–4, 174, 177;
   therapeutic effect of research on 134;
   use of research findings by 185–6
respondents' accounts 83; challenging of
   30–1, 111, 177; editing of 194;
   problematising of 30–1, 194–5
respondents' expectations 33, 109–10; of
   research 114–16, 170
retribution stories 157
revealing the researcher 21, 109–10
revelatory text 152
role: implications of gender in research
   110–11
role adoption by researchers 112
role boundaries 79, 107–10, 111–13,
   227–8; blurring of 166, 222, 229
role changing: nurse to researcher 77

selecting quotes 193–4

selectivity: in psychotherapeutic accounts
   65; at an institutional level 65–6
self, the 55–6
self-presentation: AIDS carers 97–8
sensitive topics: research on 90, 139–40,
   204–5
service provision: AIDS/HIV 165–6
service users: strategies of resistance by 174
service utilisation 166
sex workers: female 10, 39
sexual storytelling 7, 23–4
shame: Cypriot drug users 47–8
significant versus trivial 3–5, 93
silences 28–9; strategic 33–4
silencing 21, 24–5
similarities between counselling and
   therapy 63–4
social poetics 164
social versus economic models of exchange
   129–34: within the NHS 131
stigma 208–9, 215
stories 192–3; cynical 192–3; heroin
   148–9, 154, 157, 176–7; horror 160,
   208; life 207–8; retribution 157; urban
   myths 191–2
storytelling 12, 22–5; AIDS/HIV
   treatment 29–30; functions of 147–8,
   153, 155, 157–60, 168–71; sexual 7,
   23–4
strategies of resistance 33–4
street corner gatherings 148
stressors in AIDS work 78
symbolism: AIDS 5–7

target populations 37; diversity of 42
theoretical sensitivity: implications of
   researcher's personal experience for
   79–80, 91, 92
therapy and counselling: similarities
   between 63–4
topologised space 149, 150
treatment stories: AIDS/HIV 29–30
tribalising 37

urban myths 191–2

violence 151–2

welfare policy 136–9, 219–21; cost
   effectiveness of 138, 219, 220
writing: analytical potential of 197–8